D0583984

SENSORY EVALUATION PRACTICES

Third Edition

Food Science and Technology
International Series

A complete list of books in this series appears at the end of this volume.

Sensory Evaluation Practices

Third Edition

Herbert Stone and Joel L. Sidel
Tragon Corporation
365 Convention Way
Redwood City, California, USA

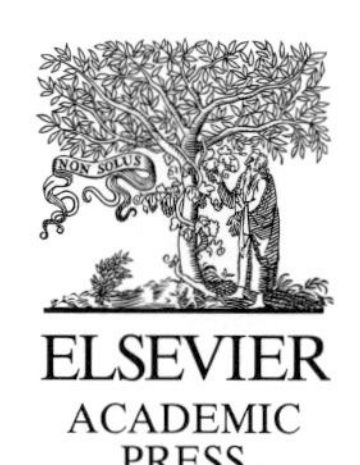

ELSEVIER
ACADEMIC
PRESS

Amsterdam • Boston • Heidelberg • London • New York • Oxford
Paris • San Diego • San Francisco • Singapore • Sydney • Tokyo

This book is printed on acid-free paper

Elsevier Academic Press
525 B Street, Suite 1900 San Diego, California 92101-4495, USA
http://www.elsevier.com

Elsevier Academic Press
84 Theobald's Road, London WC1X 8RR, UK
http://www.elsevier.com

Library of Congress Catalog Number: 2003115958

British Library Cataloguing in Publication Data
Sensory evaluation practices - 3rd ed. (Food science and technology. International series)
1. Food - Sensory evaluation 2. Sensory evaluation
I. Stone, Herbert II. Sidel, Joel L.
664'.072

ISBN 0-12-672690-6

Typeset by Newgen Imaging Systems (P) Ltd, Chennai, India
Printed and bound in Italy

04 05 06 07 08 9 8 7 6 5 4 3 2 1

Contents

Foreword

Sensory evaluation over the last 60 years has grown from an emerging area of inquiry, confined to relatively simple quality control applications in a few food organizations, to one which is considered an essential component of the research and development process in food and non-food entities throughout the world.

This growth has been reflected in the formation and increasing membership of sensory professional organizations and in sensory related presentations at national and international meetings; as well as in the emergence of sensory related journals.

Naturally this growth has been accompanied by an increase in the number of individuals who are employed in sensory positions, and who have the necessary skills and knowledge. As a result, many working in this field depend on core texts such as this one to enhance their working knowledge base.

The first and second editions of **Sensory Evaluation Practices** contributed admirably to help fill this knowledge gap both as a reference and as a textbook in educational institutions. This text was specifically designed to give practical guidance on sensory procedures that could be directly applied to the sensory issues encountered in a working environment.

The third edition updates the methods of sensory evaluation and in addition gives test design and organizational guidelines. This information can further enhance the sensory professional in performing their responsibilities at a higher level of competence.

The authors bring to this endeavor over 35 years of experience in dealing with the "real" problems of product development and quality control in both the food and non-food area.

I appreciate the invitation to write a foreword to this book and am confident that the reader will find that **Sensory Evaluation Practices, Third Edition** will contribute in a meaningful way to their development as a sensory professional.

Howard G. Schutz
Professor Emeritus of Consumer Sciences
Food Science & Technology Department
University of California at Davis

Preface

Preface, First Edition

There has long been a need for guidance in the development and application of sensory evaluation within the corporate environment. The purpose of this book is to provide this guidance and to identify principles and practices that will result in increased utilization of sensory evaluation. In recent years, there has been a considerable increase in the number of individuals working in the field who lack the necessary academic training or practical skills for sensory evaluation. Published guides have described test methods and suggested procedures for the analysis of results from sensory tests, but have not provided the rationale behind the selection of a particular procedure or test method. This book addresses this and other equally important gaps in the field, including the organization and operation of a testing program, the design of a test facility, recommended procedures for the selection, screening, and qualifying of subjects, and the communication of actionable results. We have drawn heavily from our more than two decades of research and consulting in this field. To our knowledge, no other book provides such an extended coverage of the topic.

With regard to sensory evaluation, this book expounds a particular philosophy that can best be described as one that places greatest emphasis on the concepts of planning and decision analysis in the broadest sense. For the sensory professional, the ability to provide test services should not be considered the primary goal but rather a resource that can be used if a problem warrants it. With each request, the sensory evaluation professional must decide how best to meet the needs of the requestor and what methods to apply to the problem. Considerable emphasis is placed on the quality of the information derived from a test. It is also important to have sufficient behavioral and statistical knowledge to understand the nature of a problem, to ensure that the experimental design is appropriate to the test objective, to understand results, and to communicate them in an actionable way.

The book is organized into three main parts. Chapters 1 and 2 trace the development of the field and define sensory evaluation: what it does, how, where, and for whom. Chapters 3 and 4 address the more fundamental issues of measurement, psychological errors in testing, and statistics and experimental design. Chapters 5–7 provide the reader with a detailed description of the three classes of test methods (discrimination, descriptive, affective), criteria used to select a specific method, and suggested procedures for data analysis and the interpretation of results. A final chapter and epilogue focus on a series of problems that require substantive sensory evaluation involvement: for example, storage testing, measurement of perceived efficacy, correlation of instrumental and sensory data, and systems for product optimization.

To the extent possible, pertinent literature has been referenced and discussed. However, this book is not intended as a review of the literature. In those sections with few references, the authors have drawn on their extensive experience to describe a recommended procedure or practice. For example, there is little or no published information on the design of a test facility, and the authors' experience was used to develop the enclosed diagrams and to assist the sensory professional in this endeavor.

The book is intended for sensory professionals, technical managers, product development and production specialists, and research directors considering the establishment of a program or anticipating expansion of existing resources. Marketing, marketing research, and advertising professionals will also benefit from the information in this book. The increased interaction between the technologist formulating the product and those responsible for marketing the product requires a greater awareness of sensory evaluation by everyone concerned. Individuals considering sensory evaluation as a career will also benefit from reading selected chapters of this book. In particular, Chapters 1, 3, 4, and 8 will provide both an overall perspective and specific examples of sensory evaluation applications in business. For the entry-level professional or the undergraduate taking a first course in sensory evaluation, Chapters 1 and 2 provide an introduction to the topic, while Chapters 5–7 describe the various test methods. For experienced individuals seeking to expand their perspective, Chapters 3, 4, and 8 will be especially helpful.

Numerous individuals and companies directly and indirectly provided assistance in the development of the ideas expressed in this book as well as the opportunity to put these ideas into practice. In particular, we wish to acknowledge the contributions of Jean Eggert of Kraft, Inc.; Robert Boone, Carole Vohsen, and Geralyn Basinski of Ralston Purina; Emer Schaefer of S.C. Johnson & Son, Inc.; Daryl Schaller, Jan Michaels, and Jean Yamashita of the Kellogg Company; Robert Brieschke and Lenore Ryan of Kimberly-Clark Corporation; Kaye Zook of the Quaker Oats Company; Margaret Savoca of R.J. Reynolds Tobacco Co.; Jan Detwiler of Olympia Brewing Co.; and Erik von Sydow of Nordreco AB.

Our associates also provided thoughts and assistance at various times. In particular, we wish to acknowledge the contributions of Jean Bloomquist of our staff; Professors Rose Marie Pangborn, Edward B. Roessler, and Howard Schutz of the University of California at Davis; Birgit Lundgren of the Swedish Food Institute; and Dr Richard Singleton of SRI International. We wish to express our appreciation to Marjorie Sterling-Stone who typed many of the drafts of this book and provided the comments needed to make it a more understandable text. Special thanks are due to Raymond Andersen who prepared the graphics. Herbert Stone also wishes to acknowledge the intellectual support and guidance provided by the late Professor George F. Stewart, who through the years encouraged him in this effort.

Herbert Stone
Joel L. Sidel

Preface, Second Edition

In the seven years since the publication of the first edition of this book, there have been many changes in the field of sensory evaluation. New books and journals devoted to sensory evaluation have appeared, professional associations have experienced increased membership, and there is a much greater awareness of sensory evaluation academically and in business. More universities are offering courses in sensory evaluation and more companies are recognizing the value of sensory information. This latter change created opportunities for sensory professionals that we have addressed in more detail in this revised edition. Careful consideration also has been given to the reviews of the first edition and the comments provided by numerous individuals who have written to or talked with us about the book.

In this edition we have added more background information about various recommended procedures and practices, particularly with regard to organizing and structuring resources to better operate in today's competitive business environment. Attention also has been given to methodology emphasizing developments in descriptive analysis. Several new methods have been proposed and are now in use leading to more literature on these and related topics.

As was stated in the first edition this book is not intended as a review of the literature. However, some of the literature is discussed in detail as it relates to specific methods and procedures. Attention is also given to the more practical issues of the strategy that sensory professionals use as they communicate information and demonstrate the cost benefits derived from a full-scale sensory program.

Numerous individuals contributed to the ideas expressed here, and to the opportunity to put these ideas into practice. In particular we wish to acknowledge the contributions of Patricia Beaver, Melanie Pons, and Jean Eggert (retired), of Kraft General Foods–USA; and Birgit Lundgren of Kraft General Foods–Europe; Margaret Savoca and Harvey Gordin of R. J. Reynolds Tobacco Company; Katy Word of Coors Brewing Company; and Erik von Sydow of Nestlé.

Our associates also provided helpful comments and, through their questions, enabled us to enhance our perspectives of certain problems. In particular we wish to acknowledge Brian McDennott, Rebecca Newby, Heather Thomas, Dr. Richard Singleton of SRI International, and Professor Howard Schutz of the University of California at Davis. Finally, we wish to recognize the important contributions of our longtime friend and associate, the late Professor Rose Marie Pangborn of the University of California at Davis who worked tirelessly to educate students encouraging them to pursue a career in sensory evaluation, and worked with a total commitment for the betterment of the science of sensory evaluation. This edition is dedicated to her memory.

Herbert Stone
Joel L. Sidel

Preface, Third Edition

In the decade since the publication of the second edition of this book, there have been many developments and changes in the field of sensory evaluation. However, some aspects of sensory evaluation have not changed; a continuing lack of scientific rigor, and an increased reliance on default analyses driven by the power of PCs without an appreciation for the manner in which the information was obtained or whether the output has any face validity. Despite these impediments, the field continues to grow and attract interest as a result of market forces. In addition, many books have been published and/or revised, some focused on the design and analysis of sensory tests while others provide a review of the literature. New journals devoted to sensory evaluation have appeared, and some professional associations have experienced increased memberships reflecting growth in the field especially outside of the food industry. Perhaps most gratifying has been the increase in academic programs offering course work and degrees in sensory evaluation. This has occurred in both the United States and in Europe. The latter is especially promising, in as much as 15 years ago such programs were quite rare. More course offerings will eventually lead to a more scientific approach to the testing process. In this edition, we have reviewed the organizational issues and where necessary we have made changes that we believe will help maintain programs in spite of the many changes taking place in the consumer products industries. Consideration has also been given to the reviews of the second edition and comments provided by numerous individuals who have written and/or talked with us about what is missing in the book.

In this edition, we give more consideration to methods, in part because various misconceptions have developed and recommended practices no longer appear to be practised as rigorously as in the past. The search continues for the universal scale, the perfect subject, and other sacred goals that we will discuss. Also, there have been many developments in the use of multivariate analyses, the linking of consumer and sensory information, and greater involvement of sensory with marketing research. We have expanded the discussions on the use of sensory evaluation in quality control and optimization techniques.

As we stated in the first edition, and restate here, this book is not a review of the literature. We do, however, discuss literature relevant to specific issues and cite what we consider to be pertinent to the applications of sensory resources to provide actionable information. In this edition, we continue to emphasize the importance of strategic planning and acting as a means for sensory professionals to make meaningful contributions. This is especially important as they communicate information and demonstrate the value of a full-scale sensory program.

As was mentioned in previous editions, numerous individuals contributed to the ideas expressed here, and to put these ideas into practice. In particular, we wish to acknowledge the contributions of Bruce Yandell, Heather Thomas, and Rebecca Bleibaum. We also acknowledge the comments and the suggestions from Marcia Young of the Campbell Soup Company, Josef Zach of Kraft-Europe, Birgit Lundgren of Kraft-Europe, ret.; Professor Brian Yandell of the University of Wisconsin and Professor Howard Schutz of the University of California at Davis and Senior Consultant to Tragon Corporation. We wish to express our appreciation to Ms Sylvia Heastings who typed the revised draft of this current edition.

Finally, we wish to recognize the important contributions of our longtime friend and associate, the late Professor Rose Marie Pangborn of the University of California at Davis, who worked tirelessly to educate students, encouraged them to pursue a career in sensory evaluation, and worked with a total commitment for the betterment of the science of sensory evaluation. This third edition is dedicated to her memory.

Herbert Stone
Joel L. Sidel

About the Authors

In this Third Edition of *Sensory Evaluation Practices*, the authors, Herbert Stone and Joel L. Sidel, draw from their extensive experience to provide readers with the background and understanding necessary to make informed decisions about developing and managing a sensory program. In this edition, the authors provide more current information about the applications for sensory information and operating in a more expanded business environment.

In 1974, Stone and Sidel founded Tragon Corporation, an important sensory and consulting company offering full-service consumer goods research. As a pioneering company in the field of sensory evaluation, Tragon has been able to offer unparalleled capabilities to its customers through the Quantitative Descriptive Analysis (QDA) sensory method, and Product Optimization (PROP) marketing and sensory modeling method, much greater insight into driving consumer purchase behavior.

Cumulatively, the authors have more than half a century of experience in the field of sensory evaluation and its business applications. In addition to founding Tragon Corporation, the authors have conducted domestic and international workshops; designed and analyzed, and reported on thousands of sensory tests; and have been consultants to the senior management of many major food and consumer products companies. In 2003, Herbert Stone was elected President (for the period 2003–2005) of the Institute of Food Technologists.

Introduction to Sensory Evaluation

1

I. Introduction and Objective

Since publication of the second edition of this book a decade ago, there have been many developments in the science and the application of sensory evaluation that directly or indirectly have had an impact. Today, just about all consumer products companies in the food and beverage industry as well as other industries, for example, home care and personal care industries, are aware of sensory evaluation and most agree that it has a role within their company. Marketing research and brand management professionals also are giving increased recognition to sensory information. Such recognition has yielded benefits for the profession in the form of improved status (and increased compensation), and for some, a bigger/louder voice in the product decision-making process. It is the latter which has the greater effect in the longer term. These developments have also resulted in more support for research and more course offerings at the University level. However, some fundamental, as well as some practical, issues remain to be considered or re-considered. New professionals tend to rely on pre-packed software that provides not only data capture capabilities, but also design and analyses options. While such capabilities are a significant enhancement, many also provide designs that are neither balanced properly nor relevant for anything other than a standard test. Reliance on such packages make for an easy entry for the inexperienced professional but have the potential for misapplication when the action taken is to modify the problem to fit the program. There has been a decline in understanding and appreciation for the consequences of not using qualified subjects, a tendency to limit replication (in sensory analytical tests) for cost savings purposes,

Sensory Evaluation Practices 3rd Edn
ISBN: 0-12-672690-6

and as already noted, use of statistical packages with default systems that yield results that on the surface make sense but have no real basis or there is no awareness of their weaknesses. We will explore these issues in more detail later in this book.

Using sensory information as a part of a marketing decision has given it unprecedented attention; being able to identify and quantitatively model the key drivers for a product's acceptance is now generally recognized as a core resource for any sensory program. It is acknowledged to be a powerful approach to optimizing product preference; however, this has only been possible with use of descriptive analysis to identify the specific sensory characteristics. The next logical step in this process has been to incorporate this information with other cognitive measures such as imagery. Exploiting this information to the fullest extent possible has enabled companies to grow their market share as well as implement cost savings through better use of technology, etc. All this has been possible as a direct result of use of sensory resources, better understanding about the measurement of human behavior, combined with a more systematic and professional approach to the testing process. Much of this progress has been achieved within the technical and marketing structures of those organizations that recognized the unique contributions of sensory evaluation. In the past, these activities were the exception, today it is a more common occurrence, again reflecting the increased awareness of sensory evaluation by those in and outside the field. For a summary of these developments, the reader is directed to Schutz (1998). However, much more needs to be done, in part because the link between sensory, marketing, and production is not strong, and in part because there is a lack of appreciation for the principles on which the science is based. For some, sensory evaluation is not considered as a science capable of providing reliable and valid information. This is a not so uncommon "perception," fostered in part by the seemingly simplistic notion that anyone can provide a sensory judgment. We are born with our senses and barring some genetic defects, we are all capable of seeing, smelling, tasting, etc. It certainly seems simple enough, so why should a technologist or a brand manager believe results from a test that are inconsistent with their expectations and their own evaluations? Alternatively, product experts and reporters such as those responsible for wine and food reviews in the public press have a significant impact on the success of products and businesses based on their reviews which purport to be based on the senses and by default, sensory evaluation. Myths are created and perpetuated based on hearsay simply by being in a position of authority. Suffice to say, not all of what one reads should be believed. We will have more to say about this later in this chapter and in the chapters on discrimination and descriptive analysis. As a result, demonstrating that there is a scientific basis to the discipline continues to be a challenge because the basic principles of perception are being lost in favor of quick solutions or a lack of time to do a test correctly. In the case of the latter, the authors have experienced the situation in which time restrictions take precedence over using an appropriate method even though there was a high risk of obtaining inadequate information using a method incorrectly! It is no longer a surprise to hear statements such as, "We don't have the time or money to do it right, but we will be able to do it over again later." It takes a lot of effort to overcome this kind of thinking. Since the previous editions of this book, advances continue to be made, albeit at a slow pace, not because test procedures are inadequate, but as noted previously, the science is not readily acknowledged as such. In all fairness, it should be mentioned that sensory professionals have not been effective spokespersons for their work or for the science. In one company, sensory evaluation will be used successfully, but in another it will be misused or the information will be ignored because it is inconsistent with expectation. Unfortunately, this latter situation has encouraged use of other information sources or to develop competing test capabilities in the hope of obtaining acceptable information without fully appreciating the consequences.

Over the years, numerous efforts have been made and continue to be made to develop a more permanent role for sensory evaluation within a company. Reviewing the technical and trade literature shows that progress in the development and use of sensory resources continues. There has been a noticeable increase, and much of the impetus continues to come from selected sectors of the economy, notably foods and beverages and their suppliers (Piggot, 1988; Meiselman and MacFie, 1996; Lawless and Heymann, 1999; Jackson, 2002). In their seminal textbook on sensory evaluation published almost four decades ago, Amerine *et al.* (1965) correctly called attention to three key issues: the importance of flavor to the acceptance of foods and other products, the use of flavor-related words in advertising, and the extent to which everyday use of the senses was largely unappreciated, at that time. Perhaps a secondary benefit of today's concerns about food safety has been an awareness by consumers of the sensory aspects of the foods they purchase.

It is apparent that current interest in sensory evaluation reflects a more basic concern than simply being able to claim use of sound sensory evaluation methodologies. In a paper published in 1977, Brandt and Arnold described the results of a survey on the uses of sensory tests by food product development groups. Their survey provided insight into some of the basic issues facing sensory evaluation. While the survey is dated, the information remains relevant and much of it continues to be confirmed based on more recent surveys fielded by the Sensory Evaluation Division of the Institute of Food Technologists (see below). The results were especially notable for the extent (or lack of) of the awareness of sensory evaluation by the respondents. Of the sixty-two companies contacted, fifty-six responded that they were utilizing sensory evaluation. However, descriptions of tests being used revealed that confusion existed about the various methods; for example, it was found that the triangle test (a type of discrimination test) was the most popular, followed by hedonic scaling (a type of acceptance test) and paired comparison (either an acceptance test or a discrimination test). Since these methods and the other methods mentioned in the survey provide different kinds of information, it is not possible to evaluate the listing other than to comment that the groups in most companies contacted appeared to be using a variety of procedures.

Also, there was confusion about accepted test methods and the information that each provides. For example, single-sample presentation is not a test method, yet twenty-five of the fifty-six companies responded that it was one of the test methods in use. It is, in fact, a serving procedure and such responses may reflect poorly worded or misunderstood questions in the survey. Another example of the confusion is "scoring," which was said to be in use by only seven of the fifty-six companies contacted. However, all sensory tests entail some kind of scoring. Statistical tests included in the survey elicited similarly confusing responses. The failure to define the terms confirms that the food industry utilizes sensory evaluation but there is confusion as to what methods are used and for what applications. As previously noted, sensory evaluation as a science is not well understood, methods are not always used in appropriate ways, and results are easily misused. While there continues to be a lack of qualified professionals, more are being trained. More books on sensory evaluation continue to be published; however, the science still has not achieved a status commensurate with its potential. As noted by Stone (1999), separating science from mythology is a challenge that is still with us. Similarly, its role within individual companies is far from clear. One of the goals of this book is to provide a perspective on all these issues and how one should develop resources and integrate them into the business environment. This is not to imply that the scientific basis of sensory evaluation is overlooked. In fact, considerable attention is given to the science of sensory evaluation because without it, any use of sensory information will be seriously compromised.

A focus of this book is on a systematic approach to the organization, development, and operation of a sensory program in a business environment. While emphasis is directed toward the more practical aspects of sensory evaluation and approaches to implementing a respected and credible program, attention also is given to more fundamental, underlying issues, including a comparison of specific test methods, experimental design, the reliability and validity of results, and related topics. From a sensory evaluation perspective, the twin issues of reliability and validity are of paramount importance, and are integral to developing a credible program and providing actionable recommendations within the context of that company's business and brand strategy (see Aaker, 1996). From a business perspective, it is these latter issues that loom as most important along with knowing which product formulation best meets the objective. Providing actionable recommendations is critical as it builds trust that others will place on those recommendations and the extent to which managers will act on those recommendations. The idea that volumes of data will convince one's peers and superiors is not an approach that is viable, particularly in the world of business. Sensory professionals must communicate information clearly to ensure that superiors, peers, and subordinates understand what was done and what the results mean in terms of meeting that test's specific objective.

It should be clear to the reader as to the importance of the relationship between reliability and validity of results and the credibility assigned to sensory recommendations, and in a global sense, the credibility of a sensory program itself. While it is logical to assume that a test result should speak for itself, and that quality information will be heard, understood, and, acted on accordingly; in fact, the opposite can and does occur a sufficient number of times to directly impact on the effective utilization of sensory evaluation. It raises important questions as to why sensory information is not better understood and, therefore, better used. Whether this situation reflects a basic lack of understanding of results from a test and/or a lack of understanding of the role of sensory evaluation in business, or a failure of sensory to understand the background to a specific request is not clear. It would appear that there is no single or simple answer. However, this situation can be better understood if one considers the nature of the sensory evaluation process. Product evaluation is a multi-step process in which a group of individuals respond to stimuli (a set of products) by marking a scorecard according to a specific set of instructions. These individuals are participating in this test because of their demonstrated sensory skills with that particular category of products. The responses are usually marks on the scorecard or a similar designation on a computer screen. The marks are then converted to numerical values for computation. Several aspects of this process warrant comment – the first is whether the test plan is appropriate for the problem, the second is whether the scorecard is appropriate, third is how the information will be collected (numerical or marking some type of scale), the fourth relates to the type of scale used, and the fifth is the type(s) and relevance of analysis used. Having a good understanding of why a test is being requested represents the first and perhaps most important task for a sensory professional. Failure to obtain such information is a clear sign of impending problems, beginning with establishing an objective to determining how the results will be communicated. The scorecard lists the questions and the means by which judgments will be captured, and by default, what analysis or analyses will be used. Similarly, it will determine which subjects should participate. A common problem for many is the seemingly innocuous request for subjects to provide numerical judgments because they are easy to capture (and analyze). Yet, more than 30 years ago, it was clearly demonstrated that there are number biases, some numbers have residual meanings, numbers connote a right or wrong answer, and subjects will change their use of numbers for no apparent reason, usually in the middle of a test. Scaling also warrants comment; however, there is a more detailed discussion about this topic in Chapter 3. One issue is the concept of using the same scale in all tests, another relates to using the "the standard scale" from that company (which usually has no basis in any literature) or a belief that there is a universal scale. There is no question that comparisons of results are made easier when the same scale(s) is used; however, few problems lend themselves to use of the same scale in every test. Not all questions can be answered with the same scale and this should not be a surprise. Nor should it be expected that there is one scale that is more sensitive than all other scales. Here, too, the nature of the problem and the products will help determine the most appropriate scale.

Subjects also have an impact on a program's credibility. How they were selected and what kind of training, if any, they received are important considerations as are their responses, in terms of both their sensitivity and their reliability. To a degree, a panel of subjects can be considered as functioning like a null instrument, recording what is perceived. The implication of a human (or group of humans) functioning like an instrument has obvious appeal in a technical sense, particularly to those who mistakenly envision an invariant system yielding the same numerical values time and time again. In fact, this latter concept has considerable appeal, particularly among those with a poor understanding of the perceptual process. The realities of the situation are, of course, quite different. Subjects, no matter what their level of skill or number of years of training and practice, exhibit differences in sensitivity from one another, and differences in variability that is unique (to that individual). Some training programs imply (e.g. see Spectrum Analysis in Meilgaard *et al.*, 1999) that this sensitivity and accompanying variability can be overcome through training and use of appropriate references. Such training, as much as 10 hours per week and often lasting 4 or more months, has considerable appeal (it is so special, it must be correct); however, independent evidence of the success of such an approach is not readily demonstrated nor is it consistent with our knowledge of human perception and the physiology of the senses. Such an approach is a form of behavior modification rather than a means of capturing responses as a function of a stimulus (whether that stimulus is a purified chemical or a consumer ready beverage). This ignores the fact that changing one's response does not necessarily mean that one's perceptions also are changed, nor does it recognize the variability inherent in humans and in products. In each instance, the end result is to overcome what appear to be limitations of the sensory process in the mistaken belief that they will make results more acceptable. Short of directly telling an individual what should be an answer, there always will be variability. Nonetheless, the requestor of a test expecting that test to yield an invariant result (the same response or numerical value every time) is disappointed and concerned about this unique information source. This disappointment also is accompanied by reservations as to any conclusions and recommendations; that is, the issue of credibility arises. Alternatively, when results are not in agreement with information obtained elsewhere (and often not sensory information) and no attempt is made to understand and explain the basis for any disagreement, then further erosion of program credibility will occur. The success of a program, and particularly its credibility, begins with having a plan and an organized effort, and making sure that the testing process follows accepted procedures and practices; what method was used, who the subjects were and how they were selected, what test design was used, how the data were analyzed, including the evidence of reliability, and so forth. In a business sense, it begins with an explanation of what sensory information is, how the results are communicated and whether they are understood, and ends with actionable recommendations being implemented to everyone's satisfaction. While these issues are discussed in detail in succeeding chapters, their inclusion here is to provide an initial perspective to the issue of business credibility and direct involvement of sensory evaluation in product decisions. Without an organized product evaluation effort and demonstrated reliable and valid results that are communicated in a way that is readily understood, one is returning to reliance on product experts, the *N* of 1, who made product decisions by virtue of their expertness and not because there were data to support their judgments. Decisions derived in this manner are neither new nor are they unusual; however, they make it very difficult for those individuals trying to organize and operate a credible sensory test program. As noted by Eggert (1989) and more recently by Stone and Sidel (1995), sensory evaluation must develop a strategy for success. It must reach out to its customers, it must educate them about the benefits that can be realized from using sensory information. At the same time, it must gain management support through an active program of selling its services and how the company can benefit from those services.

This book is not intended as an introduction to the topic of sensory evaluation. Nonetheless, for some aspects of sensory evaluation, considerable detail is provided in an almost stepwise manner. Readers, however, will probably derive more from this book if they have a basic understanding of sensory evaluation, experimental design, and statistics, and especially the perceptual process.

Where appropriate, background information sources are cited in this text and should be considered as recommended reading. In addition to its benefit to the sensory professional, this book is intended to serve as a guide for the research and development executive seeking to have a capability in sensory evaluation and to develop a more efficient and cost effective product development program. It should be of interest also to marketing, market research, and technical managers, all of whom have an interest in their company's products and their quality as measured by consumer responses and through sales, market share, and profitability.

II. Historical Background

Of the many sectors of the consumer products industries (food and beverage, cosmetics, personal care products, fabrics and clothing, pharmaceutical, and so on), the food and beverage sectors provided much early support for and interest in sensory evaluation. During the 1940s and through the mid-1950s, sensory evaluation received additional impetus through the US Army Quartermaster Food and Container Institute, which supported research in food acceptance for the armed forces (Peryam *et al.*, 1954). It became apparent to the military that adequate nutrition, as measured by analysis of diets or preparation of elaborate menus, did not guarantee food acceptance by military personnel. The importance of flavor and the degree of acceptability for a particular product were acknowledged. Resources were allocated to studies of the problem of identifying what foods were more or less preferred as well as the more basic issue of the measurement of food acceptance. These particular problems were apparently forgotten during the 1960s and early 1970s when the federal government initiated its "War on Hunger" and "Food from the Sea" programs. The government's desire to feed the starving and malnourished met with frustration when product after product was rejected by the recipients primarily because no one bothered to determine whether the sensory properties of these products were acceptable to the targeted groups. This is not to suggest that each country's ethnic and regional food habits and taboos were not important but rather, in the context of these government programs, there was scant attention given to the sensory evaluation of the products as they were being developed. This situation continues to exist because there remains a fundamental lack of appreciation for the importance of sensory perception on food choice behavior.

The food industry, possibly taking a cue from the government's successes and failures in sensory evaluation, began to provide support for this emerging science. Although many industries have since recognized its value in formulating and evaluating products, general appreciation for sensory evaluation as a distinct function within a company remained minimal until this past decade. In general, there is agreement on the role of sensory evaluation in industry but not necessarily how sensory evaluation should be organized and how it should operate within a company.

As with any emerging discipline, divergent opinions and philosophies on sensory evaluation exist both within and outside the field. It is not necessary that we examine all these opinions (a majority) and philosophies (a minority) in detail. However, some discussion of them is appropriate, to enable the reader to gain a greater appreciation for the problems involved in the organization and operation of a sensory program.

The food industry (as well as many other consumer products industries) traditionally viewed sensory evaluation in the context of the company "expert" (the *N* of 1) who through years of accumulated experience was able to describe company products and set standards of quality by which raw materials would be purchased and each product manufactured and marketed. Examples of such "experts" include the perfumer, flavorist, brewmaster, winemaker, and coffee and tea tasters. In the food industry, experts provided the basis for developing the "cutting sessions" and "canning bees" (Hinreiner, 1956). In the canning industry, products usually were evaluated on a daily basis and in comparison with competitive products, new products, etc. In addition, there were industry-wide cutting bees to assess general product quality. These sessions enabled management and the experts to assess product quality at their own plants, as well as to maintain a familiarity with all other company's products. This process continues today in some companies as well as in trade associations seeking to solve common problems that are usually related to product quality. In recognizing the purpose of the cutting bee and its overall function, Hinreiner (1956) described the efforts undertaken to improve the quality of the information derived from one group, the olive industry. The Processed Products Branch of the Fruit and Vegetable Division of the United States Department of Agriculture (File Code 131A-31, 1994) has updated its guidelines for approved illumination for cutting rooms, an action that recognizes the importance of providing a more standardized environment for product evaluations. In addition to the evaluation itself, record-keeping was formalized, making it possible to compare results from 1 year with another and thus provide for a great degree of continuity. It is important to remember that the industry recognized a problem, and with assistance from sensory evaluation, took some action to improve its information about product quality. This activity continues today, especially in those industries that rely on basic agricultural products that do not experience substantial value-added processing; for example, the wine industry, processed fruits and vegetables, olive oil, etc.

In addition to cuttings, product experts also have endured; however, the impact of many of these experts has been considerably eroded, or in some instances, is exerted only indirectly. In retrospect, the results accomplished (and failed to be accomplished) by these experts and the cutting sessions were quite remarkable. By and large, experts determined which alternatives, from among many alternative ingredients, products, and so forth, were appropriate for sale to the consumer. Their success reinforced their role for establishing quality standards for particular products, such as canned fruits and vegetables, and these standards, in turn, received additional support through official USDA standards that referenced these results. As long as the food industry was involved solely in the preserving of a basic agricultural crop, for example, frozen peas, canned fruits and vegetables, or a juice, then it was relatively easy (or uncomplicated) for the product expert to understand a particular product category and to make reasonably sound recommendations.

In the early stages of the growth of the food-processing industry and where competition was primarily regional in character, such standards and evaluative procedures by experts were extremely useful. In most industries, experts also created a variety of scorecards (and unique terminology) to serve as a basis for maintaining records and presenting a more scientific process. Subsequently, numerical values were also assigned to the scorecards, as described by Hinreiner (1956). These scores soon became targets or standards; for example, the 100-point butter scorecard, the ten-point oil quality scale, and the twenty-point wine scorecard all had specific numbers that connoted levels of product acceptance (equated with quality). All of these and others continue to be used. Certain values became fixed in people's minds, and they were transposed inappropriately into measures of consumer acceptance, creating a multitude of new problems. That some of these scorecards have survived virtually intact after 50 years is remarkable, considering their faults. Where they have not survived one can usually find the concept still alive, particularly that of the single number equated with quality and the associated belief of the invariance of the expert. While it is more common in quality control, the re-emergence of experts in sensory evaluation is somewhat surprising (and discouraging). Not only does it reflect a basic lack of understanding of human behavior and the perceptual process, it also may reflect a wistful desire of some to reduce response behavior to some simplistic level (or some combination of the two). The facts are that humans are neither invariant nor are their responses to products invariant above and beyond the fact that no two products are the same! Sensory professionals do an injustice to themselves and to the science when they embrace these simplistic notions about human behavior without fully appreciating the consequences. They also do a disservice when they participate as subjects, thereby perpetuating the notion of the expert, the *N* of 1 who can make these absolute judgments.

With the growth of the economy and competition and the evolution of processed and formulated foods, experts faced increasing difficulty in maintaining an awareness of all developments concerning their own product interests. As a further complication, product lines expanded to the extent that it was and is impossible for an expert to have detailed knowledge about all products, let alone the impact of different technologies. While the expert was required to continue making finite decisions about product quality, consumer attitudes were changing in ways that were not fully appreciated. With the development of contemporary measurement techniques and their application to sensory evaluation, it became evident that reliance on a few experts was questionable. To deal with this problem, some companies turned to sensory evaluation (which was often referred to as "organoleptic analysis" in the early literature). In truth, companies did not turn directly to sensory evaluation as a solution to the failure of experts, rather the marketplace created opportunities. As competition increased, and became more national (and eventually, international) in scope, the need for more extensive product information became evident. Managers were either disappointed with results from some types of consumer tests and/or costs became increasingly difficult to justify to management, and now were more willing to consider alternative sources of product information. For those companies where there were sensory resources, opportunities developed and in some instances considerable success was achieved. To that extent, sensory evaluation represented a new, and as yet, untried resource. Before discussing this contemporary view, it is necessary to further explore the earlier developments of sensory evaluation.

As noted previously, sensory evaluation was of considerable interest in the late 1940s and on into the 1950s, prompted in part by the government's effort to provide more acceptable food for the military (Peryam *et al.*, 1954), as well as by developments in the private sector. For example, the Arthur D. Little Company introduced the Flavor Profile Method (Caul, 1957), a qualitative form of descriptive analysis that minimized dependence on the technical expert. While the concept of a technical expert was and continues to be of concern, the Flavor Profile procedure replaced the individual with a group of about six experts (that they trained) responsible for yielding a consensus decision. This approach provoked controversy among experimental psychologists who were concerned with the concept of a group decision and the potential influence of an individual (in the group) on this consensus decision (Jones, 1958). Nonetheless, at that time, the method provided a focal point for sensory evaluation, creating new interest in the discipline, which stimulated more research and development into all aspects of the sensory process. This topic is covered in more detail in the discussion on descriptive methods in Chapter 6.

By the mid-1950s, the University of California at Davis was offering a series of courses on sensory evaluation, providing one of the few academic sources for training of sensory evaluation professionals. It should be mentioned that other universities, including Oregon State University, University of Massachusetts, and Rutgers offered course work in sensory evaluation but not to the extent as offered by the University of California (subsequently, many other Universities initiated independent courses in sensory evaluation producing more professionals in the discipline). These developments are reflected in the food science literature of this same period, which includes many interesting studies on sensory evaluation by Boggs and Hansen (1949), Harper (1950), Giradot *et al.* (1952), Baker *et al.* (1954), Pangborn (1964), and Anonymous (1968). These studies stimulated and facilitated the use of sensory evaluation in the industrial environment. The early research was especially thorough in its development and evaluation of specific test methods. Discrimination test procedures were evaluated by Boggs and Hansen (1949), Giradot *et al.* (1952), and Peryam *et al.* (1954). In addition to discrimination testing, other measurement techniques also were used as a means for assessing product acceptance. While scoring procedures were used as early as the 1940s (see Baten, 1946), primary emphasis was given to use of various paired procedures for assessing product differences and preferences. Rank-order procedures and hedonic scales became more common in the mid- to late 1950s. During this time period, various technical and scientific societies such as Committee E-18 of the American Society for Testing and Materials, the Food and Agriculture Section of the American Chemical Society, the European Chemoreception Organization, and the Sensory Evaluation Division of the Institute of Food Technologists organized activities focusing on sensory evaluation and the measurement of flavor. For a review of the activities of ASTM, the reader is referred to Peryam (1991).

III. Development of Sensory Evaluation

It would be difficult to identify any one or two developments that were directly responsible for the emergence of sensory evaluation as a unique discipline and its acceptance (albeit, on a limited basis) in product business decisions. Certainly the international focus on food and agriculture in the mid-1960s and on into the 1970s (it is still with us), the energy crisis, food fabrication and the cost of raw materials (Stone, 1972), competition and the internationalization of the marketplace have, directly or indirectly, created opportunities for sensory evaluation. For example, the search for substitute sweeteners stimulated new interest in the measurement of perceived sweetness (along with time-intensity measures). This, in turn, stimulated development of new measurement techniques (Inglett, 1974) and indirectly stimulated interest in development and use of direct data entry systems as a means for evaluating the sweetness intensity of various ingredients (see Anonymous, 1984; Guinard *et al.*, 1985; Gordin, 1987; Winn, 1988 for more information about this latter topic). Today, this situation has not changed and there remain many unfulfilled opportunities. Whether companies are developing new products, attempting to enter new markets or compete more effectively in existing markets, the need for sensory information remains (see Stone, 2002, *Sensory Evaluation and the Consumer in the 21st Century*). While much more could be written and speculated about these opportunities and their antecedents, it is more important that our attention be focused on how this sensory resource should be structured so it can function more effectively in the future.

After a long and somewhat difficult gestation, sensory evaluation has emerged as a distinct, recognized scientific specialty (Sidel *et al.*, 1975; see also Stone and Sidel, 1995). While the focus of this article was on the use of sensory evaluation in the development of fabricated foods, there were implications for sensory evaluation, in general. As a unique source of product information it had important marketing consequences, providing direct, actionable information quickly and at low cost. It was proposed that organizing of sensory evaluation test services along well-defined lines (e.g. formal test requests, selection of a test method based on an objective, and selection of subjects based on sensory skill) would increase the likelihood of such services being accepted as an integral part of the research and development process (or other business units within a company). It has become clearer that without an organized approach, a management-approved plan, and an operational strategy, sensory resources are rarely used effectively and are less likely to have a significant, long-term impact. More recently, some professionals have structured their sensory resources around a single method in the mistaken assumption that it will solve all problems, or that it obviates the need for a more broadly based program with specified goals and objectives and operational plan. As a general rule, reliance on a single method will create more problems than it will ever solve and hinder development of sensory evaluation as an integral part of the business decision-making process. Reliance on a single method is particularly risky because it leads one to modify problems to fit the method, and to overlook basic sensory procedures and practices. In a short course given several decades ago, Pangborn (1979) called attention to misadventures that have occurred in sensory evaluation which included this reliance on a single method. The article was one of several by this author as part of her continuing efforts to improve the quality of the sensory evaluation literature, now that its use has become more common. The three issues of particular concern to Pangborn were the lack of test objective, adherence to a test method regardless of application, and improper subject selection procedures. These three issues remain as such, even now. These are not the sole property of the sensory literature (and by default many in teaching roles) but also are quite commonplace in the business environment. It is clear that much more needs to be done to improve the quality of sensory information.

An interesting development for sensory evaluation has been the continued growth in the number of short courses and workshops being offered. When there were few University offerings, such programs served a useful purpose for individuals with responsibility for their company's sensory program. In the past decade, there has been a quantum increase in the number courses being offered, including distance learning, which suggests that University offerings are still insufficient for industry's needs. Our own experience in offering courses during the past three decades reflects a continued interest in sensory evaluation, especially the more pragmatic issues of developing a program within a technical-business environment. Some of the material presented in this book evolved from workshop material that has proven especially beneficial to participants. Newspapers and other public information sources present articles about sensory evaluation (not regularly, but often enough to be noticeable). These articles usually include some impressive revelations (to attract the reader) about the special "tongue" or "nose" of certain individuals who are claimed to have almost mystical powers. These individuals are generally associated with such products as wine, beer, coffee, fragrance, or function as wine and food writers. Still other approaches convey an impression that the sensory secrets of the subconscious mind are being tapped by some new technique, with the end result being the ideal consumer product. While sensory professionals should welcome publicity, such promotional information is not always scientifically based (in some instances it may have no basis at all). In spite of this lack of consistency, continued press coverage about sensory evaluation is helpful to the field, if only because it reaches key people who might not otherwise read about it. These changes, and a greater awareness of sensory evaluation, appear to have coincided with a dramatic shift by the food industry toward a consumer-oriented environment and away from the more traditional manufacturing/production-oriented environment. By that we mean a recognition that understanding consumer attitudes and behavior is essential information and ought to be known before one formulates a product rather than manufacturing a product and looking to others; for example, marketing, to convince the consumer to purchase that product.

Opportunities for sensory evaluation continue to develop primarily as a result of significant changes in the marketplace and to a much greater extent then changes in sensory evaluation. Mergers, leveraged buy-outs, and other financial restructuring activities, and the internationalization of the marketplace have created even greater challenges in the consumer products industry. There are numerous choices in terms of brands, flavor alternatives, convenience, pricing, new products, and combinations not thought of a decade ago; for example, yogurt beverages, etc. Many companies have determined that new products at competitive prices are essential for long-term growth and success. However, this has presented its own unique challenges and risks (see, e.g. Meyer, 1984). New product development and the proliferation of choices within a product category rapidly accelerated in the 1980s at a rate neither appreciated nor believed possible in the past. This acceleration was accompanied by considerable financial risk (Anonymous, 1989). In a publication on the topic, Carlson (1977) determined that the failure rate of new products has, at times, been as high as 98% for all new products. Since that report one can easily find similar reports in the trade literature; clearly, this situation has not changed very much and certainly not for the better. From a business perspective, this risk severely challenges creative skills and available technical resources and has provided renewed interest in other information resources such as sensory evaluation (see Stone, 2002). Companies are now more receptive to new approaches and to new ways for anticipating and measuring the potential for a product's success in the marketplace. Of course, some companies may choose to not introduce new products and thereby minimize much of that risk but to rely on brand and line extensions (Lieb, 1989). Here too, the need for sensory information is essential if such products are to be brought into the market within reasonable time and budgetary considerations. These changes should have accelerated the acceptance of sensory evaluation; however, this has not occurred to any great extent until more recently. Companies are now more aware of sensory evaluation; however, the organization and operation of sensory business units with full management support still lag other related activities such as consumer insights (a successor to marketing research?). Nonetheless, the fact that some programs are fully operational bodes well for the future.

While much progress has been made, considerably more remains to be achieved, particularly within the business environment. In the next chapter, this issue is more fully explored, with particular emphasis on structural (e.g. organizational) issues and their integration with the functioning of sensory resources; that is, how methods and subjects are developed and used to solve specific problems and maximize sensory's benefits to a company.

IV. Defining Sensory Evaluation

To more fully appreciate the situation, it is helpful if we first consider the manner in which the two words *sensory evaluation* are defined. The paucity of definitions is surprising: a perusal of various texts and technical sources reveals one prepared by the Sensory Evaluation Division of the Institute of Food Technologists (Anonymous, 1975) and quoted here, that provides insight into the subject:

> *Sensory evaluation is a scientific discipline used to evoke, measure, analyze and interpret reactions to those characteristics of foods and materials as they are perceived by the senses of sight, smell, taste, touch and hearing.*

This definition represents an obvious attempt to be as inclusive as is possible within the framework of food evaluation, with the word "food" considered global; that is, an ingredient is a food. Similarly, materials can be products for the home such as furniture polish, a product for personal care such as a shampoo, a hair colorant, or a lipstick, etc. While it may be relatively easy to find fault with the narrowness of the definition, we should perhaps look beyond the terminology and consider it in a much broader context. First, the definition makes clear that sensory evaluation encompasses all the senses. This is a particularly important issue and one that is overlooked, with the result that in some environments sensory evaluation is viewed solely as "taste testing," as if to imply that it excludes the other senses. While an individual may be asked to respond to a particular product attribute, for example, its color, but if no special care has been taken to exclude the product's aroma, then it is very likely that the obtained color response will be affected by the aroma but not in a predictable way. This will lead to a confounding of the response and potential misinterpretation of the results. A product's appearance will impact an individual's response to that product's taste, etc. Regardless of what one may like to believe or has been told, responses to a product are the result of interactions of various sensory messages, independent of the source. To avoid obtaining incomplete product information, it is important to design studies that take this knowledge into account. The familiar request to "field a test but tell the subjects to ignore the color as that will be corrected later" is a sure sign of impending disaster. This issue will be discussed in a subsequent chapter but is mentioned here to emphasize its importance in the overall evaluation process and the seemingly lack of appreciation of its consequences for the sensory professional reporting results to management who does not "ignore the color." Second, the definition seeks to make clear that sensory evaluation is derived from several different disciplines, but emphasizes the behavioral basis of perception. This involvement of different disciplines may help to explain the difficulty entailed in delineating the functions of sensory evaluation within the business and academic environments. These disciplines include experimental, social, and physiological psychology, statistics, home economics, and in the case of foods, a working knowledge of food science and technology.

As the definition implies, sensory evaluation involves the measurement and evaluation of the sensory properties of foods and other materials. Sensory evaluation also involves the analysis and the interpretation of the responses by the sensory professional; that is, that individual who provides the connection between the internal world of technology and product development and the external world of the marketplace, within the constraints of a product marketing brief. This connection is essential such that the processing and development specialists can anticipate the impact of product changes in the marketplace. Similarly, the marketing and brand specialists must be confident that the sensory properties are consistent with the intended target and with the communication delivered to that market through advertising. They also must be confident that there are no sensory deficiencies that lead to a market failure. Linking of sensory testing with other business functions is essential just as it is essential for the sensory professional to understand the marketing strategy. In recent years, other business units have expressed interest in using sensory information. For example, quality control/quality assurance professionals have initiated efforts to include sensory information into the quality equation. Here too, it has been found that sensory information is cost-effective. However, it has its own set of challenges that will be discussed in more detail later in this book. Thus, sensory evaluation should be viewed in much broader terms. Its contributions far exceed the questions of which flavor is best or whether ingredient A can be replaced with ingredient B. In this discussion and in those that follow, it should be obvious to the reader that we assign more responsibilities to sensory evaluation than just the collecting of responses from selected individuals in a test situation.

This concept is especially important in balancing the impact of consumer response behavior as developed by marketing research. In recent years, there has been a growing interest in and much greater use of sophisticated physiological and psychological approaches in measuring consumer behavior. Although the initial interest centered around advertising, it was only natural that it should also be applied to consumers' reactions to the products themselves. While such approaches can be expected to have a positive impact on the product's success in the marketplace in the long run, it would be naive to assume that such information can substitute for all sensory testing. There are those who advocate by-passing sensory testing itself, and relying on larger-scale consumer testing into which a sensory component is incorporated. Such an approach has much appeal because it could save time (and some cost) and works directly with the real consumers. This approach has considerable surface appeal; however, it comes with risk. In any population, there exists a wide range of product sensitivities. In fact, about 30% of any consumer population cannot satisfactorily discriminate amongst products they regularly consume. As we will discuss later in this book, it takes as much as 10 or more hours to teach consumers how to use their senses and as much as 10 more hours for them to learn how to verbalize what they perceive. So bypassing the sensory test by asking consumers to respond to sensory questions or having them verbalize their experiences has considerable risk associated with it. Along these same lines, the tendency to have a universal test method also presents similar challenges to the sensory professional. While it would be extremely useful to have one method to provide all needed information, it is unrealistic to assume such a solution to account for the complexities of consumer behavior. In addition, the trend toward relying on a statistical solution is equally risky when the basic information was obtained without following accepted procedures and practices.

There is no question that there are important and necessary links between sensory evaluation (and technology) and marketing research. However, one cannot substitute for the other, nor should one be designed to include the other without appreciating the risks. The contexts for both test types are different. Sensory tests focus on product formulation differences and their magnitudes, product preferences, and the relationships among the test variables. Sensory also is capable of linking these variables with consumer attitudes, purchase intent, benefits and uses, etc. While marketing research tests will obtain responses to product attributes, these responses are not a substitute for results from a trained descriptive panel. This is not to suggest they have no value, rather they are indicative of a problem when results are not consistent with existing data. This and related issues will be discussed in more detail in Chapter 7. Similarly, the results of a sensory acceptance test are not a substitute for a marketing research test with a larger population of qualified consumers. A failure to appreciate these differences has had and will continue to have deleterious effects on the growth and development of sensory resources in a company and also on the ability of a company to develop and market successful products. These issues will be discussed again in subsequent chapters of this book.

V. A Physiological and Psychological Perspective

Sensory evaluation principles have their origin in physiology and psychology. Information derived from experiments with the senses has provided a greater appreciation for their properties, and this greater appreciation, in turn, has had a major influence on test procedures and on the measurement of human responses to stimuli. Although sources of information on sensory evaluation have improved in recent years, much information on the physiology of the senses and the behavioral aspects of the perceptual process has been available for considerably longer (Morgan and Stellar, 1950; Guilford, 1954; Granit, 1955; Geldard, 1972; Harper, 1972; Tamar, 1972; Poynder, 1974; McBride and MacFie, 1990). In this discussion, we will identify our meaning of the word "senses." As Geldard (1972) has pointed out, classically the "five special senses" are vision, audition, taste, smell, and touch. The latter designation includes the senses of temperature, pain, pressure, and so forth. Numerous efforts have been made to reclassify the senses beyond the original five, but they are the ones we have chosen to consider here.

From study of the physiology and anatomy of the systems, we know that each sense modality has its own unique receptors and neural pathways to higher and more complex structures in the brain (Morgan and Stellar, 1950; Pfaffman *et al.*, 1954; Granit, 1955; Tamar, 1972). At the periphery, receptors for a specific sense (e.g. visual and gustatory) respond to a specific type of stimulation that is unique to that system. That is, a gustatory stimulus does not stimulate visual receptors. However, when the information is transmitted to high centers in the brain, considerable integration occurs. Comprehension of how sensory information is processed and integrated is important in understanding the evaluation process (Stone and Pangborn, 1968; McBride and MacFie, 1990). What this means when translated into the practical business of product evaluation is that products are a complex source of stimulation and that stimulation will not be exclusive to a single sense, such as vision or taste. Failure to appreciate the consequences of this very fundamental component of sensory evaluation continues to have serious consequences (a perusal of the current sensory literature provides ample evidence of these practices). Consider an evaluation of a strawberry jam that has visual, aroma, taste, and textural properties. Requiring subjects to respond only to textural attributes (and ignore all other stimuli) will lead to partial or misinformation about the products, at best. Assuming subjects (or anyone for that matter) are capable of mentally blocking stimuli or can be trained to respond in this way, is wishful thinking. Response to all other stimuli will be embedded in the textural responses which, in turn, leads to increased variability and decreased sensitivity. This approach ignores basic sensory processes and the manner in which the brain integrates incoming information and, combined with memory, produces a response. Probably more harm is done to the science of sensory evaluation and its credibility when procedures and practices are modified based on faulty assumptions about human behavior in an effort to eliminate a problem which usually has nothing to do with behavior. Use of blindfolds and rooms with colored lights are examples that quickly come to mind. Both practices reflect a poor understanding of the perceptual process, and the mistaken belief that by not measuring some product sensory characteristics, they can be ignored! These practices are never recommended, as they are sources of variability that lead to increased risk in decision-making. In subsequent chapters, solutions to these problems are proposed along with some practical examples.

The psychophysical roots for sensory evaluation can be traced to the work of Weber (cited in Boring, 1950), which was initiated during the middle of the nineteenth century. However, it could be argued that it was Fechner (Boring, 1950), building on the experimental observations of Weber, who believed he saw in these observations a means of linking the physical and psychological worlds that gave rise to the field of psychophysics. Much has been written about this topic as well as the early history of psychology in general. The interested reader will find the book by Boring (1950) especially useful in describing this early history. For purposes of this discussion, we call attention to just a few of these developments because of their relevance to sensory evaluation. This is not intended to be a review as such reviews are readily available in the psychophysical literature, rather to remind the reader, in an abbreviated manner, the strong ties between sensory evaluation and experimental psychology. For a more contemporary discussion about the perceptual process, the reader is referred to Laming (1986), McBride and MacFie (1990), and Lawless and Heymann (1999).

Fechner was most interested in the philosophical issues associated with the measurement of sensation and its relation to a stimulus. He proposed that since sensation could not be measured directly, it was necessary to measure sensitivity by means of differential changes. This conclusion was based on the experimental observations of Weber. By determining the detectable amount of difference between two stimuli (the just-noticeable-difference or JND), Fechner sought to establish a unit measure of sensation. He proposed that each JND would be equivalent to a unit of sensation and that the JNDs would be equal. From this point, an equation was formulated relating response to stimulus:

$$S = k \log R$$

where S is the magnitude of sensation, k a constant, and R the magnitude of the stimulus.

As Boring emphasized, Fechner referred to this as Weber's Law, now known as the Weber–Fechner Law or the Psychophysical Law. This initiated not only the field of psychophysics but also a long series of arguments as to the true relationship between stimulus and response and the development of a unified theory of perception. For many years, it was argued that one could not measure sensory magnitudes and, therefore, such a psychophysical law was meaningless. However, the most concerted attacks on the Fechnerian approach were made by Stevens (1951) and his co-workers (see Cain and Marks, 1971; Lawless and Heymann, 1999, for more detailed discussions on this topic), who advocated a somewhat different explanation for the relationships of stimulus and response. Stevens proposed that equal stimulus ratios result in equal sensation ratios rather than equal sensation differences as proposed by Fechner. Mathematically, as proposed by Stevens, the Psychophysical Power Law was as follows:

$$R = kS^n$$

and

$$\log R = n \log S + \log k$$

where R is the response, k a constant, S the stimulus concentration, and n the modality-dependent exponent.

The formulation of this law had a renewed and stimulating effect on the field, as manifested by hundreds of publications describing responses to a variety of stimuli including commercial products, and setting off numerous debates as to the numerical values of the power functions for the various sensory modalities. Certainly, the development of signal detection theory has had a major impact on our knowledge of the perceptual process, in general, and on sensory evaluation in particular. But, it too has its opponents who seek a single unified theory of perception. However, as Stevens (1962) observed, such laws generally attract criticism as well as support, and the Power Law was no exception (Anderson, 1970). In fact, the extent of criticism directed at any one theory of perception is no greater or less than that directed at any other theory and to date, there has been no satisfactory resolution. The interested reader should read the previously cited work of Anderson and Laming, and for more on this issue from a sensory evaluation perspective, see Giovanni and Pangborn (1983). The observations of Weber, however, warrant further comment because of their importance in product evaluation. Basically, Weber noted that the perception of the difference between two products was a constant, related to the ratio of the difference, and expressed mathematically as

$$K = \frac{\Delta R}{R}$$

where R is the magnitude of the stimulus and K is the constant for the JND. Experiments on a variety of stimuli and particularly those involving food and food ingredients, have shown generally good agreement with Weber's original observations (Wenzel, 1949; Schutz and Pilgrim, 1957; Luce and Edwards, 1958; Stone, 1963; Cain, 1977). As with other developments, there are exceptions and not all experimental results are in complete agreement with this mathematical expression. Nonetheless, the JND has found widespread application in the sensory evaluation of products as described in Chapter 5.

Among the contributions to sensory evaluation by psychologists, the work of Thurstone (1959) is especially noteworthy. Many of his experiments involved foods (rather than less complex unidimensional stimuli) or concerned the measurement of attitudes, both topics that are of particular interest to the manufacturer of consumer goods. Thurstone formulated the Law of Comparative Judgment enabling use of multiple paired comparisons to yield numerical estimates of preferences for different products. From this and other pioneering research evolved many of the procedures and practices used today by sensory professionals. Today, renewed interest in Thurstonian psychophysics is welcomed; however, these authors never considered it absent or not an integral part of the perceptual process.

Psychology has contributed substantially to our understanding of the product evaluation process; however, it would be incorrect to characterize sensory evaluation solely as a part of the science of psychology.

As the adherents to the various schools of psychology or particular approaches espouse their causes, it is easy to confuse research on scaling or perception with assessment of product success without appreciating the differences and the risks. It is easy to mistake developments in psychology as having immediate and direct consequences for sensory evaluation, and to blur the lines between the two. This has been particularly evident by those who implied use of magnitude estimation, a type of ratio scale, as the best procedure for obtaining meaningful numerical estimates of the perceived intensities of various stimuli (Stevens, 1960). It was claimed that use of this scaling method enabled one to obtain unbiased judgments, allowed for use of higher-order statistics, and a much greater level of sensitivity than achievable by other scales. As will be discussed in Chapter 3, attempts to demonstrate this scale superiority in sensory evaluation applications have been unsuccessful (Moskowitz and Sidel, 1971). What may be demonstrated with a single stimulus in a controlled experiment does not necessarily translate to the evaluation of more complex stimuli such as foods and other consumer products. That such superiority has not yet been demonstrated with any scale should not be surprising, particularly from an applications perspective. As Guilford (1954), Nunnally (1978), and others have noted, having a less than perfect scale does not invalidate results and any risks that such use entailed are not as serious as one might expect. As it happens, the risks are very small, particularly with regard to the product evaluation process. In Chapter 3, this topic will be discussed in more detail. Nonetheless, it should be clear that sensory evaluation makes use of psychology, just as it makes use of physiology, mathematics, and statistics in order to achieve specific test objectives. The discipline operates without the restrictions of different theories of perception competing to explain the mechanisms of perception, a task of psychophysicists and physiological psychologists. The sensory professional must be sufficiently well-informed in these disciplines to identify their relevance to the organization, fielding, and analyses of a sensory test, without losing sight of sensory goals and objectives.

The remaining chapters of this book emphasize the organization and operation of a sensory evaluation program, taking into account both the short- and long-term issues that directly affect the success of a program.

2

The Organization and Operation of a Sensory Evaluation Program

I. Introduction

An organized sensory evaluation program with full responsibility for its actions is essential for its success within a company for the short and the long term (Sidel *et al.*, 1975; Stone and Sidel, 1995). Failure to appreciate the importance of an organized approach and having a management-approved operational plan will, sooner or later, undermine the activities of the sensory professional(s) and the program itself. There is less involvement in product decision-making, a reduction in product testing requests, and generally being relegated to a minor role in the overall product evaluation process. There is no question that sensory evaluation can contribute directly and indirectly to company profitability; that is, providing actionable information at minimal expense and time. The ability to field a test in a few hours and directly advise a product manager that a particular ingredient change can be achieved at minimal or no change in preference behavior has considerable market value. However, such a response does not occur by chance; rather it comes about through an organized effort, credibility within one's company, and a reputation for being

Sensory Evaluation Practices 3rd Edn
ISBN: 0-12-672690-6

responsive to business priorities. The ability to anticipate needs, to develop appropriate resources, to assess new developments, and to be responsive can only come about if one plans and builds toward those objectives; in effect, move from a passive to an active role in the product and process development functions. Over the past decade, more companies have come to appreciate the importance of having a clearly defined sensory program with an operational strategy consistent with a company's business plans (see Eggert, 1989; Stone and Sidel, 1995). It is the authors' contention that much of the frustration with sensory evaluation encountered by product managers, and by sensory professionals themselves, comes directly from this lack of planning and an inability to provide information that is understood and actionable, at the right time.

While the concepts (and the practices) of planning and developing an organizational structure are essential for the survival of all business units, it is not yet clear that sensory professionals are fully aware of these concepts nor is it clear that they understand them sufficiently to employ them effectively. This is particularly important in the current business environment where mergers have created very large organizations with equally large and diverse product lines, and a need to be responsive to shareholders and the marketplace in ways that were unanticipated a few years ago, particularly with regard to profitability. Restructuring of large business units based on specific product categories (often associated with where they sit in a retail outlet) have resulted in the loss of resources (or their unavailability because they are now part of another business unit of the company and these units are not integrated and do not directly communicate). This creates further problems for sensory professionals, particularly if there is no organized program to promote use of the resources or serve as a role model for other business units. As Blake (1978), Tushman and Anderson (1997), and others have emphasized, companies or individual business units must be sufficiently flexible so as to respond quickly and with the full power of the available resources. While it is not our intention to provide an analysis or an evaluation of various business management practices (nor is it appropriate), there is no question that sensory professionals must be aware of their companies' business management orientation and strategies and be sufficiently flexible themselves to adjust to any changes that occur. For more background reading on these issues, the reader is referred to Blake (1978) and Tushman and Anderson (1997). In addition, the reader is directed to Aaker (1996) on brand management and related issues.

That there are different views of what sensory evaluation is, who it serves, etc., should come as no surprise. Each of these views may require a somewhat different stance (organizationally and operationally) in terms of testing, reporting, and so on. Sensory evaluation usually serves many different groups within a company and the interaction and dialog with each group will vary, depending on the problem, how the information will be used, and the extent to which sensory will participate in the planning process and in the utilization of the results. For example, tests requested by product development will be handled differently from those requested by quality control, or marketing. In fact, the entire process (from request to issuance of a recommendation) should be part of a sensory program's operational plan. Such a plan should call attention to such issues as: (a) whether a problem warrants formal sensory analysis (as distinct from bench screening); (b) what priority will be assigned; (c) what is the product source (obtained from the marketplace, production but before distribution, pilot plant, bench top); (d) what is the stage of the project (early, final); (e) what are the economic implications; (f) how will the results be used; (g) impact of other product or product-related information, and finally, (h) how the information will be communicated and to who. All of these issues must be taken into consideration by the sensory staff before a decision is made as to what will be done to satisfy the particular request. Of course, this assumes the sensory staff has the authority to accept, modify, or reject a test request. Not surprisingly, the decisions that are made will impact how the information will be received and ultimately, how the sensory program is viewed by others; that is, its responsiveness, cooperation, and its credibility.

This concept of strategic thinking is not limited to companies with a large sensory staff; a staff of one or two individuals may not have as many test requests, but the same principles apply. The key to a successful program is to identify the strengths and weaknesses of one's program (in the context of that company's corporate strategy) and to develop capabilities based on the available resources (people and support services). If capabilities are limited, then some trade-offs will be necessary until such time as the needed resources have been acquired through education, staff additions, and so forth. Regardless of the extent of one's sensory resources, if they are organized, there is a greater likelihood that the program will be considered as more credible. Of course, providing reliable, valid information that is actionable will have an even more significant impact. Each requires the other to be effective. Finally, managers will better understand sensory evaluation activities and results when presented in the context of that company's typical business structure.

In describing the organization of sensory resources, our focus is on the sensory professional developing an organizational plan and an operational strategy, including responsibility for its implementation. This approach is in contrast with those companies in which an individual not familiar with sensory evaluation decides on the organizational plan without any appreciation for its requirements let alone its unique role between technology and the consumer. Based on our experiences working with both large and small companies, it is clear that successful sensory programs use a matrix type of approach to project management (based on assigning an individual with the requisite experience rather than basing the assignment on knowledge of a specific evaluation method). This approach is by no means unique or innovative, but it has proven to be successful because it enables a sensory professional to be involved in all stages of a project. While these issues are discussed in some detail in subsequent sections, their importance to the overall success of a sensory program is such that one cannot be easily discussed without the other.

The success of this approach comes about first through a management that is aware of the value of sensory information and second because of a business-like approach by the sensory professional. It is especially important to recognize that this approach, when put in practice, will more than compensate a company for its investment, and most likely within a few months of initiation. Companies have found that every dollar invested in sensory resources returns ten dollars in savings. Conversely, highly skilled sensory professionals become frustrated and ineffective in environments that neither formally recognize the value of sensory information nor provide for an appropriate organizational and reporting structure.

II. Organizing a Sensory Evaluation Program

Organizing sensory activities begins with a plan to develop management's awareness (or raise it to a higher level) of the value of sensory information. Generally speaking, all managers have some awareness of sensory evaluation. This may have come through their own practical experience, through reading the trade or technical literature, discussions with other managers, and so forth. While such information may be useful as a starting point, sensory professionals should consider this only as background, and make no assumptions as to an individual's working knowledge of sensory evaluation. In some situations, that information could be negative; that is, a sensory test is remembered because it was unsuccessful, it did not find the problem, etc. Sensory professionals should expect to be challenged on some sensory issues.

Thus, the initial step in this process is to develop a written plan, reflecting what has been done, what is being done now and what could be done in the future (for your company). For example, Table 2.1 lists business activities to which sensory can contribute, directly or indirectly. All of these are important to a company. For some companies the emphasis may be on the marketplace; that is, on new products, cost reduction and reformulation, line extensions, etc. For other companies quality control is a primary focus. The list is intended to be quite general, with no designation as to where tests will take place, who will serve as subjects, or which methods will be used. The point is that managers first must be made aware of the different ways in which sensory information can be used. This plan also should include some technical details, proposed budgets [this will depend on how a company accounts for personnel, timing to achieve specific objectives, and some indication of the financial benefits (and risks)]. Financial benefit is a particularly important issue for sensory evaluation. While most individuals probably consider sensory evaluation as a resource that costs money to develop and operate, in fact, it can be shown to more than pay for itself. This is demonstrated through its ability to screen large numbers

Table 2.1 Sensory evaluation activities within a company
Product development
Product reformulation/cost reduction
Monitoring competition
Quality control
Quality assurance
Product sensory specification
Raw materials specifications
Storage stability
Process/ingredient/analytical/sensory relationships
Advertising claims

of alternative formulations quickly, thereby reducing the number of products requiring larger scale and more costly external testing; and secondly, in cost reduction programs through use of the discrimination model. This latter topic will be discussed in more detail in the next section of this chapter.

Before continuing with the organizational plan, it is useful to consider the appropriate location of the sensory function within a company. This usually is a political and highly controversial issue. To some people, sensory evaluation is another group competing for available funds and space; to others, it is one more potential group to manage and thereby to have a larger staff. Although such issues may seem trivial, they form part of the background from which recommendations are prepared regarding the organization and location of a sensory function.

In most companies, sensory resources are located within the research and development function; however, it is sometimes a part of marketing research or some other non-technical group. There is no rule stipulating that sensory resources must be located in a particular area; but since most sensory professionals have some technical training and most often are providing services to technical groups, sensory resources are frequently placed within the technical division. Historically, the company flavor expert was usually a part of the production and/or technical areas, thus providing additional justification for positioning of sensory activities in research and development. It was assumed that the two activities were essentially the same, a faulty perception that has led to all sorts of problems that we will discuss in more detail in another chapter of this book.

In today's environment, most requests for sensory services come from technology; however, the real source is more likely brand management. Unfortunately, the exact positioning relative to other research and development activities often provokes considerable disagreement. In some companies, sensory evaluation is positioned too low to have sufficient management effectiveness or presence relative to the information it provides, or it is positioned as part of a product development group that it also serves. This latter situation is particularly troublesome because of the pressure that often is applied to a sensory evaluation program to accommodate atypical or inappropriate problems or to hide results that are inconsistent with expectation.

As previously noted, information developed by sensory evaluation often has far-reaching implications. Consider company "A" with four plants, all manufacturing a similar line of products. Chemical analysis and purchase specifications showed that raw material and finished products were developed to one specification, yet sensory tests revealed that one plant's product was perceived as significantly different and also was significantly less preferred. If the products are all present in all markets; that is, they co-mingle, these results could have far-reaching economic and marketing implications. For example, was the difference expected, does the difference in preference translate to changes in purchase intent, were differences related to ingredients or processing conditions, etc.? Product differences could help explain atypical results obtained in a consumer test. It is possible that plant management and others will question the results or at least review them with the sensory staff. The support that sensory evaluation receives and the extent to which it actively participates in discussions such as these will reflect the program's credibility as well as its position within a company. If sensory evaluation is positioned too low, its impact will be diminished, and it also may be excluded from communications that are critical to fielding a test or understanding the implications of results.

While one would like to believe that these issues should not be of concern in the assessment of results, the realities of the situation suggest otherwise. Obviously, the experience and skill of a sensory professional will help to dispel some of these diversionary issues. Nevertheless, positioning is an important issue; it can also impact the accessibility of information, which may be crucial to the design of the test or to the true reasons for a particular request. Thus, positioning of sensory resources is a challenging and serious issue. Sensory evaluation must present itself as a unique entity within an organization and it can best achieve its goals by being independent of the groups that it serves. Sensory evaluation program must demonstrate to management the importance of this independence and the need to be treated as a unique and separate resource. In some companies, sensory resources are positioned within an R&D technical service group. This is a reasonable option provided the reporting sequence has a minimum number of levels from sensory to R&D management. In other companies, sensory resources are positioned as part of consumer affairs or marketing services. Here, too, an important consideration is its accessibility to technical management, along with other considerations, and in particular its freedom of operation.

In situations where management is undecided about the placement of sensory resources, its strategy and the professional's business skills will be tested. Management must be convinced that a final decision should be postponed until sufficient experience has been obtained, especially in relation to the contributions of sensory information to product development, marketing, sales, and quality control, to name a few. This particular approach is most desirable for those individuals who are starting their sensory programs for the first time and who have not yet provided management with sufficient evidence of the potential value for sensory information. Of course, temporary situations can become permanent unless the sensory professional maintains an active presence, keeping management informed as to the program's successes and its contributions to the company.

In addition to establishing an organizational location for sensory evaluation within a company, the resources must be capable of responding to current as well as anticipated needs. Twelve elements that form the foundation for an effective sensory evaluation program are:

1. stated and approved goals and objectives;
2. defined program strategy and business plan;
3. professional staff;
4. test facilities;
5. ability to use all test methods;
6. pool of qualified subjects;
7. standardized subject-screening procedures;
8. standardized subject performance monitoring procedures;
9. standardized test request and reporting procedures;
10. on-line data processing capabilities;

11. formal operations manual;
12. planning and research program.

For some readers, this list may simply be a re-affirmation of their own resources; however, in all probability, only a small minority will have all twelve in place and fully operational. In fact, few sensory professionals have considered their activities in this context, and even the most experienced sensory professional should find this listing helpful. The crucial point is that a successful sensory program must include all of these resources if it is to adequately fulfill its role within a company. For some, meeting the requirements is relatively easy, while for others, it will be more difficult, and could require as much as 3–5 years or more. This does not mean that an operational program will be 3 or more years away or that no actionable information will be forthcoming during this time. Rather, it means that the full and efficient use of resources often takes that long because users (of the service) do not always understand the information or do they appreciate how to use sensory resources and information to best advantage. Of course, budgetary considerations or rapidly changing management will preclude any decisions, thus, slowing program development. Similarly, sensory professionals must regularly educate their customers to ensure that there is a good understanding of sensory information, beyond the simple statement that, for example, A is significantly more preferred than B. In addition to developing and maintaining lines of communication, business priorities will change from year to year, sometimes in unpredictable ways, necessitating a shift in testing emphasis. Thus, the time span should not be considered as excessively long or unusual. The point to be made here is that test methods and the associated resources take relatively little time (a few months) to organize and provide actionable results. The proper positioning of the capability and its optimal effectiveness as a contributor to product success takes considerably longer and is more challenging. One goal of this and succeeding sections is to provide the reader with some background information about all these inter-related issues and provide ideas that are applicable to their own company.

A. Goals and Objectives

Generally, sensory professionals and their research counterparts do not fully appreciate the importance of having defined and management-approved goals and objectives for a sensory program. Goals and objectives may be likened to a license to operate, a charter that defines where and how a sensory evaluation program will operate. Perhaps the most fascinating aspect of the process of defining goals and objectives is the diversity of opinions and definitions expounded by the individuals who participate in the process. To the extent possible, the sensory professional should formulate the goals and objectives as an initial step and be able to provide supporting materials should they be required by those managers who have an input but do not necessarily understand what it is that sensory can and cannot do for them. There is a need to formulate mutually agreeable goals and objectives that reflect current company business plans as well as the overall sensory needs from a technical perspective. This process is not carried out in isolation if the result is to be workable and the impact is to be lasting. While goals and objectives can be modified if they become unworkable, such changes, if not carefully positioned, will have an unsettling effect on management (concerning whether the sensory evaluation professionals know what they are doing) and an unsettling effect on those groups that work with sensory evaluation and may cause them to question the true purposes of the function.

Therefore, the challenge is to develop goals and objectives that on the one hand provide sensory evaluation with sufficient freedom of movement to operate effectively, but on the other hand do not appear to threaten and/or replace other product information sources. For example, a purpose for sensory test results is neither to tell the technical staff how to formulate products, nor is it to replace marketing research efforts to measure the consumer's purchase intentions, nor to determine which new product should be marketed. However, it would also be inappropriate to restrict sensory goals and objectives to specific test methods or solely to measuring employee reactions to products; that is, to provide barriers based on test type or location of data source. Such barriers reflect a lack of understanding of the true purpose of sensory evaluation. It is far more useful if these goals and objectives are defined in terms of what sensory evaluation does, and what it is capable of doing, as listed below.

1. Provide quantitative information about the sensory properties of all company and competitive products.
2. Provide useful and timely information and recommendations about product sensory properties as requested.
3. Maintain a pool of individuals qualified to participate in a wide range of tests.
4. Develop methods that are unique to specific products and methods that are for general use.
5. Develop methods and procedures for relating sensory and analytical information for use in product research, quality control, and quality assurance.
6. Maintain awareness of new developments in product evaluation and their application to the company.
7. Provide assistance to other groups in the company, on request.
8. Ensure that no product of the company fails because of a sensory deficiency.

Based on these capabilities, the sensory professional should be able to develop goals and objectives that are reasonable and achievable within a specified time period. It is important to acknowledge that regardless of how these goals and objectives are stated, they do not specify a particular test method, test location, or type of individual to be included or excluded as a subject. For example, specifying that only technical or professional staff members can participate as subjects or that an individual must have worked for the company for a certain period of time is self-defeating. Such restrictions will clearly work against the development of a viable sensory testing function.

Of course, developing goals and objectives is but one step in the overall approach, a step that may prove to be more difficult to achieve than one realizes. Management will expect sensory evaluation to provide a reasonable explanation for the stated goals, a timetable, and some indication of the financial commitment. Considerable preparation will be needed, including written justification and supporting documents. The continuation of test activities during this preparation phase will help to reinforce the usefulness of sensory resources. The key to success in this endeavor resides primarily with the skill of the sensory professional in identifying the necessary information and in communicating directly with management about the goals and objectives and their benefits. When communicating, it is naive to assume that the listener, whether or not technically trained, is more familiar with sensory evaluation than any other employee of a company. In fact, many individuals have considerable misinformation about sensory evaluation that can and will create problems in establishing an adequate sensory testing capability. Inasmuch as we are all equipped with sensory receptors there exists in all of us an expert element or at the least, an attitude expressed as *de gustibus et de coloris non est disputandum*. This is further complicated by the position that an individual holds in a company; the higher the position, the more correct are one's sensory skills. Communications also are an extremely important issue, one that appears to cause considerable difficulty for many sensory professionals. Most managers have little interest in knowing the test details, rather what actions are recommended. Ultimately, of course, both management and sensory evaluation must agree on the goals and objectives for a program. A failure to do so will reduce the effectiveness of sensory evaluation and will undermine its independent function within a company. On the other hand, the establishment of goals and objectives does not guarantee a successful program!

B. Program Strategy

A sensory program (or some similar designation) must have an overall strategy for dealing with corporate issues and with the myriad of issues concerned with the everyday, sensory testing process. Of the two, the corporate issues are more general, have longer-term consequences, and most likely will take more time to formalize. To further complicate the situation, a corporate strategy will change, sometimes annually, as a company's business plans and market strategies change; for example, emphasis may shift from new products to cost reduction, an acquisition may be integrated with existing product lines, and so forth. A sensory professional needs to be familiar with corporate strategies, primarily through brand managers and through R&D managers. This information provides a basis for developing resources that will be needed but not currently available. Obviously, sensory professionals not familiar with company business plans or without their own program strategy are at a disadvantage and certainly need to correct this deficiency. This comes about through discussions with managers and with those individuals who have relevant information. Not only does the strategy information enable sensory professionals to anticipate shifts in test requests but it also provides a clearer view of a program's strengths and weaknesses. It also is a good reminder of the role that sensory evaluation plays in the business of product development, formulation, production and marketing. Everyday sensory strategy refers to management of test requests, determining what products warrant testing, how priorities are established and by who, policy and procedure for communicating results, and strategy for communicating actionable information to sales, marketing research, and other groups. A strategy is important because it provides a firm basis for an entire program's operation. It minimizes the impact of external pressures to require tests or some related activities that are inconsistent with accepted sensory principles and practices, or to involve sensory evaluation in a project for which it is not adequately staffed or qualified. For example, it is not unusual for a requestor to stipulate a method and/or the subjects to be used, or to insist on doing their own analysis and/or interpretation of results. Other undesirable practices include the insistence that a test be done regardless of merit or that a test be repeated because the result was inconsistent with a requestor's expectations.

A strategy should help define each step in the testing process; that is, the criteria by which a request is considered as reasonable and a test is warranted. Practically speaking, it should begin in the project planning process, even before a specific request is under consideration. Participating in the planning enables the sensory professional to put forward ideas about testing, to suggest alternative designs, to have an impact on what additional products could be included in a test, and so forth. As depicted schematically in Fig. 2.1, the sequence of events begins with the receipt of a request and culminates in issuing a written report (ideally this should be preceded by a presentation to the key staff).

The first level in Fig. 2.1 is the planning process; it is the responsibility of the sensory professional working with the requestor to ensure that products and test objective are consistent and that a priority has been stated on the request. It should

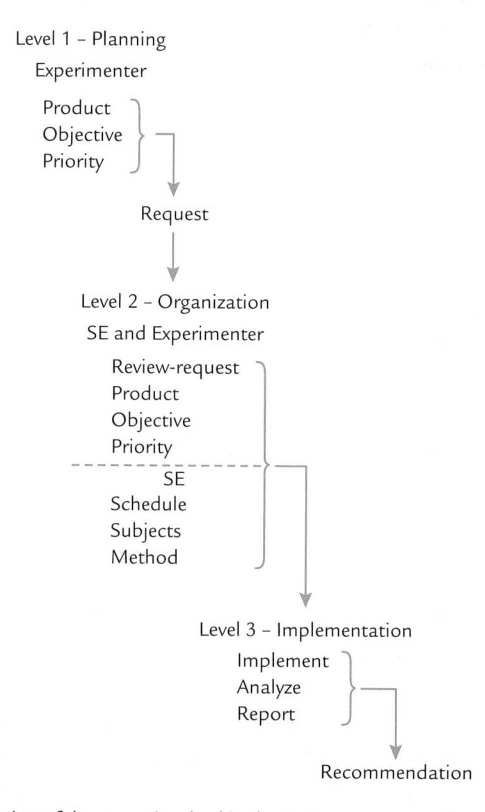

Figure 2.1 A representation of the stages involved in the testing process consistent with a defined strategy. Level 1 is the responsibility of the experimenters requesting assistance. Level 2 involves the sensory evaluation professional reviewing the request with the experimenter. On completion of this task, the test is scheduled. Level 3 involves data collection, analysis, and a written report leading to actionable recommendations.

be noted that this is a written (paper or electronic) request using a form prepared by sensory evaluation. On receipt of a request, the sensory professional reviews it and in consultation with the requestor determines that a particular test is warranted. By observing a standard protocol, the sensory professional and the requestor have ample opportunity to make changes and to increase the likelihood of a successful outcome to the request. The basis for a request must be taken into account, in its entirety. Specifically, how will results be used, is the request one of a series for this product category or is it a single request? Other important information includes where the products are located, how they were prepared (at the bench, pilot plant, production), when products will be provided for the test, and who is responsible for their delivery. On the surface, this exchange of information would seem to be both tedious and potentially intrusive and time consuming. Initially, it would certainly seem to be so; however, the success of a program is built on providing the right information and unless a thorough effort is applied, the likelihood for success is lessened. Obviously, with time, everyone involved (almost everyone – there are some who refuse to learn) in the process learns what is needed and requests proceed more quickly, with minimal difficulty, and there is a concomitant increase in the quality of the results. A strategy makes clear the responsibilities of sensory evaluation and of the requestor without serving as an impediment to progress. This procedure is important not only in establishing successful working relationships between requestors and sensory evaluation, but also between sensory and other product groups, such as brand management and marketing research (currently called consumer insights).

C. Professional Staff

Developing a capable staff is a real challenge for a company particularly when managers are not familiar with sensory evaluation or the current sensory staff lack the experience to develop needed professional skills. As noted previously, sensory evaluation is the application of knowledge and skills derived from several different scientific and technical disciplines – physiology, chemistry, mathematics and statistics, human behavior, and knowledge about product preparation practices – and few individuals have received the diverse education needed to satisfy these requirements. A professional must be sufficiently knowledgeable in all these disciplines to function effectively without constant reliance on specialists (otherwise the specialists will come to believe that they are now the sensory experts). In addition, a professional must be able to train a staff to the extent that they can perform their work and they fully understand the rationale for sensory principles and practices and to know when to seek assistance.

How does one find such individuals, and particularly a sensory professional? For a company with limited or no recent experience with sensory evaluation, this can be difficult. Initially, most look to those Universities graduating students in the discipline or recruiting an individual from another company. Once an individual has been designated, formulation of a plan must be initiated; how sensory information could be used and the program's anticipated emphasis. Ideally, such an individual will have had some courses in the science, as part of their college education, or at the least general science education. Next is the question of whether specific skills should be emphasized; for example, psychology, physiology, and statistics, or should one build a staff with individuals who have some of these skills but also have other experiences? For example, an individual with product development experience may have a better appreciation for the problems involved in product formulation and could incorporate this knowledge into the design of a test or apply it in the interpretation of results. However, this same individual may have limited knowledge of the behavioral aspects of testing and thus miss an important component of a test. Alternatively, one may start with an individual possessing a general scientific education and skill in relating to people and provide this individual with on-site training. The options are numerous; however, more practical considerations dictate that before deciding on a specialist or a generalist, there should be a program plan based on the goals and objectives and take into account the current and anticipated types of testing and the types of problems typically encountered. This information also helps to establish the number of staff members and the skills required for meaningful "job descriptions." Alternatively, one may be able to hire an academically trained sensory professional who will be able to expedite the process.

The sensory professional-manager has numerous responsibilities, all of which are equally important to the success of a testing capability. These include the following:

1. Organization and administration of all departmental/group activities (personnel and budgets).
2. Plan and develop resources (tests, subjects, and records).
3. Advise on feasibility of test requests.
4. Select test procedures, experimental designs, and analyses.
5. Supervise testing activities.
6. Determine need for special panels.
7. Ensure smooth operation of test program.
8. Train subordinates to handle routine assignments.
9. Responsible for reporting results.
10. Maintenance of all necessary supplies and support services.
11. Provide progress reports.
12. Develop and update all program plans.
13. Research new methods.
14. Maintain liaison with other departments that use sensory information.

This list clearly emphasizes management skills in addition to knowledge about sensory evaluation. Because results from sensory tests will be used in business decisions, management skills are particularly important. Sensory testing is used in a variety of situations and when and how it is applied assumes an appreciation for the particular problem and the associated business issues. For example, ingredient replacement is a typical application for sensory evaluation; however, the wording of the conclusion and recommendation from a test will reflect the source of the products (the cost implications and the risk). If the products were made in a pilot plant and not on a typical production line, the recommendation might include an appropriate cautionary statement about the potential difference between products obtained from the two sources. Another situation may involve cancellation of a test because the products are not appropriate; for example, one contains too much color due to improper weighing. The situations are almost limitless, but all require decisions, usually on the spot, and all are potential sources for confrontation or missed opportunities if not handled with skill.

In general, it is the exception rather than the rule to find a sensory professional with good management skills. Most sensory professionals are capable of organizing and fielding a test in a technical sense but experience considerably more difficulty functioning effectively in project meetings with marketing, marketing research, production, and others, where strategy and communication skills can be more important than results from a test. This does not mean that an academically trained professional is incapable of, or cannot be trained to be an effective manager. Since the activity is relatively new, there are few examples that can be cited and still fewer professionals with the experience and needed management skills. Over time, this situation will change as professionals gain experience functioning in this non-laboratory environment. Sensory professionals need to develop communication skills through their own efforts and particularly by attendance at company-sponsored training programs. It should be noted that these issues are independent of company size; that is, selecting a test method, communicating results, organizing resource, etc., are no different whether one is working in a small or large company.

Some companies may not want to wait for a sensory professional to learn how to be an effective manager and instead, assign an individual from another area, someone with proven management skills. While such a move may satisfy management, it will not necessarily satisfy the development of sensory resources or of the sensory staff, at least not in the long term. In practice, it has been observed that the manager with little or no familiarity with sensory evaluation is more vulnerable to external pressures; to accede to test requests that are not consistent with accepted sensory practices, to acquire a methodology without appreciating the risks, and so forth. However, when such a system is structured on an interim basis, to allow the sensory professional to gain the necessary skills, then it is a reasonable option. In the long term, and in the best interests of a sensory program, a professional with good sensory skills should manage the program.

The sensory professional carries out the duties assigned by the manager. These duties include the following: establish test schedules, assign responsibility on a test-by-test basis, supervise all phases of product preparation and testing, responsible for report preparation, maintenance of records, supplies, and support services, maintain the department library, coordinate new subject orientation, screening, and motivation, plan and supervise research activities, meet with requestors to review future tests as well as to discuss results, and perform all other duties delegated by the manager.

In addition to a manager and a sensory professional, a minimal (department) staff will include two analysts. While some companies might prefer the designation of technician, we believe that the responsibilities warrant a more professional designation. Responsibilities include preparation and implementation of tests, scheduling subjects, coding scorecards, serving, collecting and recording responses, data input and routine analyses, maintain records, maintenance of facilities and supplies, familiarity with technical and scientific literature, and so forth. Sensory analysts should have a science background, preferably as an undergraduate degree; knowledge of sensory evaluation principles and practices is desirable, as is training in statistics and experimental psychology. For evaluation of foods, knowledge of recipe development and product preparation also will be helpful. Individuals with these qualifications are rare, and thus a manager usually selects an individual based on potential.

In some situations, the sensory analyst position is considered interim, or entry level. Demonstrated performance leads to promotion and is considered permanent (i.e. not necessarily interim). The intention is to seek an individual who will continue in that position. We believe that the sensory analyst position should be permanent and should have a professional designation. If an individual has demonstrated the necessary capabilities, then promotion is justified and an opening for a new sensory analyst is created. The importance of the sensory analyst cannot be underestimated, inasmuch as this individual is in direct contact with subjects on a daily basis, observing their reactions before and after each test. In addition, the sensory analyst prepares and serves products, and generally functions as an "early warning system" if there are unanticipated problems during a test. Positioning the sensory analyst position as interim can lead to problems. It implies that the position is temporary, not important enough to be permanent, and could give the impression of a less professional and more casual approach to the work. The self-worth of those individuals especially suited to the position would be harmed. If employee turnover in this assignment is high, staff training costs increase and the potential for errors during a test also increases. Therefore, the emphasis should be on permanency, and hence the suggestion of professional designation for this assignment.

In addition to a professional staff, a sensory program should include an individual with clerical and data processing skills. Substantial numbers of reports with text, tables, and graphics, and large volumes of records are produced; time is needed to contact subjects, to prepare data for analysis, to ensure that supplies are ordered and received, and to manage databases. While these tasks can also be performed by the professional staff, it is an inefficient use of their time.

A typical staff should consist of a core group of five persons: a sensory professional-manager, a sensory professional, two analysts, and a clerk. Companies familiar with the use of sensory testing procedures and having an extensive product line may have a sensory evaluation staff consisting of five or more professionals and an appropriate number of analysts. Companies new to sensory testing may have only two individuals – a sensory professional-manager and an analyst. This latter group is minimal and its overall impact will, of necessity, be limited. Either fewer tests are done each week or the amount of dialog with requestors (before and after a test) is limited. Obviously, no single formula or rule can apply to all situations; thus, one cannot state the optimal number and type of staff necessary to operate a sensory program. Some companies may chose to contract with external services for most testing needs, in which case the staff needs are adjusted accordingly; however, there can be no compromise on their sensory knowledge.

As previously mentioned, it is possible to gain another perspective on the number of professional and technical personnel needed in a program and by preparing high and low estimates of the number and types of tests that would be expected to be requested. Obviously, a new program has few criteria to use in this latter effort, nonetheless, it is surprising how much valuable information can still be obtained. For example, one can use three levels of test volume and from that result gain a reasonably accurate estimate of staff requirements. Considered in another way, if a program starts out with a limited service; for example, four or five tests per week and then expands to about eight to ten tests per week, what are the initial and final staff requirements? How many tests can one individual expect to handle in a week before it impacts on the quality of the results? This discussion assumes there are no limitations on subjects, facility, or data processing capabilities; however, these will have a direct effect on volume. Their impact on test volume will be discussed later in this chapter, but for current purposes they are considered available.

A modest program, capable of providing about 200 tests per year (equivalent to four or five tests per week) will require a full-time staff of a sensory professional and an analyst. Clerical support of about 25% also will be required. The professional's time is spent meeting with requesters, planning tests with the analyst, data interpretation, report preparation, and reporting results. The analysts' time is spent organizing and fielding tests, contacting and qualifying subjects, scheduling subjects, data entry and analysis, and maintaining records. A volume of 200 tests per year assumes an average distribution in terms of the types of tests – discrimination, descriptive, and acceptance, as follows:

Discrimination	15%
Descriptive	45%
Acceptance	40%

This listing of test volume by type is an average and each test type requires different amounts of effort (subjects, time for data collection, analysis). The amount of staff time and the total test volume will change, if, for example, there are more descriptive tests and fewer discrimination and acceptance tests. Increasing volume to about 300 tests per year will create considerable pressure on a staff of two; first by increasing the time between request and report, and second, by decreasing the amount of time given to each request and to discussing results. From a management perspective, the issue of staff growth must now be addressed if the services provided are to continue to grow (assuming the demand is there). In general, one sensory professional should be able to supervise the work of two or three analysts and the addition of a second or third analyst would be a reasonable next addition. The reader should note that an increase in test volume is expected at this stage because the usefulness of the information and its contributions to overall company profitability is recognized and the demand is there. Increasing volume beyond this (e.g. to 400 tests or more) requires the addition of a second professional, for a total staff of four. The increased volume of tests demands more professional attention, hence the staff need for the professional rather than another analyst. As test volume continues to increase, more attention also must be given to the nature of the tests themselves (e.g. descriptive, discriminative), the amount of time which the sensory professional needs for project planning, discussing results, and the extent of involvement in related activities such as those that incorporate marketing research information, advertising, and so forth. All these activities are incorporated into the department's growth plan as originally developed (and revised), and is used as a guide for further staff expansion.

Once testing volume exceeds 500 per year, growth can be expected to accelerate up to 700 tests (or more) per year. This acceleration occurs in larger companies directly as a result of previous work; that is, familiarity with sensory information increases its demand. Obviously, this expansion will produce considerable pressure on the staff; however, a properly prepared plan will minimize disruption and allow for an orderly growth of the sensory evaluation staff.

Basically, staff development and growth result from the need for sensory information, which should be directly related to the quality of the information and to test volume. As noted, with each sensory evaluation professional supervising two analysts, this core group of three should be capable of handling about 300 tests per year. A doubling of test volume will require a doubling of this core group, but with a need for the management responsibility to be separated from day-to-day test activities. In effect, there would be a manager, two sensory professionals and three analysts. The manager should be designated as early as possible in the development of the program. This individual serves as the focal point for the program and "sets the stage" for all test services, as well as determines the rate at which staff additions are made. Of course, the type of testing will require staff additions that favor one type or another (sensory evaluation professional or analyst) to satisfy a particular need. For example, increased use of design studies and larger numbers of products per test with a concomitant increase in complexity of the analyses and interpretation will require more professional level involvement. This will lead to an obvious growth in the sensory professional staff rather than increasing the number of analysts. Some efficiencies are possible through use of direct data entry systems, a topic discussed later in this chapter.

D. Facilities

One of the more fundamental requirements of a sensory program is the availability of a facility dedicated to testing. A specific area should be set aside for this purpose, just as space is allocated for other company activities, such as a chemistry laboratory or data processing center. Most companies recognize the need for a facility for sensory evaluation and have provided some space for this purpose. Over time, a variety of structures have been constructed, but few have included all the elements necessary for an efficient operation. The literature on sensory facilities has been limited (see Amerine *et al.*, 1965) and has not proven to be helpful except in a most general way, thus leaving sensory professionals to fend for themselves when working with architects and building contractors. In 1986, ASTM published a monograph (Eggert and Zook, 1986) on the design of a sensory facility, including guidelines for size of a facility, suggested booth dimensions, and related information. Several schematic diagrams are included as a supplement to assist in the planning of a facility. Before making any final plans, sensory professionals should read this document and the information in this and the following sections. As with any major capital expenditure, it is very difficult to convince management that additional funds are needed to "correct" mistakes due to inadequate design. We believe that the sensory facility is as important as any instrument used by the scientist and therefore warrants serious consideration. Of particular importance are ventilation, lighting, traffic patterns and locations, product preparation, subject communications, and experimenter comfort. Deficiencies in most facility designs come about for several reasons. In most cases, a facility is ideally described as a quiet area free from distraction, with controlled lighting, partitions between subjects to minimize visual contact, neutral colors for the walls, and odor-free surfaces wherever possible. However, many facilities constructed today continue to have structural deficiencies that become evident only after testing is initiated.

It is not unusual to observe two companies having comparable numbers of staff but with large differences in test capacity; or the reverse, that is, a similar test volume but with different numbers of staff. In each instance, facility design is the difference. In some food companies, inadequate ventilation necessitates a long delay between tests to allow for removal of cooking odors, which reduces test capacity. Over the past 30 years, we have observed that architects and building contractors appreciate receiving as much assistance as possible in the design and construction of a facility. The objective is to have a facility that is flexible enough to handle current and future testing activities, as well as to provide a workable environment for the staff.

Before making a commitment to actual drawings, it is important to develop an information base about testing in your company. This information base should include amount and location of space available, current and anticipated volume of testing on a daily and monthly basis, current and anticipated types of products, current and future availability of subjects, and types of tests. With this information, one can identify some of the other details and prepare drawings that will be useful to an architect. In Table 2.2, we have prepared a guide relating space, number of booths, number of tests, staff, and number of subjects.

Basically, a certain amount of space is necessary for a sensory evaluation facility; the space requirements ranges from a minimum of 400 to ~2000 ft^2 (or more, in some instances). However, the number of booths and number of staff do not increase

Table 2.2 A guide for allocating space for sensory testing[a]

Area (ft^2)	Number of booths	Number of staff	Annual volume of testing	Number of subjects
400	5–6	1–2	200–300	100–200
600	6	2–3	300–400	200
800	6–8	4	400–600	300–400
1000	8	5–6	700–800	400–500
1500–2000	2 × 6	8–9	≥1000	>500

[a] The entries are estimates of the amount of space, booths, and staff that are capable of doing a specified number of tests. Additional information about the use of the table can be found in the text.

in relation to the space allocation. Obviously, efficiencies are to be gained through size, but the greatest advantages are realized in terms of the types of tests that are possible within a larger facility. In fact, it is often more efficient if sets of booths are located in different areas of a facility, rather than in a single bank of twelve or fifteen. Of course, having booths in two locations does not mean two physically different parts of a building, which is quite a different arrangement (referred to as a satellite facility with its own reception and product preparation areas). While an arrangement of twelve booths in a single bank may have initial appeal, it could prove to be inefficient particularly if there are an insufficient number of servers. Serving requires more than one staff person unless one uses rollerblades! If products are heat sensitive, temperature control will be difficult; keeping track of when subjects arrive for a test is not easy, and generally the preparation area must be oversized (this can be inefficient and a costly use of space). Finally, since most in-company testing is small panel testing, rarely exceeding 40 subjects per test, there may be little need for more than eight to ten booths in any one location (serving as many as 24–32 subjects in 60 minutes, assuming 15 minutes per subject).

Another comment regarding the guidelines relates to the availability of subjects. With few people available, one must consider alternative approaches, including satellite facilities where the people are located, having the testing done in an external location, and so on. Some companies make use of local residents for their pool of subjects for internal testing. If this is a possible option, then accessibility from the outside and from a centralized reception area becomes very important. It should also be emphasized that the guidelines make no differentiation between types of products or types of tests (both of which are discussed below). Each of these considerations will alter the input–output listings in the table. Nevertheless, one can proceed to develop the basic information according to the five primary criteria.

Space may be a problem only if the area is already designated and if total space is less than that estimated to be needed for the current testing volume, or if it is located at some distance from subjects. The emphasis on locating the facility in a quiet area is secondary to accessibility. A location on the fifth floor in one corner away from most people is undesirable. No one wants to walk for 15 minutes to take a test that can be completed in 5 minutes! One should begin with a map (or blueprint) of the building and make notations on the number of people in each location (this may require a little extra effort, but it is worthwhile). The primary purpose of this exercise is to locate the facility as close as possible to the largest concentration of potential subjects. It also may be necessary to trade some space for accessibility. Management may offer twice the area in a location adjacent to a pilot plant or some other out-of-the-way place. While the offer may be tempting, sensory staff should review its proposal with management to make clear the importance of accessibility. One may even accept less space with the knowledge that in 5 years it will be too small. By then the program will have more than proven its value and additional (or new) facilities will be more easily justified.

When considering space, it is useful to be able to characterize it in some detail. When plans are in preparation, the ability to provide detailed requirements including dimensions for booths, counter height, and so forth, will demonstrate sensory responsiveness and help to minimize faulty designs. The typical facility can be separated in six distinct areas, as shown in Table 2.3. Also included are approximate amounts of space for each of these areas. The space allocations in square feet are realistic for most food and beverage testing activities. With limited cooking, the preparation area can be reduced and some other area expanded. If extensive product preparation or storage is necessary, then this area would be expanded. For product requiring no or only limited preparation, the area could be reduced and the space used elsewhere in the facility. A panel discussion area also may not be available and a nearby conference room may be proposed for this purpose. This is feasible provided it is accessible and has adequate ventilation, lighting, and so forth.

Another consideration is the pattern of subject movement to and from a facility. Subjects should pass through the reception area on their way to a test, but should not pass through or see into the preparation area. Similarly, visitors to a facility should have separate access to the offices and preparation area of the facility. Thus, the issue of space has many ramifications beyond the specific question of total area.

Finally, some comments about the use of direct data entry should be noted here. Most companies have installed direct data entry systems, thus obviating the need for the traditional paper scorecard. The relative merits of such systems are discussed later in this chapter (section on data processing), and are mentioned here only as it relates to the space and wiring requirements. This must be thoroughly investigated so as to minimize future disruptions as well as the costs involved.

Most tests involve limited numbers of subjects, usually twenty or fewer per test. Thus, in a day one could field as many as four tests and use about eighty subjects. Since it is possible for an individual to participate once a day, 5 days a week, a potential maximum volume can quickly be estimated at 20 tests per week $\times$ 50 weeks $=$ 1000 per year.

It should be obvious that twenty tests per week will require a reasonably large panel pool (more than 500) to minimize subject overuse and management complaints about an individual's time spent away from their regular work routine. Ideally, an individual should expect to participate about four times per week, with holidays

Table 2.3 Individual areas in the test facility and the approximate square footage[a]

	Approximate space allocated (ft^2)
Subject reception	50
Six booths	100
Preparation, holding, and storage	300
Panel discussion	350
Data processing/records	75
Experimenter desk/office	125
	1000

[a] The allocation of space is relative and will change depending on the types of products and the daily volume of testing. See text for further explanation.

of about 2 weeks every 6 weeks. In practice, most individuals participate two or three times per week with occasional periods of several weeks of no participation and other times when a test design requires daily participation for 2 or more consecutive weeks. The issues of how large the pool should be and frequency-of-use are explored in more detail in the section on subjects. The numbers used here are for illustrative purposes, relative to facilities design.

Assume the following:

Ten tests per week use twenty subjects per test.
Ten tests per week use forty subjects per test.
Ten minutes residence time per booth per subject.
Six booths.

Thus, the total booth time is determined to be

$$\frac{(10 \text{ tests} \times 20 \text{ subjects} + 10 \text{ tests} \times 40 \text{ subjects}) \times 10 \text{ minutes/test}}{6 \text{ booths}} = 1000 \text{ minutes/booth/week}$$

If we assume 5 hour test time per day $\times$ 60 minutes = 300 minutes/day test time, then 3.3 days are required, which is well within the typical work week.

Therefore, we conclude that six booths would be adequate for up to 1000 tests per year. As noted in Table 2.2, however, eight booths are recommended once volume reaches about 800 tests per year, and two banks of six booths each are recommended when the volume reaches 1000 tests per year. This increase in the number of booths reflects the practicalities of depending on large numbers of volunteers. But perhaps most important, the requirement for replicate responses in many tests will increase the number of visits to the booth by each subject. To minimize potential scheduling problems and to increase flexibility, the additional booths are recommended.

As previously noted, the types of products that will be evaluated are a related issue. The more different types of products that are to be tested, especially those that require preparation, the more space must be allocated for this purpose. For example, frozen prepared foods will require freezers as well as heating and controlled holding equipment. This equipment will reflect the primary methods by which the products will be prepared (by the consumer, the food caterer, or others). Sensory evaluation should prepare a list of needed equipment with space and power requirements so that it can be reconciled with the space and power allocations. Installation of such equipment at another location is not acceptable, since it will mean transporting products from one area to another. In addition to an evaluation of product preparation, one must also consider the available areas for test preparation; that is, sufficient storage space must be allocated for serving containers, utensils, and so forth.

The types of tests also will have an effect on the allocation of space as well as on subject requirements. If there is an equal distribution between small and large panel tests, then the previously mentioned numbers may be used as a guide. However, in situations where product acceptance tests are rarely done, an increase in test volume with no increase in number of subjects could be expected. Discrimination tests require a maximum of twenty subjects per test; thus, three tests per day could be done in 3 or 4 hours. The sensory professional must consider past history relative to the test pattern; anticipated requirements must be reviewed, and then a plan prepared.

From this inquiry, sensory evaluation should develop a comprehensive plan, describing basic information about the test program, desirable space requirements, a listing of equipment, and appropriate schematic drawings. Once management has given approval to this preliminary plan, the next step is the development of working plans that can be incorporated into the architect's drawings that serve as the basis for the eventual construction.

Working with an architect requires considerable patience and a tremendous amount of preparation. It is not a matter of doing the architect's work so much as delineating the specialized nature of a sensory evaluation facility. This preliminary effort will facilitate the development of plans, the bidding, and the actual construction. If the facility is to be located in an existing structure, then it must be visited and regularly inspected. Of course, if the facility is to be located in a new structure, one works from blueprints, but attention to detail is just as important and an effort made to visit the site during construction. Once dimensions are known, one develops schematic diagrams including dimensions for each piece of equipment, for all cabinets, and so forth.

1. Booth area

Most product tests are fielded using individual booths. Of course, some products do not lend themselves to booth evaluation; for example, some a personal care products. In this latter situation, the subjects might be doing their evaluations at home or using an alternative environment. A booth consists of a counter top with walls that extend from ceiling to floor on three sides and ~18 in. beyond the serving counter surface (so subjects cannot view their neighbors), with a small door at the counter surface. The subject, seated facing this door, signals the experimenter to serve the product. Figures 2.2 and 2.3 are schematic diagrams of a booth and booth area, including recommended dimensions.

We recommend the dimensions shown in Fig. 2.3 and find that they are quite adequate for all products. The booth depth of 18 in. is adequate except when "bread box" openings are used, which will require an additional 6–8 in. The booth width of 27 in. is sufficient without producing a claustrophobic effect; increasing this width beyond 30 in. may be a waste of space. Note that the counter is between 30 and 36 in. from the floor. This height is desirable because it makes serving easier and reduces server problems with lower back pain. Adjustable chairs enable the subject to select a comfortable height for a test. The length of the booth room will depend on the number of booths, but if possible additional space (2–3 ft.) should be allocated as a buffer from the reception area. The partitions extend from floor to ceiling and 18 in. beyond the booth counter. About 4 ft. above these counters is a soffit that extends the length of the booths and out ~18 in. (even with the counters). This soffit accommodates booth lighting fixtures and ventilation ducts. The booth room should be not less than 6 ft. wide, with 3 ft. allocated for partitions and counters and the remaining space allocated for passage by the subjects. Additional space is unnecessary. Having a small sink for oral rinsing in each booth is not recommended. Sinks are a potential source

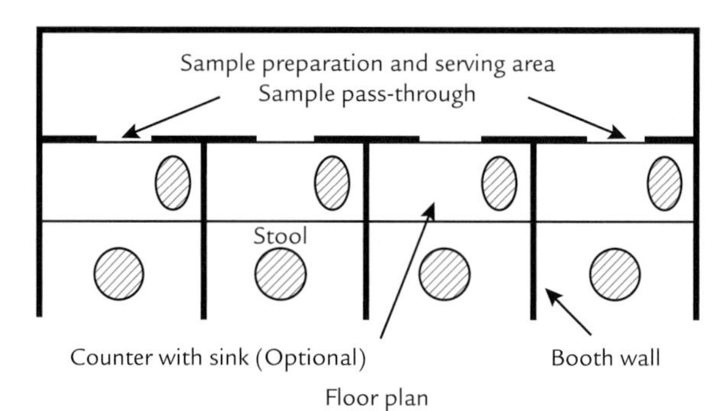

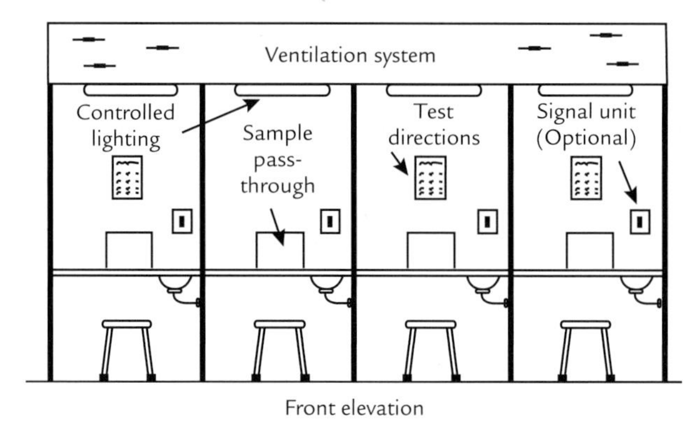

Figure 2.2 Schematic diagrams of the booth area in a sensory evaluation facility (not drawn to scale). See text for more details.

of odors and noise, require regular maintenance, and will increase construction costs. Where possible, the use of covered, disposable containers for expectoration is a more acceptable alternative.

Lighting in the booth area is fluorescent, except in the booths themselves, where incandescent lighting is recommended. This lighting should be sufficient to provide 100–110 ft-candles (or their equivalent) of shadow-free light at the counter surface. These incandescent lights are located slightly to the front of the soffit and are tilted toward the seated subject to minimize shadows on the products. Opalite diffusion glass can be placed beneath the bulbs to eliminate any spotlight effect. Off–on and dimmer switches for the booths are located in the experimenter area.

The use of various types of colored lights (e.g. red, yellow, and blue) for alternative booth illumination is not recommended. Typically, use of these lights is intended to mask color differences between products not associated with the variable being tested. Use of other than conventional lighting is not recommended because it causes more problems than it solves. Colored lighting increases subject variability (it is an intervening variable) because it is different from typical lighting and the color differences may not be masked but only altered. Perhaps the strongest argument that can be made in opposition to the use of colored lights is the indirect impact on management. Suppose that a test has been done using red illumination and there is no difference between products. It is not unusual for these results to be discussed by management

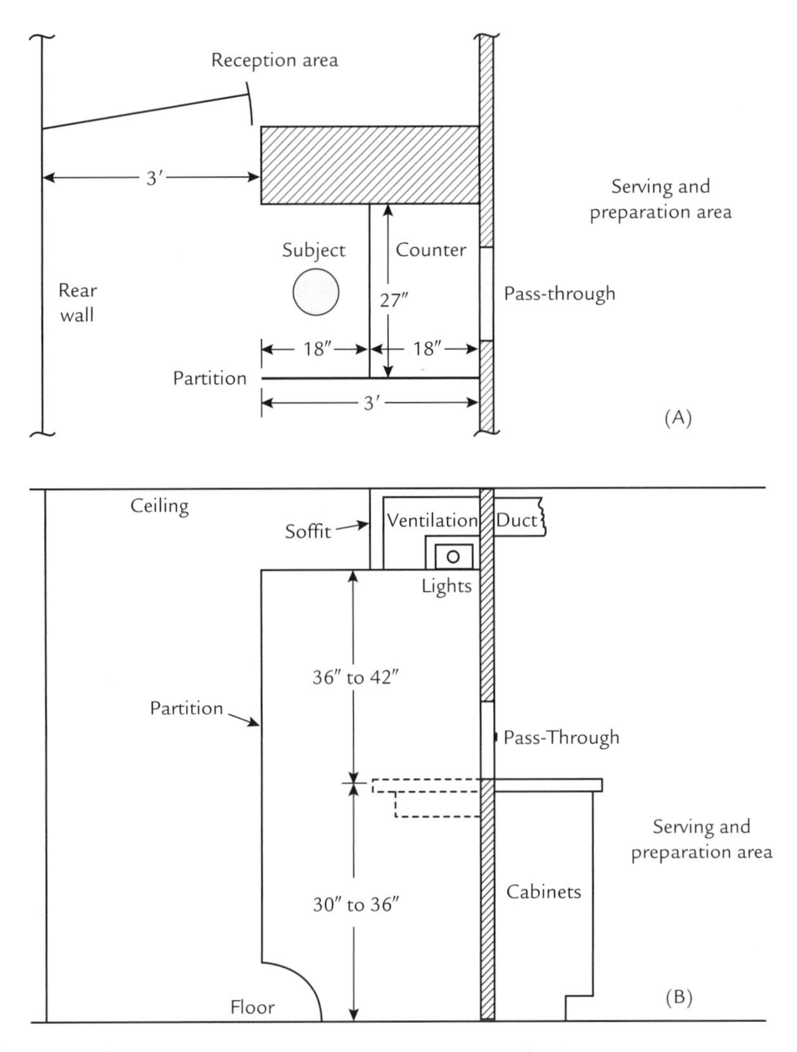

Figure 2.3 Detailed description of the booth area including recommended dimensions: (A) shows the booths from an overhead view; (B) is a side view of the same area. See text for more details.

with products available. Management will look at the products under normal illumination and will conclude that there is a difference. Despite reminders that the test was done under red illumination to mask this difference, there will be doubt expressed about the credibility of such a result and the long-term credibility of sensory evaluation questioned. While there are numerous procedures and practices that are unique to sensory evaluation (e.g. three-digit coding, balanced designs), the idea of hiding a difference represents a very difficult concept for managers to accept (or at least it should be!). Assurance by product specialists that this difference will be corrected is rarely ever achieved, and managers will continue to question why the particular test was done. Alternatively, masking illumination may be recommended by a manager but the request forgotten when results are reviewed at some later time. We also have observed situations in which red illumination was used in the booths, but white illumination in the preparation area enabled the subject to see the difference each time a pass-through door was opened. In some situations, colored containers have been used as a means of neutralizing product differences; however, one must be very confident that the difference can be masked. In Chapter 5, we will describe use of a paired procedure in which a monadic serving procedure can be used. This permits use of the typical white illumination in the booth, and as we will describe, is applicable to many product situations. Finally, we believe that the short-term benefits of using alternative lighting will be overwhelmed by the long-term credibility consequences for sensory evaluation.

In some instances, the product preparation area will be used as a primary location for bench screening prior to testing. In this case, the lighting should be based on the United States Department of Agriculture guidelines for approved illumination (see File code 131-A-31, January, 1994).

The ventilation for this room and especially for the booth area is quite critical and is probably the single most costly (and most important) investment that is made. If one aspect of a facility needs special attention, it is the ventilation. Most architects and engineering personnel cannot be expected to appreciate this need and will generally state that the building ventilation is more than adequate – do not believe it! For example, the ventilation requirements must take into account such variables as all booths will be occupied, the number of people in the preparation areas, the likelihood that all heating equipment (ovens, steam tables, etc). will be in use throughout an 8-hour time period, etc. The booth area must have a slight positive pressure relative to other areas; in addition, individual exhaust ventilation ducts should be located in each booth (in the soffit, if part of the design). Air turnover in the booths should occur every 30 second as a minimum; however, this timing can vary depending on the product category. For example, a more rapid turnover of every 20 second will be needed for tobacco and for flavors and fragrances, with a special exhaust in case of spills or excess smoke buildup. By confining the improved ventilation to the booths and booth area, the capital expenditure should be reasonable. Obviously, for products that do not contribute odor, no additional ventilation may be necessary; however, the facility should still have good ventilation. Since ventilation systems also have filters, every effort should be made to ensure that they are accessible for frequent changing. By frequent changing we recommend at least once per month unless the filters are very dirty, in which case weekly changes will be necessary.

Facing each judge seated at a booth will be a small door, referred to as a "sample pass-through door." The door opens either up or to one side, allowing samples to be passed to the subject (Fig. 2.4). A variety of designs has been developed, and while most look attractive or appear simple to operate, they have the potential to create problems. For example, horizontally sliding doors or those hinged at the top usually stick, catch papers, or have a tendency to fall on the samples. Another type is based on a lazy-susan design, but with a center barrier so that when it swings around there is space for the product. Unfortunately, these units loosen and after a while they move like a merry-go-round and can spin product out, causing spills. The most commonly used door types are the "bread-box" and the balanced guillotine. The breadbox is so constructed that when one side is open, the other is closed. This minimizes the likelihood of the subject having any view of the preparation area. Major disadvantages of the breadbox include the increased amount of space required on the subject's side

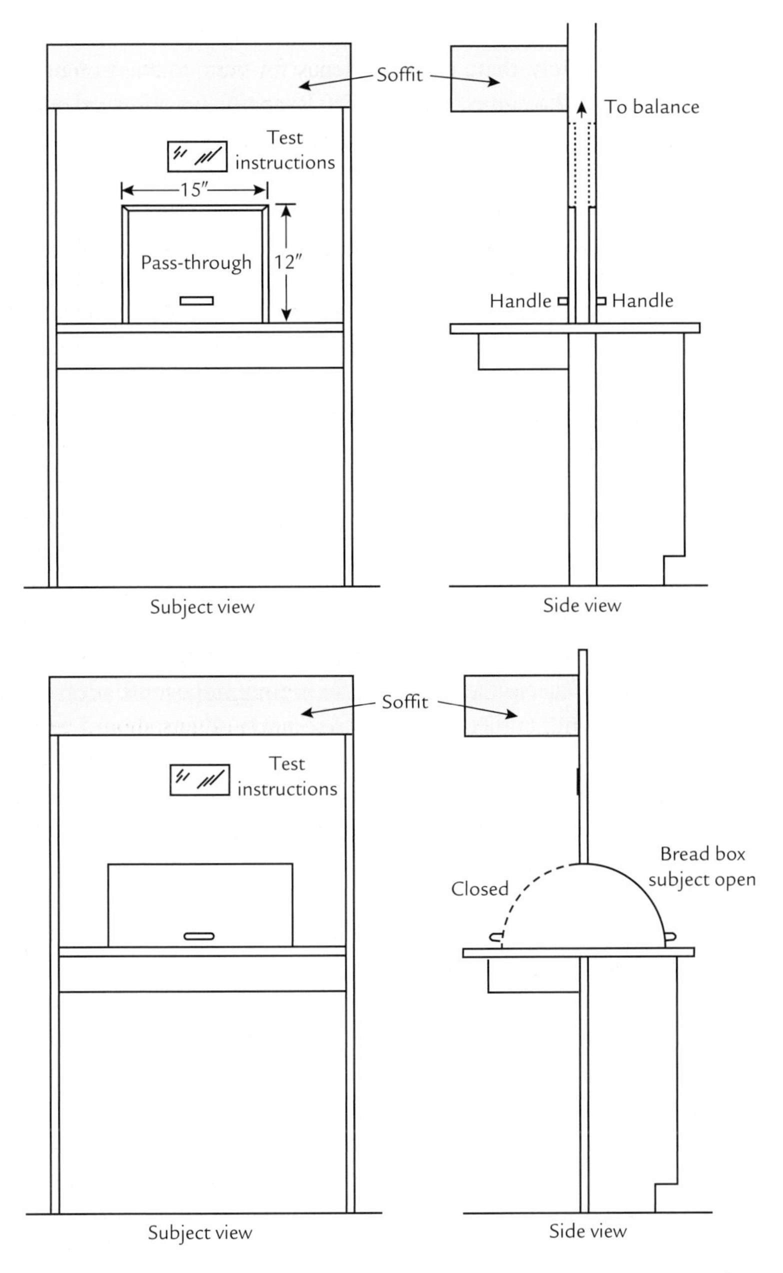

Figure 2.4 Schematic diagrams of the two most common types of product pass-through doors.

when the door is down, the height of the box relative to serving containers, and the inability to easily communicate with subjects. Since these containers are made of stainless steel for durability and ease of cleaning, they are costly. The use of the breadbox delivery will require a deeper counter (from 18 to 22–24 in.). Before fabricating, however, it will be necessary to check the height of all serving containers to make certain they will fit. Because of these disadvantages, we do not recommend use of the breadbox door and find that they are losing favor.

The balanced guillotine-type door is newer; earlier versions were held open with blocks or pegs. Unfortunately, there was a tendency for them to crash on one's fingers or on the products (hence the name "guillotine"). Recently, we observed considerable success with a guillotine door that is counterbalanced and suspended with high-quality wire (airplane) cable to minimize breakdowns. The use of food-grade, white plastic belting material for the door, about 3/8 to 1/2 in. in thickness, makes them easy to clean. For ease of removal for washing and maintenance, the experimenter-side trim is bolted. Alternatively, one can create a door without the wires that is not counterbalanced and uses a small ledge on which to rest the door, when open. Such a door is quite inexpensive to make and will last for decades. These comments regarding door opening and closing design could be impacted in those situations where there are laws regarding safety. We recently encountered such a problem designing a facility in the European Union (EU), necessitating a change in how the doors are to be operated. In these latter situations, the sensory professional should be able to accommodate such restrictions by referring to the function and what are the advantages of a particular design.

The booth arrangement is primarily intended for products that lend themselves to this type of evaluation. Some products such as furniture polish or skin conditioner require a different test environment; however, there should be no visual contact between subjects, minimal contact with the experimenter, ventilation to remove odors, and constant lighting. For example, the evaluation of a room air freshener may require construction of a series of containers of known volume (e.g. 27 ft^3) with small doors to enable the subject to open and sniff the contents without disturbing subjects at adjacent test stations. In addition, subjects can move from station to station, thus making more efficient use of the facility. The key to a successful facility design is to develop an understanding of the reasons for the various parts and to then incorporate them into the particular booth design.

The booth area should be adjacent to a subject reception area. This multipurpose area provides a sound barrier to outside noises and enables the experimenter to monitor arrivals; it is a space for posting test results and for serving rewards for test participation; it serves as a barrier to subjects wandering into the product preparation area or prematurely disrupting other subjects.

The traffic pattern also is important. Subjects must be able to get to the booths, check on their specific assignment, and determine in which booth they are to be seated. The experimenter (or some designated individual) should also be able to monitor arrivals. Once preliminary drawings have been completed, the sensory staff should review them relative to the flow of people and to the location of specific equipment and so forth. This state of preparation may even require development of a mock-up to be sure that there is adequate space.

2. Preparation area

The preparation area is more difficult to define, since it is highly dependent on the types of products and equipment, and on the amount and type of preparation required. Figure 2.5 shows two schematic diagrams for an entire sensory facility with six areas, designated as reception, product preparation, panel discussion, and so

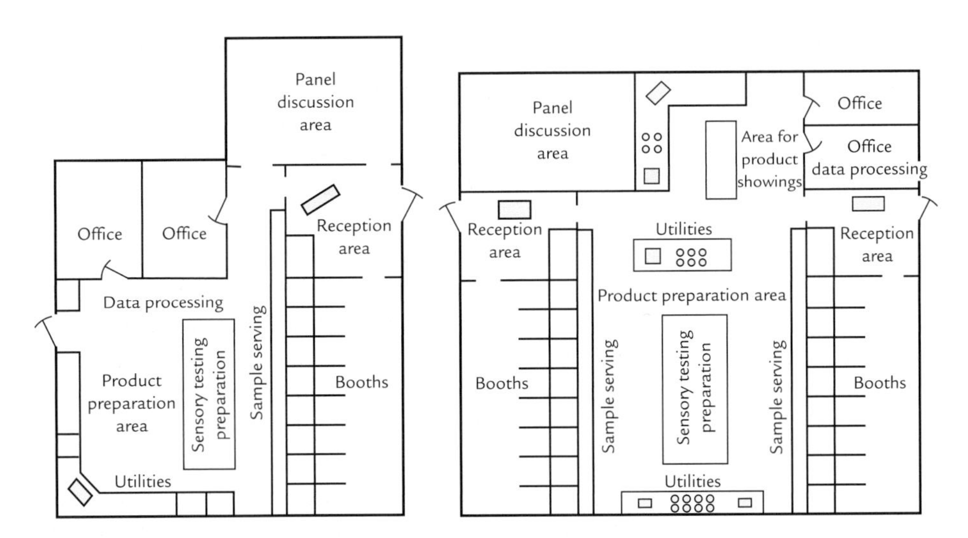

Figure 2.5 Two examples of sensory test facilities showing the various activities within the department.

forth. Of the six, three are continuous (reception, booths, preparation) one with the other, while the others can be moved around to fit the available space. The design on the right has two product preparation areas to reflect sharing space with a recipe development/home economics function. About 300–400 ft^2 should be allocated to the area. Critical factors in determining the size of the preparation area include the expected amount of cooking and the size of the units necessary to achieve this, and storage requirements for these products. As noted previously, this space can be modified for products such as tobacco, fabrics, chewing gum, and candy, where product preparation is minimal and limited to storage and test setup arrangements. However, the individual confronted with a limited amount of space must be even more resourceful in the use of space. It is not so much a question of the space being too small but rather of organizing it to allow for the most efficient operation. For example, the space below the serving counter (on the experimenter side) can be used for storage of supplies as well as for refrigerator and freezer space. Similarly, the space above this counter can be used for storage, provided the cabinets are not so low as to constitute a hazard to the experimenter when serving. Counter space is especially important and there can never be enough of this type of space. In areas with minimal space, it may be useful to have drop-down counters set in place for product setup or to prepare scorecards and products on stacking trays. For products that require heat or refrigeration, one must be sure there is adequate equipment and space.

Storage cabinets and counters should be made from any polymeric material that is easily cleaned and maintained. While the booth area requires careful attention with regard to selection of color, one can be more relaxed with regard to the preparation area; counters continuous with the booths should be of the same color, because a contrast in color could effect the appearance of a product as it is served to the subject.

Ventilation in the preparation area is especially important for those products with aromatic properties. All heating areas should have individual exhaust units (about 350–400 CFM) and estimates of environmental and electrical load requirements should always be based on the "worst case" point of view (all heaters operating at once). Use of three-phase wiring for heating outlets is highly recommended, as is minimal use of shared wiring for these outlets. Lighting in the preparation area should be such that products can be examined with ease and where appropriate, special lighting should be available, for example, northern, supermarket, and so on.

3. Data processing

The sensory area will include space for data capture and processing. A typical arrangement of equipment is shown in Fig. 2.6; however, much has changed over the past decade regarding data capture and analyses. Current PCs and laptops are capable of handling just about all possible needs for sensory programs, large or small. This provides for a real time operating environment. Any system should have a digitizer or direct data capture system (usually by means of a touch screen), a PC for the analyses, graphics and reporting, and data archiving, a printer/plotter, and Internet connection. These systems are relatively low cost except for the direct data entry which has a significant capital outlay and continuing maintenance requirements. Regardless of what kind of a system one has, the ability to function independently has important benefits for sensory programs. For an historical background on the uses for computers in sensory evaluation, see Aust (1984), Brady (1984), Pecore (1984), Russell (1984), Savoca (1984), Brady *et al.* (1985), Stone and Drexhage (1985), Guinard *et al.* (1985), Gordin (1987), and Winn (1988). As the Internet becomes more accessible, the potential for its use in sensory evaluation (and in larger scale consumer testing) increases and could totally change the ways in which responses are obtained.

If one continues to use paper scorecards, then a digitizer system (as depicted in Fig. 2.6) is most efficient and least costly while providing maximum flexibility in terms of scale types and scorecard format. The cost of the hardware and software is recovered in less than 1 week of use. A digitizer is nothing more than a pad (an oversized paper tablet) with a wire grid and a sensor, the size and shape of a pen. When the pen touches a mark (on the scorecard), it converts it to a numerical value and transmits it to a data file. Alternatively, if one chooses to use direct data entry, there are several options including pads the size of a digitizer with their own memory that, in effect, are an electronic scorecard, and there are touch screen systems which have proven to be most popular. The latter are now in use in many companies and provide a wide range of added features, including test design and analyses options. As noted above, they do represent a significant capital investment and some re-construction requirements for older facilities. For sensory professionals lacking background knowledge in test design and analyses, the current systems are very appealing; however, they often operate on a default system that may not be appropriate for every problem. When using these features, the sensory professionals must be especially thorough in their preparation of a design and fully understand the specific analysis or analyses being done. This issue will be explored in more detail in Chapter 4. The reader should keep in mind that these systems provide a means of impressing management with sensory professional's commitment to using the latest technology and exploiting its efficiencies. This is valuable as one promotes a program.

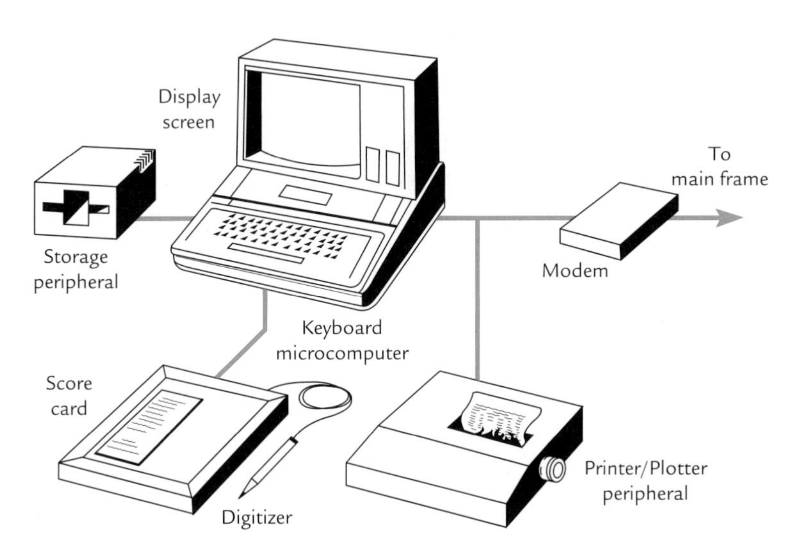

Figure 2.6 Schematic diagram of a satellite data processing system for sensory evaluation. The digitizer coverts the marks on scorecards to numerical values; each value is displayed on the screen of the microcomputer and then transmitted to storage (e.g. floppy disk). After all data are entered and hard copy obtained from the printer, the appropriate software is entered into the microcomputer and the analysis is completed and the results printed. If the data require use of the mainframe computer, then it is accessed by way of the modem. When the analysis is complete, the results are printed. For plotting data, files in the peripheral storage are accessed.

4. Satellite facility

The basic elements that are essential to the sensory facility within a company can also be achieved at an external location. Such a situation is not atypical; one's internal resources may be physically limited or constrained, usually by an insufficient number of subjects available for testing. The use of satellite facilities represents a degree of freedom that is often overlooked in the development of resources. Such facilities can be located in areas where there are large numbers of potential subjects, for example, corporate offices or off-site in a shopping mall. These sites are usually not intended as an exact duplicate of the existing unit, but rather designed for specific uses, such as primarily for acceptance tests that require relatively large numbers of subjects (more than twenty-five) per test. Lighting, ventilation, booths, and the other structural requirements remain valid for this facility, although there may be some modifications to meet the particular testing needs.

A satellite facility may be nothing more than a table with portable booths. Obviously, the more portable the facility the less the degree of environmental and lighting controls that is possible. Such a facility will not be ideal; however, it will be suitable if the conditions are similar from session to session and from day to day. Each situation must be considered within the context of the overall plan for sensory evaluation. Are the reductions in controls and the potential reduction in sensitivity offset by the need for information; are the expected product differences of sufficient magnitude to be perceived in this test environment? Will management consider the satellite as a more permanent solution? The sensory professional must give consideration to all factors that will influence the current facility before deciding on the contents of a satellite facility.

Another factor that is often overlooked is the extent to which a facility is used as a public information/public relations activity (e.g. tours and promotional photographs). Sensory evaluation is one of the few technical activities in a company that most visitors and consumers can "understand." With this knowledge in mind, the facility, whether it is a single unit or has several satellites, should be designed accordingly. It may be helpful to discuss this with public relations and personnel representatives.

E. Test Methods

In addition to an appropriate facility, sensory evaluation must have tools with which to work, including the methods used to evaluate the products (e.g. difference tests and acceptance tests). There are a substantial number of test methods (for a description, see Amerine *et al.*, 1965; American Society for Testing and Materials (ASTM), 1968, 1992; Sidel *et al.*, 1975; Stone and Sidel, 1995). In recent years, fewer methods have been described and most of those described in the literature are proposed modifications to existing methods. However, the recent work by Schutz and others (Cardello and Schutz, 1996; Schutz and Cardello, 2001) on the development of enhancements to the acceptance/preference model shows substantial promise. This latter topic will be discussed extensively in Chapter 7. As shown in Table 2.4, the methods are assigned to three broad categories. This classification, which is just one of many that have been proposed, is used here for illustrative purposes and to make the reader aware of the different kinds of test methods that are available. In more recent years, we have chosen to reduce the classification by one and talk in terms of two categories, analytical and affective, but consider the discriminative and descriptive as warranting separate consideration because of their importance. In subsequent chapters, each test type is described in detail. The sensory professional must be familiar with all of the methods in order to apply them properly. A thorough understanding of all test methods will also reduce unwarranted reliance on a single method to solve all problems.

F. Selection of Subjects

Besides test methods, the sensory professional needs subjects. In most companies, employees serve as subjects; in some circumstances, subjects may be recruited from the local community and remunerated as part-time employees. The latter practice is becoming more common and both approaches are discussed. Regardless of the source,

Table 2.4 Categories of tests and examples of methods used in sensory evaluation

Category	Test type
Discriminative	Difference: paired comparison, duo trio, triangle
Descriptive	Descriptive analysis: Flavor profile, QDA
Affective	Acceptance – preference: nine-point hedonic

all subjects participating in a sensory test must be qualified to participate. This requirement is often overlooked and does have serious consequences in terms of the decision-making based on those results. Failure to use appropriately qualified subjects is one aspect of the sensory process that has a significant impact on credibility of the program. We will have more to say about this issue later in this discussion.

A successful testing program should involve employees from all parts of the company. To attract volunteers and maintain their interest requires careful planning and a commitment on the part of one's company management. Employees should never be made to feel that they volunteer as a requirement for employment or promotion depends on their participation. Individuals are selected for a specific test based on their skills rather than their proximity to the test facility. There must be a formal program for subject selection, so as to improve the general level of sensitivity, to match panel with problem, and to increase one's confidence in the conclusions derived from the results. Such programs are not created overnight, and once in place, they require maintenance to ensure that subjects are neither over- nor under-used (easier stated than practiced). Subjects need regular contact to ensure that their interest remains high. Before describing recruiting procedures, some guidelines on working with people as test subjects are appropriate:

1. Sensory skills vary from person to person.
2. Most individuals do not know what their ability is to smell, taste, or feel a product.
3. All individuals need to be instructed on how to take a test.
4. Not all individuals qualify for all tests, nor should they be expected to.
5. Subjects are rewarded for participation, not for correct scores.
6. Skills once acquired are forgotten if not used on a regular basis.
7. Skills can be overworked or fatigued.
8. A subject's performance can be influenced by numerous factors unrelated to the test or the product.
9. All subject information should be treated in a confidential manner.
10. Employees should not be paid to participate in a sensory test.
11. Test participation should always be on a volunteer basis.
12. Subject safety is of paramount importance and should precede all other considerations.

These guidelines should be in writing and available to the sensory staff. Since there is a regular inflow and outflow of people (new employees and employee attrition), the value of a written guideline is obvious. Developing the subject pool requires a special effort, regardless of past experiences or assumptions as to an individual's skill. In most companies where testing has been in progress for many years, the problem can be especially difficult. From management's perspective the need for more subjects may be viewed with disinterest or an inability to understand the need for any program to get more subjects. Ideally, an individual should not participate more than three or four times within a week, for not more than about 4 continuous weeks followed by 1 or 2 weeks of rest. While there will be situations where an individual could participate every day for 5 or 10 days for a special project, continued use on a daily basis can lead to problems both in terms of maintaining subject interest and the effect of the absences on that individual's primary job responsibility. These issues are discussed in the section on motivation; the current emphasis is on attracting the employee to serve as a subject.

The initial goal of the sensory professional is to develop a plan for both management and the sensory staff, describing the importance of recruiting and screening subjects and how it will be achieved. Obviously, the documentation for management need not be detailed, but should be sufficiently clear to be understood. The first task is a clear statement of the objective for seeking employee volunteers; for example, why all employees should be encouraged to volunteer, what benefits are accrued, and how this participation might disrupt their regular work activities. As many employees as possible should participate, to minimize dependence on a few and to provide greater options in selection for tests. The larger the subject pool, the more tests can be done and the more rapid a response can be achieved. For example, a pool of 100 subjects could limit testing to only 300–400 tests per year (and put considerable pressure on the subjects to participate). While it is possible to complete more tests with a pool of 100, there is a greater risk that subject bias will develop and/or their management may resent the time away from their regular work. With more subjects to draw from, for example, 200, it will be possible to increase the number of tests, reduce the frequency of testing for an individual, as well as use less time from request to report or to field the same number of tests. The ability to respond quickly, to meet a deadline, and provide rapid feedback will secure many benefits for a sensory program, hence, the importance of having a large pool of subjects.

Employee participation has some side benefits as it relates to the individual's regular work activities. This break is a welcome diversion from regular work activities, provided it is brief, and is often found to have a positive effect on motivation – contributing to success of the company. While this benefit is more difficult to measure (as compared with the increase in the total number of tests), it is a benefit and should be identified as such to management.

All of these benefits and others that accrue to the company should be a part of any plan presented to management. The goal is to have management approval such that one can approach individual department managers and, ultimately, the potential subjects. While manager participation (as subjects) is desirable, it is unrealistic to expect their regular participation. However, their willingness to permit solicitation of their staff is crucial to any permanent program.

The estimated time necessary to build a subject pool should also be taken into consideration. It usually takes about 12 months to build and maintain a pool of about 200 subjects. If there already is a core group of about fifty, it could take less time to convince former participants to return or that a new program will be worthwhile. The time needed to reach people through memos, electronic mail, or in face-to-face meetings should be minimal; however, the major time constraints are the screening tasks before a subject is considered qualified. In addition, all subjects who volunteer cannot be screened within the same time period nor would it be reasonable or practical to attempt such an effort. Typically, one starts with about 20–25 individuals for discrimination and descriptive tests so that there will be enough of them qualified to satisfy initial test requests. Once this group completes screening, a second group can begin the process. In this way, test requests can be satisfied without long delays, the subjects have immediate opportunities to participate in a test and gain some sense of contributing to the program's success. Too long a delay between the end of screening and the start of testing; for example, 4 or more weeks, will likely have many subjects thinking they are no longer needed or they will forget the process. The concept is to structure activities so they can be managed to best advantage by the sensory professional and at the same time, to not discourage the subjects.

Once individuals have been recruited, it is time to begin the screening process, keeping in mind that not everyone will meet the qualifying criteria either because they neither use nor like specific products or cannot demonstrate a minimum level of sensitivity or of reliability. Typically, about 30% of those who volunteer will not meet the minimum level of sensitivity and reliability; hence, the need to start screening with more subjects than is needed. In addition, there should be a schedule for regularly new subjects. This issue is discussed in more detail in the next section.

Once the screening program is in operation, it can be very useful to work with one's human resources department to include in a new employee's packet of information, documents that describe the company's testing program. A card or e-mail contact indicating interest also can be included. In this way, there can be a flow of potential subjects available on a continuing basis.

Previously it was noted that in some companies, sensory testing cannot be done solely with employees; either there are too few, or work schedules, or job performance criteria makes it necessary to use local residents. Recruiting this latter group can be done using a local recruiting service, advertising in local newspapers and shopping guides, or some combination of these.

For background reading on this topic, the booklet by ASTM (Anonymous 1981a) and Resurreccion (1998) may be helpful.

G. Subject Screening Procedures

Once individuals have indicated a willingness to participate, they are required to participate in a series of screening tests to determine their level of skill. This screening process has two basic stages, the first being completion of a product attitude survey, and second, participation in a series of selected sensory tests. Once subjects start participating, their performance is based on actual test results. The first step is to have each individual complete the survey form. The information, shown in Fig. 2.7, includes a limited amount of demographic and background information (age groupings, general job classification, gender, and special product requirements such as a food allergy, in the case of a food company). Responses to the latter questions are intended for use in meeting specific test requirements or eliminating specific individuals). The survey also lists a wide variety of products (not necessarily by brand) of current or of future interest. This listing could include several hundred products; the idea is to be comprehensive such that the survey does not have to be repeated each time new product categories are tested. Associated with each product is a

SENSORY EVALUATION PRODUCT ATTITUDE SURVEY

To match your product preferences, usage, and sensory skills to the samples to be evaluated, please complete this questionnaire. All information will be maintained confidential.

PLEASE PRINT

Name ____________ Department ____________

Telephone Ext. ____________ Date ____________

General Information

Female ________ Male ________

Under 34 yrs. 11 mos ____ 35 to 50 ____ Over 50 ____

Married ________ Single ________

Children 0 ________ 1 ________

2 ________ 3 ________

4 or more ________

1. Please indicate which, If any, of the following foods disagree with you. (allergy, discomfort, etc.)

   Cheese (specify) ________ Poultry ________

   Chocolate ________ Seafood ________

   Eggs ________ Soy ________

   Fruits (specify) ________ Spices (specify) ________

   Meats (specify) ________ Vegetables (specify) ________

   Milk ________

2. Please indicate if you are on a special diet.

   Diabetic ________ Low Salt ________

   High Calorie ________ No Special Diet ________

   Low Calorie ________ Other (specify) ________

The following is a list of products of current, or perhaps of potential interest, arranged in categories. Each product has descriptive terms from *won't eat* or *never tried* to *like extremely* or *dislike extremely*. Using these descriptions as guidelines, please **circle** the number under each phrase that most closely describes your attitude about that particular food.

Categories	Won't Eat	Never Tried	Food Item	Like Extremely	Like Very Much	Like Moderately	Like Slightly	Neither Like nor Dislike	Dislike Slightly	Dislike Moderately	Dislike Very Much	Dislike Extremely
Baked Products & Desserts	11	10	Cakes	9	8	7	6	5	4	3	2	1
	11	10	Cookies	9	8	7	6	5	4	3	2	1
	11	10	Puddings	9	8	7	6	5	4	3	2	1
Breakfast Foods	11	10	Pancakes	9	8	7	6	5	4	3	2	1
	11	10	Toaster Pop-Ups	9	8	7	6	5	4	3	2	1
	11	10	Donuts	9	8	7	6	5	4	3	2	1
Beverages	11	10	Carbonated Soft Drinks	9	8	7	6	5	4	3	2	1
	11	10	Coffee	9	8	7	6	5	4	3	2	1
	11	10	Tea	9	8	7	6	5	4	3	2	1
Juices	11	10	Citrus	9	8	7	6	5	4	3	2	1
	11	10	Non-Citrus	9	8	7	6	5	4	3	2	1
Canned Foods	11	10	Chili	9	8	7	6	5	4	3	2	1
	11	10	Fruit	9	8	7	6	5	4	3	2	1
	11	10	Spaghetti	9	8	7	6	5	4	3	2	1

Figure 2.7 Example of the Product Attitude Survey (PAS) for use in screening prospective subjects.

nine-point hedonic scale (dislike extremely to like extremely) as well as two additional categories, "never tried" and "won't try" (see Peryam *et al.*, 1954).

Obviously, completion of this form will take a reasonable amount of time and volunteers are usually allowed 2–3 weeks to return them. This is a first step in screening process; those individuals who do not elect to complete it are usually not worth having as subjects. Chances also are very good that these are the same subjects who will not report for testing as scheduled or will in some way fail to follow instructions. Responses are then tabulated and processed such that one can easily identify a particular subset of people, for example, all those individuals between the age of 21 and 35 years who like cola beverages and whose degree-of-liking mean score is between five and seven on the nine-point scale (nine is like extremely). Alternatively, if the panel mean score is 6.3, it should be possible to identify all those individuals (by name and location) whose score is ±1 SD around that mean. This information has proven to be extremely valuable in screening subjects; identifying individuals who dislike a product or those who exhibit atypical behavior; that is, they like and/or dislike all products in the extreme. In the latter situation, both types of behavior are not desirable inasmuch as they introduce more variability than is typically observed. In effect, such individuals are not discriminating and subsequent behavior in actual product tests confirms this. In effect, one is selecting individuals who will be more representative of the typical consumer for a particular product. This latter point is especially important when one is selecting the subjects to measure product acceptance as a prelude to larger scale consumer tests. Selecting a more homogeneous group also increases the probability for obtaining a more consistent scoring pattern.

The usual procedure has been to maintain a spreadsheet that can be easily accessed. Since the subject pool will be dynamic, with some leaving and others just beginning, the program must have provision to allow for changes. Current computerized systems are particularly sophisticated, able to not only identify individuals, their location, and telephone contact, but also able to send reminder notices electronically and in a hard copy, if desired.

As a general guide, one should expect about 75–80% of the survey forms will be returned, as requested, within 2 or 3 weeks. Once these forms have been received and processed, orientation and screening tests should be scheduled, with minimal delay. Otherwise, there is dramatic decrease in interest in participation and the program will experience considerable difficulty in attracting sufficient numbers of subjects to be effective. From a practical viewpoint, screening tests should involve not more than about twenty people at a time. This will depend, in part, on the size of one's staff and facility and, in part, the scheduled plan for full testing operations. Assuming a 75% rate of return of survey forms and screening accommodations for about twenty people, about thirty forms should be distributed at any one time.

At orientation, the testing should be described and all those present should directly participate in one or two practice tests. This second stage of screening is particularly important insofar as concerns the selection of subjects qualified for analytical testing; that is, the discrimination and descriptive tests. The methods use a limited number of subjects and assume a homogeneous subject population; homogeneous in terms of their skills. Also, the mathematics involved in data analysis makes certain assumptions about response behavior that, in turn, is directly related to subject skill. Failure to use qualified subjects increases the risk of decision errors, hence the importance assigned to qualification. These issues will be discussed in more detail in the chapters on methodology.

Screening for sensory skill can be achieved in several ways, all of which are derived from the subject's ability to discriminate differences among products. Before discussing the actual screening procedures, it is useful to briefly summarize the research background to this activity. The early literature was helpful in identifying approaches that were not recommended as well as some that suggested a more successful approach (see Giradot *et al.*, 1952; Mackey and Jones, 1954; Sawyer *et al.*, 1962; Dawson *et al.*, 1963b). Based on the cited research, it was clear that selecting individuals for a test based on availability, their knowledge about the products, years with a company or their titles yielded unreliable and/or invalid information. It also was clear that an individual's sensitivity to simple aqueous solutions of sweet, sour, salty, and bitter stimuli had no meaningful relationship to subsequent performance in the evaluation of typical foods and beverages. What is particularly interesting (and surprising) about this latter finding is the extent to which threshold tests continue to be used. Unfortunately, much effort is expended on measuring thresholds to various stimuli for no useful purpose, unless one is marketing threshold testing as a business. The early research also suggested that predicting performance in a difference test based on results from a preliminary series of difference tests was encouraging, provided the products used were from the same category as those being tested. With this background in mind, we initiated a program in which all subjects for sensory analytical tests had to demonstrate their skill on an empirical basis (after completing a survey as the initial barrier). This approach recognized that an individual had to first learn how to use his/her senses and second, learn how to take a test. So the protocol began with a replicated series of easy comparisons that were made progressively more difficult. Once these tests were completed one could classify people in terms of their sensitivity and their reliability and expect them to perform better; that is, more sensitive and more reliable, than the unscreened individual. In fact, this is precisely what has been observed in thousands of tests. While this approach does not guarantee that an individual, so qualified, will always detect differences, it does eliminate individuals who are insensitive, unreliable and/or unable to follow directions.

One could use ranking, and/or scoring procedures; however, primary reliance should be on the difference test. It provides a measure of correct (and incorrect) matches and in most situations, it does not require knowledge of the difference between product pairs. This protocol makes no *a priori* assumptions about an individual's level of skill and requires all individuals to participate (regardless of prior test experience or years of employment). One assumes that all individuals have never participated in such tests and, therefore, the initial tests must be sufficiently easy so that 90–100% correct decisions are achieved. The initial goal is to encourage individuals to continue to participate, to motivate them. In this way the subjects develop a sense of accomplishment without the frustration that comes with early failures. Determining which product comparisons are easy and which are difficult (to detect) is based, initially, on professional judgment. Products should be screened by the sensory staff; however, the true level of difficulty will be determined empirically (once the first few groups have completed screening). It is usually easy to select pairs of products for a difficult test, for example, two products from the same production line, selected a few minutes apart. Over a series of about 20–30 trials, it will be possible to rank the subjects based on their skills. It is interesting to note that about 30% of those persons who volunteer will not qualify; that is, will not be able to achieve at least 51% correct matches across the thirty trials. What is particularly interesting is that this experience extends across all ages from children (age 8–12 years) to adults (age 60–65 years), and across many countries and regions of the world. However, this observation should not be interpreted to mean that this percentage of the population cannot discriminate any differences, only the level of sensitivity is not adequate or response is unreliable from one trial to the next. If one were to extend screening over several weeks, it is possible that some individuals will qualify. However, practical considerations dictate that repetitive testing with no end can and will lead to altered response behavior thus obviating any beneficial effects achieved by qualifying a few more subjects who may not be representative of the discriminating segment of the population. Some individuals take longer to learn how to participate, how to follow instructions, but as noted, this extra effort may not be cost effective. The orientation includes information about the duration of screening without suggesting that there are winners and losers. Finally, the screening process should be limited so that actual testing can be initiated without delay (or at least within 1 or 2 weeks at the most), otherwise those that were qualified will lose interest and their sensitivity will decline. Remember, the learning curve is shallow and the forgetting curve is steep!

On completion of the screening tests, individuals are categorized according to performance, with those having the greater number of correct scores, available for analytical tests (discrimination and descriptive tests). The others could either participate in re-screening or be put in the pool of subjects available for acceptance tests. This latter task requires a different kind of judgment, one that almost everyone is capable of providing. We will have more to say about this latter issue in Chapter 7. The performance measure from discrimination tests would be the percentage of correct decisions, and depending on the test type, hence level of chance probability, would be either >33% or >50%. Thus any individual who achieves at least 51% correct decisions would be considered as qualified; however, the usual practice has been to select individuals who achieve at least 65% correct. The criterion of 65% is arbitrary, the sensory professional must decide what skill level is appropriate for that product category. In addition, one might categorize an individual as qualified based on 55% correct, but the correct matches were achieved with difficult pairings, etc. Once regular testing begins, and then performance is monitored based on the results (see Chapter 5 for more discussion on this topic).

To reinforce the importance of following directions, several types of discrimination test procedures could be used, and different sensory modalities included. This approach also helps to establish whether all methods can be used with their products, as well as to identify appropriate products to use for screening future subjects. It is important to note that screening and qualifying of subjects always makes use of products rather than model systems – for example, aqueous solution of sweet, salt, sour, and bitter or specialized "reference," etc. Use of model systems will create problems in the form of different perceptions once the subjects are presented with finished products, and also, will send the wrong sensory messages to the subjects. For example, when developing a descriptive language, a panel is more likely to repeat the sensory messages (and experience "phantom perceptions") from the model systems/references rather than what they actually perceived. This occurs because of the context of the various stimuli presented at the start of the testing process.

For companies that manufacture many different types of products, the selection of appropriate screening products can be challenging. However, there are no shortcuts and one might find it most appropriate to use the product category for which there is a business priority. This problem cannot be entirely resolved as business priorities can change; however, one could develop groups of subjects screened for specific product categories, provided there is a need. Another option is to screen subjects using a variety of products. Once again, the decisions about how many people to screen, and with what products, depends on business priorities and the potential number of people available for testing. In practice, one often finds that subjects sensitive to one product category will do equally well on many other categories.

Sequential analysis is another approach to the selection of subjects for a discrimination test. The procedure is described in a number of publications; however, the description in Amerine and Roessler (1983) is quite readable. An early application of the method for selection of a taste panel was described by Bradley (1953). Basically, it requires the sensory professional to establish statistical limits on a graph for accepting, rejecting, or continued testing of a subject. The maximum number of trials to be given to a subject in the test can also be established. The technique is mathematically quite rigorous; however, the problem of product and variable selection has to be established by the experimenter. The sequential procedure does not appear to yield a more skilled subject and can require time-consuming repeated tasks before one can unambiguously select subjects.

The major point to be emphasized with regard to subject qualifying is not the rigid adherence to one product or test procedure exclusively, but rather the provision of some diversity and making the task enjoyable for the subject. The importance of teaching individuals to gain confidence in their ability as subjects is of paramount importance. Once this confidence has been established, it is easier to teach individuals to follow test directions and to focus their attention to the particular task. As already mentioned, subjects should be given an easy task initially to gain their confidence. Only with continued testing is it possible to determine how well the skills are developed and maintained.

Screening should always involve products of interest to that company. A series of test methods could be used to broaden the individual's experience and to assist sensory evaluation in identifying whether a specific procedure is appropriate for a product. Results should become a part of the individual's performance record and should be kept confidential. At the conclusion of screening, each employee should receive a notice acknowledging participation and advising about future testing.

In recent years, there has been an interest in and discussion on the use of standardized materials for screening and training. By standardized, we mean a series of materials one could obtain that would represent, like a standardized test score, stimuli that an individual would have to detect and/or recognize in order to be considered a "qualified" subject. The assumption of identifying those individuals with improved performance using specially prepared samples certainly sounds appealing, almost "too good to be true." The reality is that it is too good to be – it lacks merit. Just as threshold testing provided no good indication of product performance, so to will the use of standardized sets of externally obtained samples. Each product category has its own requirements and subject screening should be specific to that company. There is little to be gained and much to lose spending time screening subjects to be generalists. In any screening, the use of a stimulus that is not relevant to the interests of company's products be a distraction and is not recommended.

Initially, screening may be time-consuming, but once a sufficient pool of subjects is available, screening can be reduced to once or twice a month depending, of course, on staff availability and the backlog of requests. This organized (and controlled) effort causes the least disruption of regular testing activities and provides for continued but controlled introduction of new subjects. The frequency of the process is dependent on the influx of volunteers; if there is a high rate of change (employee turnover), it will be necessary to determine whether the problem is peculiar to specific areas of the company and plan accordingly. This knowledge, in turn, should be taken into account when seeking new subjects. In practical terms, it should be possible to initiate and complete screening within 2 or 3 weeks and have a panel available for routine testing directly thereafter. If one is using non-employees, the time requirements can be reduced by at least a third.

H. Performance Monitoring and Motivation

The two additional subject-related activities that warrant special attention are performance monitoring and motivation. Performance monitoring is an integral part of every testing program and requires an accessible and easily understood record system. Each time a subject participates, the date, the product, and the performance measure(s) are recorded. For each subject, there is a file listing performance by test type that can be accessed by name, test type, etc. These records constitute the basis for subject selection for subsequent tests. The chapters on specific methods provide more details on the use of performance records. In any operation, record keeping is easily accomplished using any spreadsheet format. The key is for the information to be retained and monitored after each test. The system needs to be kept current and performance records older than 3 or 6 months are probably best removed from the active file.

Subject motivation is an issue of concern to all sensory professionals. The most common problem of an established subject pool is sustained motivation, that is, maintaining an individual's interest such that the activity is welcomed regardless of the number of times that person has participated. Unfortunately, no foolproof solutions to the problem exist and an approach that is successful in one situation may prove unsuccessful in another. Since testing is done on a continuing basis, the staff need to develop a variety of practices to maintain interest. While the use of electronic noses and tongues is increasing (Bleibaum *et al.*, 2002), they are still in their infancy and will probably have greatest application in environments in which repetitive testing is required, for example, quality control, rather than be used in place of individual tests.

As with other aspects of testing, there are some general guidelines on motivating subjects. The following guidelines have proved to be especially useful:

1. Subjects should be rewarded for participation, not for correct scores.
2. Subjects should not be given direct monetary rewards, unless they are non-employees.
3. Subject participation should be acknowledged on a regular basis, directly and indirectly; food and/or beverage rewards (direct) should be available at the conclusion of each test and should be varied (be imaginative, do not serve the same treat every day!).
4. Management should visibly recognize sensory evaluation as a contributor to the company's growth as an indirect source of motivation.
5. Subjects should be given "vacations" from testing; for example, for a week every 4 weeks.
6. Sensory evaluation should hold an open house during selected holidays for all subjects, using the occasion to acknowledge participation and identifying some special accomplishments. Management participation in these activities is important.
7. Memos acknowledging special assistance should be included in the subjects' personal files.
8. The sensory evaluation staff should exhibit a positive attitude and should display a friendly but professional approach to its work.
9. The sensory professionals should never suggest that sensory testing involves "right" or "wrong" answers.
10. Subjects should be allowed to examine the summary sheet from a discrimination test, to identify which samples are the same.

The problem of sustaining subject motivation is especially difficult if the frequency of participation is high, once or twice each day or every day. Development of a sufficiently large pool minimizes reliance on the same group of subjects, boredom is minimal, and the subject's management is less concerned about work absence and so forth. As previously mentioned, sensory evaluation must develop a balance between frequency of participation, which sharpens sensory skills, and motivation, which tends to decrease with frequency of testing, and the effect of time away from regular work.

Another issue that warrants comment is the matter of direct compensation in addition to regular wages for motivating subjects. While the concept appears to have merit, from a practical viewpoint it leads to a multitude of problems, most of which become evident only after the compensation program is well underway.

Money has high initial impact but rapidly loses its appeal. There is no evidence, to our knowledge, that financially compensated subjects perform more efficiently, are more prompt, or express greater interest in their work as panel members. All subjects do not maintain their skills; some improve, and some do poorer than chance and should not continue as subjects. Providing brief vacations from testing may still require payment (as well as orientation and screening). Thus, considerable money is needed without having collected much useful information. Eliminating non-performers may prove very costly and a few subjects may create problems, even legal challenges. For example, some subjects may demand to see performance records, complain to the personnel department, and so on. It may be necessary to continue their payments although they do not participate. Should this occur, it could create motivational problems for the other subjects. Finally, the cost of direct compensation can be quite substantial and would appear to be a less than efficient use of company funds.

The other motivation problem for the sensory staff is the amount and content of the information given to the subjects, directly after a test, and over the long term. As noted in the guidelines, directly after some tests (e.g. discrimination), it is useful for each subject to have an opportunity to compare his or her decisions with the sample serving sequence. Note that no one is advised "you were wrong on the first set." This latter situation is unacceptable; it is a value judgment, which will in turn decrease motivation. Subjects should be reminded that there are no "real" correct responses; all information is of equal value.

Over the long term, one can also provide each subject with a performance record, for example, comparing each subject's performance with change performance and assessing the individual's performance relative to that of the panel as a group. Sensory evaluation should develop specific procedures for displaying performance (see the procedure developed by Swartz and Furia, 1977), especially given the availability of graphics capabilities in today's software environment.

I. Requests and Reports

When program development evolves to the stage where the various basic elements are in place, it is appropriate to focus on the issue of how tests are initiated and the results communicated to the requestor. There is an anecdote in sensory evaluation that describes the requesting process as follows: Returning from lunch you find 2 qt. of juice (or whatever product) on your desk with a note that requests that you "do a quick 200-consumer test for my meeting tomorrow morning, and let me know if sample A really is better" or some similar request. This continues to occur (since publication of the first edition) and is especially unfortunate that some sensory professionals consider this typical and proceed to do the test. Our attention here should be directed not to the issue of the test, but to the nature of the requesting process itself. Sensory staff must develop a standard protocols, approved by management, that stipulates that no testing be initiated without receipt of a paper or electronic request and appropriate authorization. While some individual may find these requirements to be tedious or unnecessary, the issues are of sufficient importance that they cannot be ignored.

The objective is to obtain a record of the request to make certain that the test purpose is correctly stated, that products are properly identified by code and by location, and a priority has been assigned. The assignment of priority is not a sensory responsibility; that is, sensory can state the backlog of work but cannot properly assign a priority to a request. The requestors and/or their management must decide

REQUEST FORM

To: Date:
Approval:
From: Priority:

Test Objective:

Product with Code: Project No.:

Product Description and History:

Product Location and Amount:

Preparation Procedures:

People to be Excluded: Report Distribution

For SE Use Only

Test method: ______	Sample quantity: ______
Suggested test date: ______	Sample temperature: ______
Design: ______	Carrier: ______
Number and type subject: ______	Serving container: ______
Method of sample presentation: ______	Lighting conditions: ______
Number of replications: ______	Other: ______
Serving conditions: ______	Experimenter comments: ______

Figure 2.8 Example of a form for use in requesting a sensory test.

on priority. This, of course, assumes that management has agreed on a procedure for assigning priorities.

The form should be relatively simple in its use and should provide space for sensory staff to add sufficient detail so that it can be used in actual test planning and implementation. As shown in Fig. 2.8, those requesting a test provide information such as the objective(s), date of request, priority, product source and location (e.g. whether products are commercial or experimental), and who should receive copies of the report. Based on this information, sensory staff record receipt of the request, examine the request, and, if warranted, schedule a meeting with the requestor.

Generally, several meetings (several test requests) are required to educate requestors on the important issues of test objective and product history. An objective is not "to do a triangle test," "to do a 200-consumer acceptance test," etc. An objective must define the purpose of the test (e.g. to determine whether product A containing a replacement ingredient is perceived as different from the current product). Alternatively, the requestor may explain the background of the request and define the objective in conversation with the sensory professional. For the former, the requestor may inform sensory that the company would like to replace a particular flavor (for any of a variety of reasons) used in certain products, and based on this sensory evaluation can formulate the objective. Also, confusion about the objective of a test may have come about as a result of the brand manager asking questions about sales decline, or consumer acceptance information that is not clear as to product acceptance: "Our product has been losing market share at a rate of 2% per month for the past 4 months, it's not delivering, improve the flavor… and so on." By the time such directives reach sensory staff in the form of a request, the test purpose may be vague or contradictory. The sensory staff must recognize the potential risk of unclear requests, and through discussion with the requestor, must ascertain whether more information about the test is needed, and if so, identify who initiated the request and how the results will be used. Ideally, sensory staff should be involved at the earliest possible time or notified about the situation before actual product work is initiated. This early involvement will facilitate the testing process and, where appropriate, sensory professionals may be able to recommend an alternative test plan as an aid to the requestor.

The dialog between the requestor and the sensory professional is important for both. It minimizes the selection of an inappropriate test, eliminates an unwarranted test, and ensures that products will be available when needed and that priorities will be met. Sensory professionals will establish lines of communication with their customers, who in turn will benefit from an understanding of sensory testing activities and the kinds of information that will be available. Over time, requests will become more informative and discussions will be primarily limited to problems that have a more complex background; however, as we will discuss in Chapter 4, the dialog is never totally eliminated. One additional aspect of this dialog, important to sensory evaluation, is the financial benefit derived from a test result. If, for example, a test result enables a cost reduction to be made, or minimizes additional testing, and so forth, then these benefits must be credited to the sensory program. In this way, the sensory staff can demonstrate to management the benefits that accrue from an organized sensory program.

Reports represent a special opportunity for sensory evaluation, primarily because test results in the form of numbers and statistics may not be as informative and can be easily misunderstood, but tend to form an important basis on which a sensory program is judged. Sensory staff must develop ways of communicating results that make them understood and actionable. While test results are only one basis for evaluation, they should not detract from the overall accomplishment. Reports are prepared by the appropriate sensory professional and not by the requestor or by some other individual. Allowing others to prepare reports will seriously undermine credibility and lead to other problems. Occasionally one encounters situations in which sensory evaluation provides everything including a report, but offers no interpretation. This procedure would work only in special situations, for example, during the preliminary stages of a research effort, and only if it has been agreed to by sensory evaluation.

With regard to the report itself, the first issue is to not write a report as if it were a manuscript for a journal, but to consider it as the recommendation based on the test objective; that is, was the objective satisfied and what is its meaning, what is the next course of action, if any? All numbers, including statistical significance, should be relegated to the back of a report or made available on request. As shown in Fig. 2.9, the first section of a report should summarize results and the conclusion-recommendation

REPORT FORM

To: Date:

From: Project No.:

Objective:

Sample Description:

Conclusion and Recommendations:

Results:

Product Preparation:

Test Procedures:

Test method: ______	Serving conditions: ______
Design: ______	Sample quantity: ______
Number and type subject: ______	Sample temperature: ______
Sample presentation: ______	Carrier: ______
Replication: ______	Other: ______

Figure 2.9 Example of a form for use in reporting test results.

in a few sentences. It should identify the products, objective, test request and date, distribution, and author of the report. For results of a discrimination test, one can develop a similar report format. As shown in Fig. 2.10, the format closely follows the request format, thus facilitating report preparation by the appropriate sensory staff member. Subsequent pages containing more detail can be added as needed; however, it is unrealistic to expect that a long and tedious report will be read, except by a very few individuals. While the technical staff may feel that they require all of the information, including computer printout (if a part of the analyses), sensory evaluation should not confuse this documentation with the purpose of the report (and particularly, the conclusion and recommendation).

A report that successfully summarizes the results in a few sentences is more likely to be read and appreciated. A long and involved discussion should be viewed with concern; there is a problem with the results, and the author is trying to explain them. While management will welcome brief, concise reports, some frustration may be experienced by the technical staff. Familiarity with the format of scientific journals and a sincere desire to have everything available for examination may prompt the scientist/technologist to request all of the study details. However, this concern for detail should gradually diminish with an increase in sensory evaluation credibility.

A standard format should be developed to facilitate report preparation as well as ease of reading. The standard format should be modified for reports that cover a

DIFFERENCE TEST REPORT FORM

To: Date:
From:

1. Product Description:

2. Objective:

3. Conclusion and Recommendation:

4. Results:
 Date of Test ______

Sample	Number of Judgements	Number of Correct Judgements	Significance

5. Test Procedure:

Number of subjects ______ Different sample: ______
Subject type ______ Carrier, if any: ______
Replication ______ Interval between sets ______
Sample temperature ______ Rinse water ______
Sample quantity ______ Mouth cleanser ______
Container ______ Lighting ______

Figure 2.10 Example of a form for reporting results of a difference test.

series of tests, for example, for storage or for a research project. For example, each storage withdrawal should not require a full report, but possibly an interim document, and should incorporate elements of previously reported data where reasonable. Sensory evaluation should determine the type of report best suited to their particular business activities and where necessary, obtain management approval for the format, and so forth. In some environments, use of PowerPoint® presentations are prepared and distributed electronically to everyone involved in a project thus enabling individuals to examine the details at their leisure.

J. Operations Manual

An operations manual should be available in every sensory department. The document describes all activities of the department, including development of program objectives, how tests are requested and reported, job descriptions for each staff member, examples of scorecards, and subject selection procedures. The manual often includes information on product preparation procedures and amounts required for different test types. Such documents are extremely important in that they serve as a basis for the orientation and training of new staff members, ensure that standardized procedures will not be inadvertently modified, minimize recreation of procedures already developed, and aid in the efficient use of resources.

Preparation of the manual takes a reasonable amount of time and is modified as new information is developed. We have found that the actual preparation should be undertaken only after sensory staff members have at least 1 year of experience and have sufficient familiarity with all procedures that are likely to be encountered. The important point is the need to document the purpose and procedures of all sensory evaluation activities.

K. Planning and Research

Planning in sensory evaluation is important to prepare for and/or anticipate special needs, to identify specific gaps such as a declining subject pool, and to propose alternative procedures for overcoming them. Each year the budget process requires attention so as to identify the needs for the forthcoming year; however, this attention is usually focused on financial rather than operational needs and should, therefore, be separate from the business planning effort.

The planning document should identify sensory evaluation's accomplishments to date, anticipated skills requirements, the basis for each need, and how these capabilities will enhance the department's activities in the coming years. For the supplier of ingredients (flavors and fragrances), information provided by a potential customer is often limited, as is the time allowed to submit a sample. The supplier's sensory resources may be unable to provide adequate assistance because it did not develop the necessary specialized capabilities. Such procedures are not developed on short notice, but require planning. If one department is providing more than half of all test request in the most recent 12-month period, then it is desirable to determine if this trend will continue. It will also be useful to meet with potential customers to describe services available to them and assess their interest in these services.

The development and/or evaluation of new methods or the modification of current methods are activities that also need attention. The literature on sensory evaluation appears in a variety of sources. Sensory staff should have funds available in its budget to monitor the literature, to identify new developments, and to provide an assessment of those that have possible application (the Internet connection is an excellent way of keeping current).

Planning documents should be concise, preferably not more than four pages. It may be useful to characterize the previous year's accomplishment; for example, the number of tests by month and by requesting group, total number of responses, and any other pertinent information. Coupled with typical budget requests, the planning document constitutes a business statement about sensory evaluation and its contributions to the company's growth in the marketplace.

III. Conclusions

In this chapter, we have identified and characterized the individual elements that make up a sensory evaluation department in a company. Numerous activities were identified, including management-approved goals and objectives, professional staff, program strategy, facilities, test methods, identification, screening and selection of subjects, subject performance monitoring, test requests and reports, data processing, operations manual, and planning and research. Recognition of these specific activities is an integral part of a fully capable sensory evaluation department. This approach assumes a reasonable level of management skill in addition to familiarity with sensory evaluation principles and practices on the part of the sensory staff. It can be argued that this exercise is unnecessary, as well as demanding of the sensory staff; nonetheless, without this background and the individual elements in place, the full potential of sensory evaluation cannot be realized.

The development of sensory evaluation resources as described herein can take as much as 2 or more years, based on a plan that is both realistic in terms of staff skills and consistent with the long-range needs of the individual company. This should not be construed to mean that no actionable sensory information will be available for this time period (actually information can be available within 1 month), but rather it takes that long for a program to establish its credibility, to develop a record of successes, and for the sensory professional(s) to know how best to use resources. A first step in the process, after identifying the need for sensory resources, is to establish a dialog with management and with potential test requestors that identifies how the sensory program will be a benefit to them. Matching this expressed need with available resources enables sensory evaluation to develop a realistic plan for the company. This approach is consistent with a management-by-objective philosophy; however, there is no evidence that other management approaches would not work equally well. The key is to recognize the need for a formal, business approach to all aspects of a sensory program.

Throughout this discussion, considerable emphasis has been placed on a need for a formal approach to the development of sensory resources, to develop a pool of qualified subjects, use procedures that are scientifically sound, document requests and reports, maintain subject performance records, and establish direct lines of communications with technologists and brand managers. Sensory information is a unique information source that has significant value in the marketplace. Ultimately, however, the success of a sensory program will depend on the individuals involved, the sensory professionals, and their ability to make meaningful contributions to the decision-making process.

Measurement

3

I. Introduction

The definition of sensory evaluation described in Chapter 1 emphasizes the importance of measurement for treating sensory evaluation as a scientific discipline. Measurement is critical to quantifying responses to stimuli for the purpose of utilizing descriptive and inferential statistics. Such statistics provide a rational basis for decisions about the products that are evaluated and the subjects who did the evaluations. The value of measurement and the requirement for valid scales of measurement are not, however, unique to sensory evaluation. Physics, with its impressive list of achievements, provides an excellent example of what can be accomplished through measurement.

Psychology, in its evolution from philosophy to laboratory science, devoted much attention to developing methods and scales for measuring behavior. Many different types of scales were developed, and each was accompanied by controversy regarding the appropriateness of the various scales and how best to measure behavior. This controversy continues into the present and the interested reader will find the early publications by Boring (1950), Guilford (1954), Eisler (1963a,b), Ekman and Sjoberg (1965), and Carterette and Friedman (1974) most helpful in describing the

Sensory Evaluation Practices 3rd Edn
ISBN: 0-12-672690-6

issues and providing a detailed history of measurement. The more recent publications by Marks (1974), Nunnally (1978), and Laming (1986) bring this discussion to the current state, but by no means is this the end of the discussion. Guilford (1954) in his book *Psychometric Methods* credited the early development of behavioral measurement to investigators involved with the two distinctly different research areas; mental testing (e.g. the intelligence quotient) and psychophysics (i.e. the mathematical expression describing the relationship between changes in the physical stimulus and perceived intensity).

Ekman and Sjöberg also discussed the development of scaling theory and methods as proceeding along these two distinct yet parallel courses of test theory and classic psychophysics. They categorized the two lines of development according to different research interests and the application of scaling to two entirely different kinds of studies, one to measure preference for a product and the other to study the psychophysics of perception. Representative examples of scaling theory related to preference measurement are found in the published works of Thurstone (1959), and examples of psychophysics and scaling theory are found in Stevens (1957, 1960). While this literature is more than 40 years old, it provides an excellent perspective to current practices. Unfortunately, one still encounters scale use based on faulty or no assumptions, a lack of awareness of the earlier literature, other than a long history of use in a particular company without any evidence of the sensitivity or the reliability of the scale. Still others search for the universal scale as if it represents some kind of special instrument.

Major developments in scaling from the Thurstonian school included assumptions and procedures related to comparative and categorical judgments, and from Stevens, ratio scaling methods such as magnitude estimation. It is well documented that the data obtained from category and ratio scaling experiments are different (Stevens and Galanter, 1957). However, as Marks (1974) reported, Stevens' belief that only ratio scaling could yield valid scales of sensation has been challenged (Anderson, 1970; Weiss, 1972).

Eisler (1963a,b) suggested that discrimination was the basis of category scale judgments, and because discrimination changed with the magnitude of the stimulus difference, category scale data could be expected to deviate from magnitude scale data. However, output from the two types of scales have been shown to be related, although the relationship is nonlinear. Marks' (1974) view of this relationship was not that one scale was derived from the other (one explanation), rather that both category and ratio scales were valid and also were different types of scales. He postulated that for any given sensory attribute, there are two basic underlying scales; a scale of magnitude and a scale of dissimilarity.

The position of the sensory professional regarding this controversy about category versus ratio scales should be pragmatic and eclectic (unless one is engaged in research). Appropriately constructed category scales will enable the sensory professional to determine whether a product is more or less liked or the magnitudes of differences for specific sensory attributes (e.g. color, aroma). To derive a mathematical expression describing the relationship between ingredient concentration and perceived intensity, a ratio scaling procedure such as magnitude estimation might be an appropriate choice. However, that mathematical expression has value only if it has a practical application for the sensory professional. Hence, the selection of a scale will be based on very practical considerations. Philosophical arguments and claims that certain scales are more or less linear when compared to one another must be viewed in the context of research hypotheses and not embraced without fully understanding the basis on which such a conclusion was reached. Differences in subjects, instructions, measurement techniques, choice of stimulus, and objective will influence results. Finally, the reader is reminded that studies with simple stimulus systems often do not yield similar conclusions when the stimulus is a more complex product.

In this discussion about measurement, primary emphasis is placed on descriptions of various (but not all) types of scales, suggested applications, and methods for analysis.

II. Components of Measurement: Scales

Selection of a scale for use in a particular test is one of several tasks that need to be completed by the sensory professional before a test can be organized and fielded. Determining test objective, subject qualifications, and product characteristics will have an impact on and should precede method and scale selection. These issues were discussed in Chapter 2 and are considered in more detail in Chapter 4. For purposes of this discussion, it should be kept in mind that these issues are, for the most part, interdependent; that is, a decision on one task will influence the next decision. In the case of scale selection, knowledge of the test objective, who will be the subjects, and the type of information desired must precede choice of scale. Before examining the different types of scales available, it will be useful to review some practical issues. To derive the most value from a response scale it should be:

Meaningful to subjects. The words used for questions and/or to scale the responses must be familiar, easily understood, and unambiguous to the subjects. The words must be readily related to the product and the task, and they must make sense to the subject in how they are applied in the test. Words that have specific and useful meaning to the requester and/or the sensory professional may be much less meaningful to subjects, especially if they are not qualified subjects; that is, typical consumers. Assuming that a consumer will understand terminology that is specific to project team members is, at best, risky. In some situations, it is essential to add an explanation to a particular question as an aid for that consumer.

Uncomplicated to use. Even where questions and words describing the task and response scale are understood and meaningful, the task and scale must be easy to use. If not, it will result in subject frustration, increased measurement error, and provide fewer differences among products. Although a particular scale may be better from a theoretical perspective, it may produce less useful results than a simpler scale that is easier to use. Other issues to consider include the practice of switching scale direction from one question to another, switching number of scale categories for similar scales, or changing scale magnitude. Unfortunately, consumers do not necessarily read every instruction and switching scale structure and direction without clear delineation will cause problems (e.g. decreased sensitivity) that cannot be corrected after a test is completed. We will say more about this later in the chapter.

Unbiased. It is critical that results not be an artifact of the scale that was used. Ideally, the scale is a "null" instrument that does not influence the test outcome. Where products are perceived as different, we want to know this; where they are not, we want to know this as well. Unbalanced scales easily bias results because they decrease the expected probability for responses in categories that are under-represented. They introduce a bias for which no obvious advantage has been demonstrated. The most typical explanation is to learn more about negative responses, as if knowing this enables products to be better liked. Number and word biases have been well documented in the literature, yet one continues to encounter their use, particularly in the measurement of quality; for example, "best quality, good quality, poor quality," or 1 is best quality and 5 is worst quality. These latter scales are unique to a company, having been developed years earlier without any research or awareness of the measurement literature and have taken "a life of their own," that is, they have been used for so long that no one is able to not use them. It makes it very difficult for the sensory professional to change these practices. For more on this topic, the reader is referred to a later chapter on special problems.

Relevant. This relates to scale validity; that is, the scale should measure that attribute, characteristic, attitude, etc., that it is intended to measure. For example, preference scales should measure preference, and quality scales should measure quality; and it is unwise to infer one from the other. Where the subject or the requester does not see the relevance for a particular scale or task, test credibility is lessened for data collection and eventual presentation of results. Simply stated, if the scale is not relevant for the task or issue, do not bother using it. This particular problem extends well beyond the measurement process itself. It derives in part from a lack of understanding of the perceptual process and a belief that humans will act in certain ways contrary to our knowledge of behavior. The typical situation arises when a request is made to save time by having the subjects respond to questions about differences (the magnitude, the nature of the difference, whether it is good or bad quality, etc.). The subjects are at the test site so why not ask these questions! Unfortunately, the matter of subject qualifications is not appreciated nor is the halo effect of one response on the other, etc.

Sensitive to differences. Not all scales are equally sensitive for measuring differences. Scale length and number of scale categories are major variables that have an effect on scale sensitivity. For example, one continues to encounter disbelief that there are differences in scale sensitivity based solely on the number of categories available. This is purely a mathematical issue without any impact of words or numbers (numerical scales). In effect, a three-point scale is less sensitive than a five-point scale (by about 30%), and both are less sensitive than a seven- or nine-point scale. This topic will be discussed in more detail later in this chapter.

Provides for a variety of statistical analyses. Statistical analysis of responses is critical to determining whether results are due to chance or to the treatment variables. The more powerful the statistics that can be applied, and the more of them, increases the opportunity for identifying significant events that have occurred. This does not mean that scales that use less powerful statistical analyses are of no value; they are less flexible and may be less sensitive, thereby making it more difficult to demonstrate their usefulness.

For those situations where new scales or words for a scale are required, it will be prudent to first do a small pilot test to eliminate potential problems with their use.

Just as there are different types of test methods, there also are different types of scales that provide different kinds of information. For clarification purposes, the classification of scales proposed by Stevens (1951) will be followed here. While Coombs (1964) challenged the classification as being too restrictive, it remains a frequently used system that is relatively easy to follow. It should be noted that Stevens presented the idea that a particular scale determines the permissible mathematical operations for the responses (from that scale). Whether this latter restriction about permissible mathematics must be followed precisely cannot be stated unequivocally, inasmuch as there are scales that are not easily classified or that yield responses consistent with results from scales in other categories. Nonetheless, this system is useful for discussion purposes. The different types of scales are distinguished on the basis of the ordering and distance properties inherent in measurement rules; that is, the property of numbers based on how they are assigned. Stevens postulated four categories of scales:

1. Nominal scales for use in classification or naming.
2. Ordinal scales for use in ordering or ranking.
3. Interval scales for use in measuring magnitudes, assuming equal distances between points on the scale.
4. Ratio scales for use in measuring magnitudes, assuming equality of ratios between points.

A. Nominal Scales

In these scales, numbers are used to label, code, or otherwise classify items or responses. The only property assigned to these numbers is that of non-equality; that is, the responses or items placed in one class cannot be placed in another class. Letters or other symbols could be used in place of numbers without any loss of information or alteration of permissible mathematical manipulation.

In sensory evaluation, numbers are frequently used as labels and as classification categories; for example, the three-digit numerical codes are used to keep track of products while masking their true identity. It is important that the product identified by a specific code not be mislabeled or grouped with a different product. It is also important that the many individual servings of a specific product exhibit a reasonable level of consistency if the code is used to represent a group of servings from a single experimental treatment.

An example of a use for a nominal scale is shown in Fig. 3.1. In this particular application, no actual product is involved; however, the results would identify the rooms in which air fresheners are used most frequently. This information will be useful for identifying appropriate types of fragrances and alternative positioning statements for further product research.

Nominal scales also are used to classify demographic data about respondents such as age, gender, and income, as well as to classify product usage behavior (see Fig. 2.7).

Name ______________________ Code ______________ Date ______________

In which location(s) in your home do you most often use air fresheners? Please check as many as necessary.

- ❑ Bathroom
- ❑ Kitchen
- ❑ Bedroom
- ❑ Closet
- ❑ Hall
- ❑ Garage
- ❑ Family room
- ❑ Dining room
- ❑ Living room

Figure 3.1 Example of a scorecard that uses a nominal scale to obtain information about product usage characteristics.

Another feature of nominal scales is the total independence of the order among the various categories. The order can be changed without altering the logic of the question or the treatment of the results.

In general, subjects have little or no difficulty in responding to questions that use nominal scales (this assumes the questions are understood). This is an obvious advantage when a problem has a large number of alternatives; for example, developing a test protocol that best reflects the most frequently used preparation and consumption mode for the product. Or, if one wanted to obtain responses from a large number of respondents without taking a substantial amount of time, the use of a nominal scale might be quite appropriate.

Responses to open-ended questions such as "What did you like about this product?" are used in a *post hoc* manner to develop a nominal scale, in contrast to *a priori* scale development where all response categories are present at the beginning of the study.

Once open-ended data have been collected, all responses are read and categories for responses are developed to reflect some minimal number of independently appearing response comments. A frequency count then is obtained to represent the number of times a particular comment was made.

Because the same words may have different meanings and different words may have the same meaning to the respondents and to the experimenter, there exists substantial opportunity for responses to be incorrectly assigned to a category. Since this would be a violation of the restriction for using nominal scales, the mathematical treatment and value of open-ended data is seriously questioned. It has been suggested that one or two individuals could categorize the data independently; however, this approach would neither alter the meanings of the words nor be helpful in situations where disagreements between the two classifiers existed. On occasion, the sensory professional may use an open-ended question as an aid in the construction of categories for use in subsequent testing. In this situation, the open-ended question may have application; however, it should not be used as a direct guide for product development. Open-ended questions should not be used as a substitute for focus group or descriptive panel information.

Mathematics permissible for nominal scale data include frequency counts and distributions, modes (the category containing the most responses), chi-square (χ^2), and a coefficient of contingency. Of the permissible computations, χ^2 is probably the most helpful. It allows for a comparison of frequency distributions to determine whether they are different, comparison of frequencies for data that can be categorized in two or more ways to determine whether the actual responses are different from some expected values, and comparisons of two or more groups relative to a series of categories. Data derived from the scorecard shown in Fig. 3.1 would be consistent with this category. For a detailed description of the various applications of χ^2 to nominal responses, the interested reader will find the discussion by McNemar (1969) helpful.

The coefficient of contingency may be viewed as a type of correlation or measure of association between different variables having nominal scale information and is derived from the χ^2 computation. The computation is possible if the same objects have been classified on two variables or attributes, each having two or more categories. For example, to determine whether there is dependence between two income groups and sex of the respondents, the formula is

$$C = \sqrt{\frac{\chi^2}{\chi^2 + N}}$$

and the contingency table would appear as follows:

	Income	
Sex	**Low**	**High**
Male	A	B
Female	C	D

C will have a value <1.0, and will depend on the number of categories involved in the computations. As noted by McNemar, for a two-by-two table the maximum of C is $\sqrt{1/2}$ or 0.7071, and the closer the computed value to this maximum, the stronger the degree of association.

It is possible to convert nominal scale data by assigning ranks or percentages based on frequency. This conversion permits use of statistical analyses usually restricted to ordinal data and proportions (e.g. t test for proportions). In this case, it would be prudent to identify that scale conversion was done prior to using these inferential analyses.

Although considered a "low-order" scale because of the limited permissible computations, nominal scales are a valuable resource to the sensory professional. They are easy to use by the subject, require limited test time, and with limited computations provide rapid results to the requester. Other than the potential for misclassifying responses, the other serious limitation is the ability of respondents to contribute differentially to the database. Some subjects respond to open-ended questions (e.g. what did you like most about the product?) with many comments compared to other subjects that give terse replies or have difficulty answering. As Payne (1965) noted many years ago, the open-ended questions have value in the early phases of research but close-ended questions are more informative and thus, serve more useful purposes, in subsequent stages of any testing.

B. Ordinal Scales

Ordinal scales use either numbers or words organized from "high" to "low," "most" to "least," etc., with respect to some attribute of a product set. The categories in an ordinal scale are not interchangeable. No assumptions are made regarding the distance between categories or the magnitude of the attribute represented by a category. Other than direction, all that is assumed is that a category is either greater or less than another category. Ordinal scales are considered to be the first or most basic scale for measuring perceived intensities and as such have more in common with other magnitude scales than with nominal scales.

Ranking is one of the most commonly used types of ordinal scale. It is a relatively easy behavioral task and a number of procedures have been developed for ranking products. The most direct procedure is to have respondents arrange or sort a set of products so that each succeeding product has more (or less) of an attribute; for example, rank products from most to least sweet or from most to least liked. This procedure works well for products that can be easily manipulated by hand, such as a series of fabrics or a series of bottled liquids. However, for products that are not in closed containers and especially foods and beverages, the risk of spills may require some modification in the test procedure. For example, having subjects list the products by their codes rather than rearranging the products would be an acceptable step, as shown in Fig. 3.2.

The paired-comparison test is a special use of the rank-order test, as are the directional discrimination (e.g. which sample is sweeter) and the paired-preference tests. Chapter 5 is devoted exclusively to the discrimination test and its applications in sensory evaluation. For purposes of this discussion, attention is directed to the binary form of the data derived from these two-product rank tests. In Guilford's (1954) discussion about paired tests, there are procedures for transforming binary data to interval data. In multidimensional scaling, Shephard (1966) described procedures for deriving "partially metric" data from multiple paired comparisons. Such approaches take advantage of the fact that there is a constant interval or distance between the first and second rank in a two-sample, forced choice situation. These latter computations are not typical of the use of ranking in a laboratory sensory test. Nonetheless, they offer opportunities where there are a large array of stimuli (e.g. products or concept statements), all stimuli are compared to one another, subjects are limited to forced choice responses, and results are described in terms of interval data. This methodology is more likely to be encountered in consumer research when there is interest in determining product preference under different purchase options, for example.

With simultaneous product presentation, ranking is considered a direct method; it does not depend on memory. The products serve as their own frame of reference before

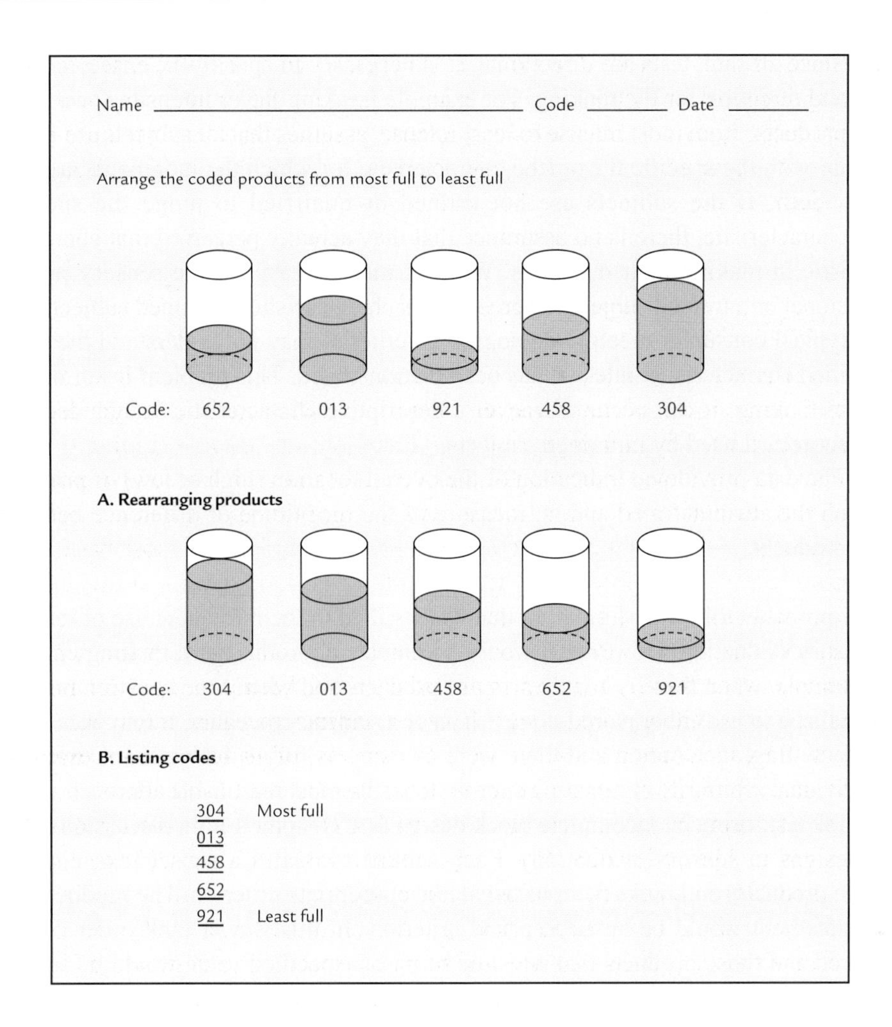

Figure 3.2 Examples of a direct ranking test in which the respondents can (A) rearrange the products or (B) list the codes. In the former procedure, the products are moved; in the latter, the subject records the order and no product movement is required.

any response is obtained and they require uncomplicated statistical assumptions and applications. Beyond ranking, the subject does not provide a number or score for each product or mark a word scale. Both of these tasks have some bias associated with them. However, there are limitations to the more widespread use of ranking in product evaluation, and only the paired comparison for directional difference or preference finds much use in sensory evaluation. Limitations include the following:

1. All products in a multi-product ranking test must be considered before a judgment is made. This can easily result in sensory fatigue and interactions, a problem that is most acute with products having a lingering flavor or odor or when a large number of products are to be evaluated. In paired-comparison tests, the number of pairs increases at a rate of n^2 for each additional product beyond the first two. Of course, in a visual test, sensory fatigue is not an issue.

2. Since all rank tests are directional, it is necessary to specify the characteristics and direction for the ranking. For example, ranking flavor intensity for a set of products, from most intense to least intense, assumes that all subjects are familiar with the specific flavor (the characteristic for which the judgments are provided). If the subjects are not trained or qualified to judge the specific characteristic, there is no assurance that they actually perceived that characteristic in making their decisions. While it may be easy for the sensory professional or a trained subject to perceive this characteristic, untrained subjects (the typical consumer meeting demographic criteria) may not understand the specified characteristic unless it has been demonstrated. This problem is not unique to ranking; it can occur whenever a descriptive characteristic is included in a scorecard used by untrained subjects.
3. The data provide no indication of the overall location (high or low) of products on the attribute rated and no measure of the magnitude of difference between products.

It is probably this latter limitation that has resulted in the infrequent use of ranking in sensory evaluation. However, it would be unrealistic to disregard ranking entirely. For example, when there is a large array of products and when time constraints make it unrealistic to use either paired-comparison or a scoring procedure. If one were seeking a new fragrance option and there were as many as fifty submissions. Other than an individual arbitrarily eliminating submissions, the most reasonable approach would be a rank test, using an incomplete block design (see Chapter 4 for a discussion about test designs in sensory evaluation). Each subject evaluates a subset (e.g. eight of sixteen products) and ranks them based on the appropriate criterion. The product concept statement would be an appropriate criterion. In this way, a rank order can be achieved and those products that equal or surpass a specified value would be subject to further evaluation. We have employed this specific approach quite successfully and hence our insistence that ranking should not be disregarded as a test method. It is most helpful for screening a large array of products to a smaller more manageable product subset. In a "round robin" procedure, where an incomplete block has been used, only the highest ranked product(s) from each segment is selected for inclusion in follow-up testing. Informal ranking procedures are used for benchtop screening to reduce the number of product alternatives submitted for sensory tests.

Analysis of rank data can be accomplished by several different methods, including those appropriate for nominal scales and in particular those referred to as nonparametric methods. Methods that will be helpful include Wilcoxon signed ranks test, Mann–Whitney, Kruskal–Wallis, Friedman two-way analysis of variance, χ^2 and Kendall's coefficient of concordance. A detailed description and worked examples of the various tests can be found in Hollander and Wolfe (1973), Daniel (1978), and O'Mahony (1986). Kramer (1960, 1963) also developed a set of tables for ease in determining whether there was a significant difference in the ranks for a set of products; however, some errors were identified in those tables and the publications by Joanes (1985) and by Newell and MacFarlane (1987) provide more precise directions and analyses for ranked data.

An alternative to the limited information obtained from direct ranking is provided by the use of rating scales. These scales provide subjects with an unbroken continuum or with ordered categories along a continuum. As a group, they are perhaps among the most widely used and oldest scales of measurement in sensory evaluation. This durability is attributable primarily to the ease with which they can be formulated and administered, the large number of statistical tests that can be used to analyze results, and empirical evidence that they work.

Numerous examples of rating scales can be found in the literature as evidence of their diversity and application (Baten, 1946; Hall, 1958; Amerine *et al.*, 1965; Ellis, 1966; Lawless and Heymann, 1999). Scale categories varied from as few as five to as many as twelve, although the majority of the scales had eight or ten response categories. Some scales had a word and/or number for every scale category while others were anchored only at the extremes. The most difficult of issues appeared to be the number of categories and the specific words used to anchor them. Cloninger *et al.* (1976) used results from a series of rating scales, and after applying various normalization and transformation techniques concluded that a five-point scale was more suitable than scales with more categories.

Contrary to this conclusion, there is extensive literature on scaling and information theory that supports the nine-point rating scale as being more useful and optimal for information transmission (Garner and Hake, 1951; Bendig and Hughes, 1953; Garner, 1960; Cox, 1980). Two examples of ordinal scales are shown in Fig. 3.3, both representing methods that use words, numbers, and/or categories for the measurement of intensity. The first example (A) represents a type of hybrid consisting of five word and ten numerical categories. Obviously, more weight is given to some categories (associated with the word "strong" are three numerical categories) than to others ("none" has only one numerical category). The second example (B) represents a less complicated scale with no numbers and only two word anchors. The use of fewer words is intended to minimize bias. As mentioned earlier in this chapter, one can easily demonstrate an advantage in sensitivity for the scale with more categories. Taken to an extreme, one could envision greatest sensitivity to a scale with 100 or more categories; however, the reality is quite different (as reported by Bendig and Hughes and Garner and Hake, op cit). As the number of categories increases from two to about ten, sensitivity increases reaching an optimum at about nine to ten, and then decreases as the number of categories increases (beyond ten). This inverted "U" is explained by having either too few or too many categories; either leads to reduced sensitivity and lack of product differentiation.

Selection of the word anchors for rating scales often appears too arbitrary, providing opportunities and especially pitfalls. By opportunities, we refer to the use of words that are meaningful and unambiguous to the subjects relative to the specific scale. An example of ambiguous words would be a scale of overall reaction to a product having anchors of excellent to poor, good and bad quality, best tasting ever and worst tasting ever, etc. These are general quality terms, not personal preferences, and do connote different perceptual meanings to different people, opportunities for confusion in scoring (and a concomitant loss of sensitivity) increases dramatically when such words are used. Finally, measures of product quality might not be equivalent to

Name ______________________________ Code ______________ Date __________

Check one of the boxes that represents your opinion about the taste intensity of the product you are evaluating.

Intensity of taste		Product	
		487	924
		Taste	Taste
None	10		
Slight	9		
	8		
Moderate	7		
	6		
	5		
Strong	4		
	3		
Extreme	2		
	1		

A

Name ______________________________ Code ______________ Date __________

Check the box that represents the relative intensity for that characteristic you are evaluating.

Characteristic A

Light ... Dark

❑ ❑ ❑ ❑ ❑ ❑ ❑ ❑ ❑

Characteristic B

Weak ... Strong

❑ ❑ ❑ ❑ ❑ ❑ ❑ ❑ ❑

B

Figure 3.3 Two examples of ordinal-type rating scales that have been used in sensory evaluation. The first (A) represents a structured scale that contains both numerical and word categories, some of which have been weighted. The second (B) is a less complicated scale with no numerical values and only two word anchors.

specific product differences; that is, there could be perceived preference differences between two products, yet the judgments on the "quality" scales may not be sufficient to yield a significant score difference. It is possible to have different preference for products that are perceptually different but of equal quality.

The use of scoring is intended to determine the magnitudes of the differences between products. If products are being evaluated based on quality, it will be quite difficult to determine in what ways a product should be modified. In addition, it would be quite risky to have a sensory panel of ten to twenty provide judgments of product quality, a task for which it may not be suitable (Sidel *et al.*, 1981, 1983). A more detailed discussion about the use of sensory evaluation for measuring quality is presented in Chapter 8; however, our interest here is in the use of word anchors that are least likely to be misinterpreted and to not use words that connote quality. As we will show in the discussion on descriptive analysis, the use of intensity measures, usually from low to high combined with word anchors that can be demonstrated to subjects (given examples of products that represent those sensory measures), is a very successful procedure in the sense that one can achieve optimal sensitivity and minimal variability without extensive effort devoted to training of subjects. This does not mean that there is only one ordinal scale or that scales that do not follow this pattern of development will not be useful. As with the use of any scale, it is a question of risk on the part of the sensory professional considering the problem, the products and the extent to which the subjects are familiar with the use of the scale.

In addition to responsibility for selection and/or development of a specific scale, it should be kept in mind that ordinal scale data may exhibit interval properties. In fact, the same scale under different operations may exhibit more or less equality of intervals between scale points. The degree to which the distance between intervals is equal has some bearing on the risk involved with using various statistical techniques to analyze results. However, we agree with Guilford (1954), Labovitz (1970), and Nunnally (1978) that violation of the assumption of equality of intervals between points on these rating scales usually is sufficiently tolerable to have minimal effect on the use of parametric statistical analyses of these data. Later sensory evaluation literature (McBride, 1983; Land and Shepherd, 1988) provide further support for this conclusion. However, the reader is cautioned that such violations can be quite risky if the rules are stretched to excess. While it may be difficult to specify what is "to excess," some degree of protection is afforded if a conservative approach is taken in scale construction and selection and data interpretation. There are operational (Anderson, 1970) and mathematical (Guilford, 1954) procedures for producing intervals sufficiently equal to be treated as equal interval data. For the sensory professional, little is to be gained and much is to be lost by following an unnecessarily restrictive policy that would classify all rating or category scales as ordinal scales, limit their analyses to nonparametric techniques, and sacrifice any internal quality that they contained. Although we recommend a more flexible point of view than that of O'Mahony (1982), this should not be interpreted as disregarding the order and interval requirements consistent with the use of parametric statistics. Rather, it is to allow the professional to take full advantage of the interval component of properly constructed and used rating scales.

According to Nunnally (1978), "when rating scales are used to obtain interval responses ... they are said to constitute the method of equal-appearing intervals." Furthermore, Guilford (1954) indicated that the task of sorting stimuli into equal-appearing intervals produces category values as interval-scale values, which then can be treated statistically as such. It is this procedure with its theoretical and mathematical foundations attributable to Thurstone that has produced useful scales such as the nine-point hedonic scale (Jones *et al.*, 1955). Because of its widespread use, this particular scale is discussed in a separate section of this chapter.

Analysis of ordinal and rating scale data falls into two broad categories: parametric and nonparametric. The application of the latter was described in the section "An Analysis of Rank Data." The parametric methods are applicable given adequate equality of intervals of the scale data and assuming the results are consistent with a normal distribution. For parametric data, there are numerous methods for analysis, including *t* test, analysis of variance, and correlation, as well as typical summary statistical measures such as mean, standard deviation, and so on. These tests and suggested references are described in more detail in the statistics discussion in Chapter 4.

No discussion on ordinal scales would be complete without some comments about the relative sensitivity of paired-comparison versus rating methods. The statement is often made that the paired-preference test is the most sensitive method for measuring consumer acceptance–preference attitudes. This belief may be supported in part by the psychophysical axiom that states that man is a better discriminator than a judge of the absolute. It is also believed that presenting the consumer with both products simultaneously makes the choice decision easier because the respondent has simultaneous access to both products. In sensory evaluation, however, few responses are absolute, even if they involve a single product, because product memory plays an important role when no other product is available. The ability to "go back and forth" between products, when served simultaneously, is certainly not an advantage for products that have strong aroma and flavor characteristics. This technique maximizes the potential for sensory fatigue and increases the likelihood of a loss in differentiation between products, which is the most probable outcome when product differences are relatively small.

As Seaton (1974) concluded, in a review of the comparative merits of the two procedures, rating and comparison methods were comparable; however, the former offered substantial additional information not possible with the latter, the comparative procedure. In particular, he was referring to the score for each product, which provides a measure of location on the scale, a measure of the magnitude of difference between the products, as well as the opportunity to convert the responses to ranks and proceed with an analysis of the comparative information as was used in the direct paired comparison. Also, obtaining scaled responses from products served monadically is more typical of consumer behavior; that is, evaluating one product at a time. These are most useful measures that are not directly obtainable with a comparative method. While Laue *et al.* (1954) concluded that direct comparative methods were more sensitive to small differences when the dimensions of difference were known to the subjects, this is most unlikely in a consumer test. Considering the potential for sensory fatigue and sensory interaction and the limited output of information, we see no advantage or demonstrable evidence for the paired comparison, and we recommend the use of rating scales for measuring product acceptance–preference. However, there can be situations such as an advertising challenge in which the message is based on the direct comparison, in which case the paired method would be appropriate. Children above a certain age (usually about 7 or 8 years), also find it easy to use a scale for stating their reaction to a product. As discussed in Chapter 7, Kroll (1990) found that children used rating scales as effectively as they did paired comparison. This has been our experience, as well; however, there will be situations in which the paired-comparison procedure would be the method of choice; for example, with children whose cognitive skills were not sufficiently developed to understand the scaling concept. These issues are discussed in Chapter 7.

C. Interval Scales

An interval scale is one in which the interval or distance between points on the scale is assumed to be equal and the scale has an arbitrary zero point, thereby making no claims about the "absolute" magnitude of the attribute measured. Interval scales may be constructed from paired-comparison, rank, or rating scale procedures, or by the method of bisection, equal sense distances, and equal-appearing categories. For a description of each of these procedures, see Guilford (1954).

An example of an interval scale is the monthly calendar in which each day constitutes an equal interval of time. A true or rational zero is not necessary for effective use of the calendar, and the interval between days is independent of whether that interval occurs early or late in that month. For example, the interval between the third and fifth day of the month is the same as that between the thirteenth and fifteenth day. Any x day interval is equivalent to any other x day interval.

In the foregoing discussion, we made note of the equal-appearing intervals with some ordinal scales and the need to be cautious about always assuming that any ordinal rating scale is an interval scale. Relatively few interval scales have been developed by directly setting out to formulate a scale with equal intervals. The two interval scales with which most sensory professionals should be familiar are the nine-point hedonic scale and the graphic rating scale. The hedonic scale will be considered later in this chapter.

The graphic rating scale was developed from the work of Anderson (1970, 1974), utilizing a procedure described as functional measurement. In this procedure, the subjects are exposed to the stimuli they will measure in pretest sessions and are provided practice with stimulus end anchors, that is, as examples of scale extremes. These two steps when coupled with a line scale result in response behavior that can be stated mathematically as equal interval. In descriptive analysis, use of a line scale has proven to be very effective (Stone *et al.*, 1974; Stone and Sidel, 1998), and their use in descriptive analysis will be discussed more extensively in Chapter 6. Analyses of hundreds of tests using this type of scale have made clear the equal interval nature of the scale. With untrained subjects, Lawless (1989) and Lawless and Malone (1986a,b) found line scales to be at approximate parity with other standard scales

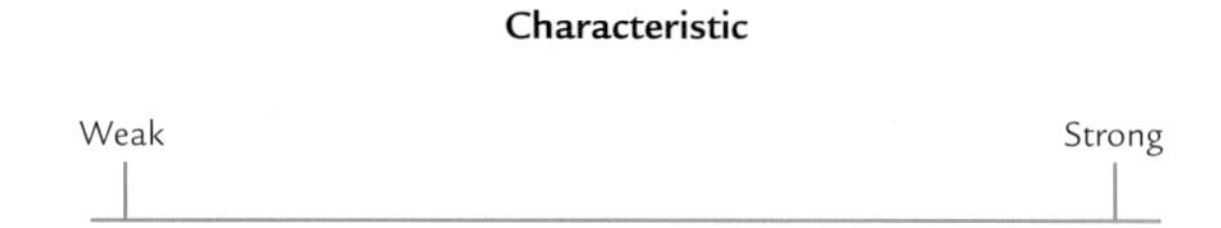

Figure 3.4 An example of a line scale – graphic rating scale. The subject places a vertical line across the horizontal line at that place that best reflects the intensity of that characteristic. Typically the two anchors reflect a continuum from weak to strong intensity.

used in sensory evaluation. Since best use of the scale requires subjects' experience in using the scale, we would expect it to be more sensitive when used by experienced subjects. An example of a line scale is shown in Fig. 3.4. One distinct advantage of the line scale is the absence of any numerical value associated with the response plus the limited use of words to minimize word bias. Measuring the distance from the left end of the line to the vertical line yields a numerical value for computational purposes.

Interval scales are considered to be truly quantitative scales, and most statistical procedures can be used for their analysis; these include means, standard deviations, *t* tests, analysis of variance, multiple range tests, product–moment correlation, factor analysis, regression, and so forth. Numerical responses also may be converted to ranks and standard rank order statistics may be applied to the data.

D. Ratio Scales

Ratio-scale data exhibit the same properties as interval-scale data, and in addition, there is a constant ratio between points and an absolute zero. Stevens (1951, 1957) described four operational procedures for developing psychophysical scales having ratio properties. These procedures are magnitude estimation, magnitude production, ratio estimation, and ratio production. Of the four, magnitude estimation is most frequently used for developing ratio-scale data. This is primarily because of organizational issues, that is, the relative ease with which the experimenter can organize the test and the absence of an elaborate scorecard. In addition, minimal amounts of product are required compared with the methods of magnitude production and ratio production. In a magnitude estimation experiment, the respondent assigns a numerical value (neither less than zero nor a fraction) to each stimulus. This numerical value should represent the perceived intensity for that stimulus or more specified attributes (e.g. loudness, brightness, sweetness, odor strength, etc.). When presenting subjects with a series of different stimulus concentrations, using any of the ratio-scaling procedures described above together with a specific method for treating the obtained responses, researchers found that equal stimulus ratios produced equal response ratios. Stevens (1957) called this the "psychophysical law" and expressed it mathematically as

$$\psi = ks^n$$

where ψ is the geometric mean response to a stimulus, k a constant, s the concentration of the stimulus, and n the exponent of the function, equivalent to the slope of the line. Engen (1971) and others refer to this equation as the power law or Steven's Power Law. When data from ratio-scaling experiments are plotted on log–log coordinates, a linear relationship is obtained between stimulus concentration and perceived intensity. From this background, Stevens (1957) concluded that scales other than ratio were biased and should not be used for measuring prothetic continua. By prothetic continua, we are referring to stimuli that are additive; for example, loudness and brightness. Metathetic continua are those stimuli that involve substitution or change; for example, location between two stimuli. These concepts relate to scaling and scaling theory; a discussion on the subject is provided by Stevens and Galanter (1957).

Ratio scaling has had a significant impact on psychophysics, but there is considerable controversy concerning its role in measurement and especially in relation to its claimed superiority to other scales. The interested reader will find the discussions by Anderson (1970), Cartarette and Friedman (1974; see the chapters by Anderson, Jones, and Stevens), Nunnally (1978), and Birnbaum (1982) especially helpful in characterizing the various issues associated with this controversy about scale superiority. The literature (Birnbaum, 1982; Land and Shepherd, 1988) of the past 20 years suggests no such superiority. For the sensory professional, the impact of ratio scaling and especially the use of magnitude estimation in sensory evaluation has been controversial and almost chaotic. Proponents of the method (Moskowitz, 1975) emphasized advantages in the use of magnitude estimation, including a means of circumventing the problem of word selection associated with most other scales, and provided direct numerical measures in response to products. It also was claimed that task instructions were so easy as to make it possible for any individual to participate as a subject without benefit of any detailed instructions, and that the elimination of numerical restrictions would further reduce number biases. For the past two decades starting in the early 1970s, few publications on sensory evaluation failed to make use or mention of the methodology. However, it was soon realized that subjects, especially consumers, required more instruction, that the procedures were no easier to learn than other methods and for some consumers it took more than the usual amount of time to learn the task. In addition, the use of numbers was not as anticipated. For example, some individuals will use a relatively narrow range of numbers (1–10, in equal increments) while others will use a very wide range (1–1000). In effect, each subject may settle into a specific pattern in the use of numbers, and the issue of bias has not been removed at all.

The issue of scale superiority, as noted previously, has never been demonstrated satisfactorily insofar as sensory evaluation of products is concerned. Studies involving different products have not shown any substantive advantage compared with standard sensory test methods (Moskowitz and Sidel, 1971; Warren *et al.*, 1982; Giovanni and Pangborn, 1983; Vickers, 1983; Lawless and Malone, 1986a,b). The fact that ratio scaling does not exhibit superiority is not surprising. It was developed in the context of inquiry into the measurement process, which, in turn, was hoped would better explain the stimulus–response relationship. The fact that the shape of a psychophysical function relating responses to a series of stimuli could be stated mathematically opened new research vistas. However, it tells us nothing about the validity of that function (Shephard, 1981) and it tells us nothing unique about similarities and differences for complex products, which are of primary concern to the sensory professional. The fact that responses are numerical does not alter the situation, because all other sensory rating methods also yield numerical values! Thus, it is not surprising that the use of ratio scaling has not proven to be superior. It is important for the sensory professional to be aware of the scaling option afforded by ratio scales; however, there should be no expectation that it will result in more or better results.

Traditional analysis of ratio-scaled data involved computation of an exponent, or slope of the line, representing the increase in sensory magnitude as a function of an increase in stimulus magnitude. Numerous examples of ratio-scaled data are available in the literature. The publications by Stone and Oliver (1969) and Engen (1971) are especially clear in describing the analysis of magnitude estimation ratio data.

Data analysis usually is accomplished by first normalizing the obtained responses to eliminate inter- and intra-subject variation. The most frequently used normalization procedure requires initial transformation of raw stimulus and response values to logs, where the means of the logarithms for each subject on each sample is equivalent to a geometric mean. Log transformations compress the range of data values and it could be inferred that extreme positive skewness is expected. To avoid this criticism, Powers *et al.* (1981) described normalization procedures that do not require the log transformation. In either case, the concept of normalization is consistent with the view held by Stevens (1951, 1957) that variability represents measurement error and as such should be eliminated from the analysis. Fortunately, not all researchers hold this view, and many choose to utilize variance measures in establishing confidence levels for the responses obtained. This is an extremely important point not to be overlooked. Products vary as do subjects, and our reason for using a panel of subjects and evaluating an array of products is intended to help quantify responses to variables of interest and to better understand and account for variability that may be inherent in the test or non-test variables.

Once the entire data matrix from a magnitude estimation experiment has been transformed and normalized, curve fitting commences. The method of least squares is used to determine the line of best fit. The resulting equation takes the form of

$$\text{Log response} = \text{log intercept} + (\text{slope} \times \text{log stimulus}).$$

The slope is equivalent to the exponent as described earlier where $\psi = ks^n$ and n is the exponent of the function. The data are then plotted on log–log coordinates where the ordinate represents the log mean response and the abscissa the log of the stimulus.

Analysis of variance (AOV) and other statistical analyses as described for nominal, ordinal, and interval scales may be applied to ratio scale data. However, responses obtained using a magnitude estimation procedure present practical problems when models such as the AOV are used to determine statistical significance. Raw magnitude responses generally are positively skewed, which can translate into very large variance measures as mean intensity scores increase. In the example reported by Engen (1971, see p. 76), the highest concentration received raw scores ranging from 7.5 to 150, with a mean of 45.95 and an SD of 38.66. The lowest concentration sample had raw scores ranging from 0.5 to 75, with a mean of 6.68 and an SD of 13.6. This type of situation is susceptible to significant violations of the homogeneity and distribution assumptions on which AOV models are based. In addition, the large standard deviations that are possible with the high mean values can result in large error terms, increasing the likelihood of Type 2 errors.

To eliminate the effects of inter- and intra-subject variability, the data can be normalized prior to using the AOV. This will result automatically in non-significant interactions between subjects and products, a measure that could be critical in making a decision as to which product formulation warrants further attention. Thus, normalization prior to use of an AOV will weaken the analysis of the data; yet without it, some critical information could be lost. By weaken, we mean the aforementioned interactions will be lost as will the information it tells us about the products, as perceived by the subjects. Of course, this dilemma can be avoided by using any other scoring method. Ratio-scaling methods may be well suited to determining the form of a relationship between perceived and stimulus magnitude (which can be predicted); however, they are not well suited for measuring differences among products that vary according to different sensory modalities and attributes. Additional discussion about psychophysics and scaling in sensory evaluation is found in Frijters (1988), Land and Shephard (1988), and Lawless and Heymann (1999).

A recent development is the Labeled Magnitude Scale (LMS) described by Green *et al.* (1993). The LMS scale is considered a hybrid, having characteristics of both a labeled category scale and a ratio scale. Labeled categories are not automatically spaced at equal intervals, a contrast to how one constructs a traditional category scale. Each category is labeled and spacing for the individual categories is determined from previously collected ratio-scaling data. The end anchors use extreme statements such as "strongest imaginable" and "not at all detectable." In Chapter 7, we will discuss this type of scale in more detail.

III. Selected Measurement Techniques

In this section, we describe some scales that have special appeal. This appeal may be based on popularity of a scale, ease of use, or simply habit, without an appreciation for why it is used, which can be risky.

A. Hedonic Scale

Of all scales and tests methods, the nine-point hedonic scale occupies a unique niche in terms of its general applicability to the measurement of product acceptance–preference. The scale was developed and is described in detail by Jones *et al.* (1955) and by Peryam and Pilgrim (1957). As part of a larger effort to assess the acceptability of military foods, these investigators studied a number of different scales of varying length and number of categories as well as selection of most appropriate words used as the anchors for each category. This research yielded a scale with nine points or categories and nine statements. As shown in Fig. 3.5, the hedonic scale is

Name ______________________ Code ______________ Date ______________

Please circle the term that best reflects your attitude about the product whose code matches the code on this scorecard.

Like extremely
Like very much
Like moderately
Like slightly
Neither like or dislike
Dislike slightly
Dislike moderately
Dislike very much
Dislike extremely

Figure 3.5 An example of the nine-point hedonic scale. The subject's task is to circle the term that best represents their attitude about the product. Boxes adjacent to the terms could also be used. The responses are converted to numerical values for computational purposes: like extremely, 9; dislike extremely, 1.

simple to describe, and as it turned out, it is equally easy to use. We believe that this latter feature is a major reason for its general usefulness in assessing product likes and dislikes for all types of foods, beverages, cosmetics, paper products, and so on, and used on a worldwide basis (when translated).

The scale was developed to assess acceptability of several hundred food items (Peryam *et al.*, 1960), and since then has been reconfirmed by further studies of foods served to the military (Meiselman *et al.*, 1974). These investigations demonstrated the reliability and the validity of the scale to a degree that has been especially satisfying. Of particular value has been the stability of responses and the extent to which such data can be used as a sensory benchmark for any particular product category. A product may have a mean score and standard deviation of 6.47 ± 1.20. Tests with an array of competitive products will typically yield an ordering of the products with mean values within this range that is quite stable; that is, independent of panel size and region of the country. There is no question that for some products a subset of the population of consumers may alter the ordering; however, the usefulness of the benchmark is not lost. This degree of stability is especially important for companies that seek to develop a database for their own products as well as to have a means for rapid assessment of formulation changes and/or track competition. In addition, knowing that a particular product category has an average score of 6.02 ± 1.50 provides a frame of reference as to what scores might be possible. This is especially useful if management has an expectation that the product should receive a score >7.5. Or, alternatively, marketing guidelines might require a particular product score, for example, 7.0, for the project to proceed. In this latter instance, the sensory database could be used as a warning system that the action standard might not be met. While the sensory acceptance test result is not intended for use in this kind of a situation, nonetheless, it is not surprising to learn that it often is the only acceptance information available. The usefulness of the method with employees is discussed in more detail in Chapter 7. Parametric statistical analysis, such as the AOV, of nine-point hedonic scale data can provide useful information about product differences, and data from this scale should not be assumed to violate the normality assumption (contrary to O'Mahoney, 1982; Vie *et al*., 1991). Figure 3.6 shows the results from an acceptance study where 222 consumers evaluated twelve products using the nine-point hedonic scale. The sigmoid shape of the curve indicates that the scores are normally distributed. In many other tests involving thousands of consumers, the method has proven to be effective in ordering of preferences and the scale comes as close as one would like to being an equal interval scale.

Where there is interest in converting hedonic scale data to ranks or paired preference data, this too is readily achieved. It is only necessary to count the number of subjects scoring one product higher than the other and analyze the result using a $p = \frac{1}{2}$, or binomial distribution, as discussed in Chapter 7.

Periodic efforts to modify the scale by eliminating the midpoint (the category of "neither like nor dislike") or some other categories ("like moderately" and "dislike moderately" have been suggested) have generally proven to be unsuccessful or of no practical value, even where children are test subjects (Kroll, 1990). A frequent comment has been that there is avoidance of the midpoint; however, there has been no systematic study demonstrating the existence of such a bias or that it results in a loss of significance between products. Similar arguments about the moderate categories have been equally unsuccessful. Still another concern for some sensory professionals is the

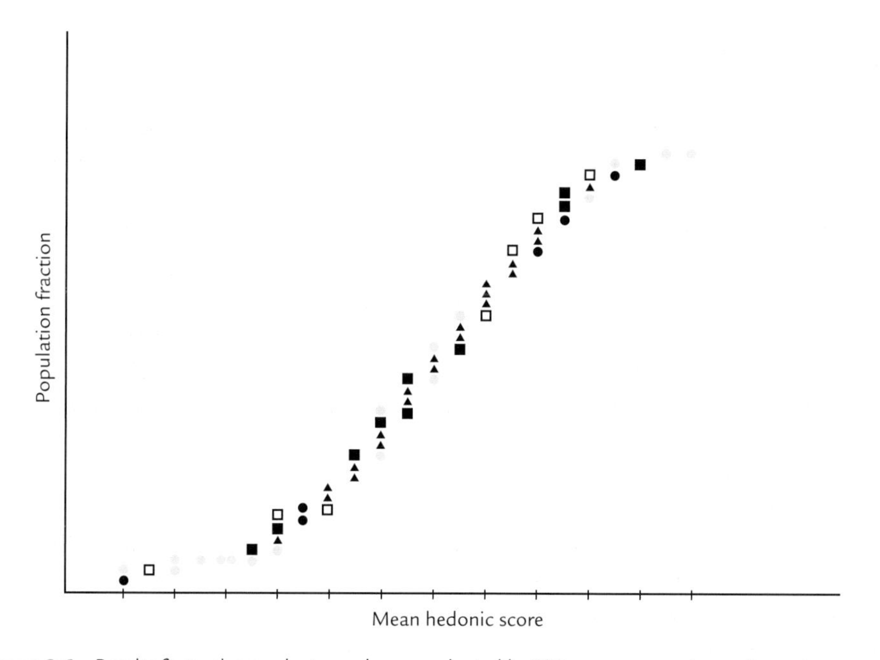

Figure 3.6 Results for twelve products, each was evaluated by 222 consumers using a nine-point hedonic scale. Note that the *Y*-axis is the consumer population fraction in cumulative percent and the *X*-axis is that portion of the scale from 2.0 to 7.5 in 0.5 units.

bipolarity of the scale from the experimenter's viewpoint and its treatment mathematically as unidirectional. Whether consumers consider it bipolar cannot be easily determined nor should it necessarily be so. Empirically, consumers respond in ways that make clear they are using it in a way one can describe as equal interval. While it is reasonable to expect subjects to experience difficulty with bipolar scales (generally more variability because of the avoidance of the neutral- or midpoint of such a scale), there is no adequate evidence of this problem from our experience. The computational issue seems to be equally trivial; the numbers used are of less importance than the significance or lack of significance in the difference in scores.

Efforts to demonstrate that magnitude estimation is a more useful scale for measuring product acceptance–preference have also proven to be less than successful. The earliest comparative study by Moskowitz and Sidel (1971) concluded that magnitude estimation was not a superior test method, as does the more recent research by Pearce *et al.* (1986) and Pangborn *et al.* (1989). The authors for the latter study concluded that magnitude estimation may be inappropriate for scaling liking. McDaniel and Sawyer (1981) provided a contrasting conclusion; however, their study had design flaws that make it difficult to conclude much about the question.

In conclusion, it would appear that the nine-point hedonic scale is a unique scale, providing results that are reliable and valid. Efforts to either directly replace or improve this scale have been unsuccessful, and it should continue to be used with confidence. In recent years, research by Schutz and Cardello (Cardello and Schutz, 1996; Schutz and Cardello, 2001) on extensions to the scale have proven to be very promising and these will be discussed in some detail in Chapter 7.

B. Face Scales

These scales were primarily intended for use with children and those with limited reading and/or comprehension skills. They can be described as a series of line drawings of facial expressions ordered in a sequence from a smile to a frown, as shown in Fig. 3.7, or they may depict a popular cartoon character. The facial expression may be accompanied by a descriptive phrase and may have five, seven, or nine categories. For computational purposes, these facial expressions are converted to their numerical counterparts and treated statistically, as in any other rating scale. Little basic information on the origins and development of the face scale is available. A sensory test guide prepared by Ellis (1966) provided an example of a face scale similar to the one shown in Fig. 3.7. It was identified by the author as having been used successfully; however, no details were provided.

The face scale is the type of scale that is frequently used and would be expected to have considerable merit; however, it will create more problems than it will solve. Very young children (6 years and younger) can be distracted by the pictures, and can even be disturbed by the mean look of the frowning face. The scales may add undesirable and possibly complex visual and conceptual variables to the test situation. Matching a product to a face representing the respondent's attitude is a complex cognitive task for a child, and may in fact be more complicated than some other more

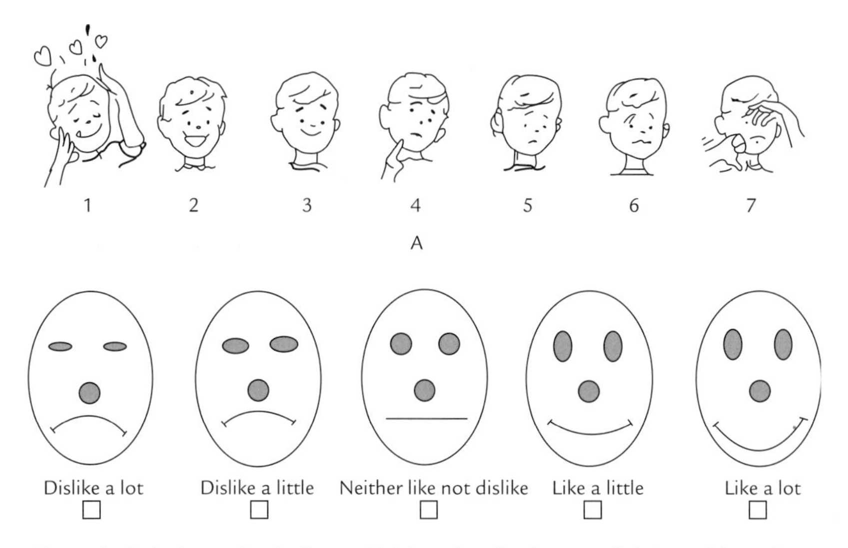

Figure 3.7 Two examples of face scales that can be found in the literature and appear to have been used for measuring children's responses to products.

typical scaling procedures. For example, in a study of flavorings for use with children's medication, it was observed that the children tended to use the happy smile portion of the scale because they thought that they should feel better after taking the medication. This information was derived from post-test interviews necessitated by the lack of differentiation of the products and a desire by the investigators to reformulate the products. As a result, it was necessary not to reformulate the product but to develop a scale that was not subject to misinterpretation by the children.

There is no question that children's testing is challenging. The ability to read and to comprehend test instructions is not uniform among children of the same age. This does not necessarily mean that typical scales cannot be used; rather, it suggests that some changes may be necessary in the test protocol and especially with the oral instructions given at the time of the test. It is interesting that the face scale would be proposed for use with individuals having limited reading and comprehension skills when one of the basic requirements of its use is the ability to interpret reaction to a product represented by a face. There is no question that with instructions some children can learn the task. However, this would defeat the claimed, primary advantage for the scale – the ease with which it can be used by the child. Finally, if one must train an individual to use a scale, it would be more reasonable to work with a scale that does not require transformations. In our experience working with children 8 years and older, we obtain reliable acceptance information using the nine-point hedonic scale provided all the children can read and, most important, can understand the meaning of the words. It should not be a surprise that many adults also do not understand the meaning of all of the statements. However, this is overcome through an appropriate orientation such that the children (and adults) develop an understanding of the scale's direction and what will be their task. Alternatively, if there are doubts about the use of individual experimenters or the subjects' ability to follow instructions then it is recommended that some version of the paired preference model be used. As noted elsewhere (see Chapter 7), this is a very basic task and minimal reading or comprehension skills are required.

While there exists considerable anecdotal information about the use of face scales, little research appears to have been done with them (or little been published). In her study with children, Kroll (1990) found no advantage for face scales over other category scales. Until more positive evidence is available, we do not recommend use of face scales. Sensory professionals should give consideration to modifying test instructions and using more typical measurement techniques. Chapter 7 contains additional discussion about children as subjects.

C. Just-About-Right Scale

The just-about-right (or jar) scale is one of the most frequently encountered in larger-scale consumer testing. These bipolar scales, as shown in Fig. 3.8, have three or five categories (the three categories is usually the preferred mode), usually anchored with statements of too much, too little, or about right for each product attribute.

We do not recommend this type of scale for sensory evaluation tests. Jar scales are championed as a diagnostic tool for consumer tests, but are an ineffective substitute for designed experiments (e.g. DOE) or good sensory descriptive data. Reliance on these scales is usually an indication of limited resources or limited knowledge about sensory descriptive methods, or both. These scales combine (or more correctly, confound) attribute intensity and preference in a single response, and are highly susceptible to interpretive and/or semantic errors because the product attribute to be measured is given a name. This particular risk is common to any scale that uses word anchors; however, consumers are especially vulnerable. Even if the consumer does not understand the particular descriptive word, a response is still obtained. As a

Name ______________________ Code ______________ Date ______________

Make a mark in the box that represents your reaction to the product.

Aroma
- ❑ Too strong
- ❑ Just about right
- ❑ Too weak

Sweetness
- ❑ Much too strong
- ❑ Strong
- ❑ Just about right
- ❑ Weak
- ❑ Much too weak

Figure 3.8 Two examples of just-about-right scales. Both types of scales would not be placed on the same scorecard. They are presented here for illustrative purposes.

result, there is a preponderance of judgments placed in the middle category of the scale. Enterprising investigators have proceeded from this experience to formulate these scales with five or even seven categories. The difficulty arises when trying to anchor each category: leaving blanks typically results in consumers avoiding the unlabeled categories.

Analysis of data from these scales also presents numerous problems. Frequently, only the percentage responding in each category is reported without any rule for determining how much of a difference between percentages is to be considered significant. Although we do not advocate use of these scales, data from them may be treated as follows:

1. Option A

Establish an agreed-on "norm" or "minimum" response percentage for the "just-about-right" category (a reasonable number may be 70% just about right). When the minimum is achieved, ignore the other responses. If the minimum is not achieved, use a table for $p = \frac{1}{2}$ to determine whether there is a significant difference between responses in the remaining two categories. Do not treat the "just-about-right" response as tie scores; the total number of observations is the sum of the two extreme categories only. Obviously, a large proportional difference will be necessary for significance when total N is small (as it should be).

2. Option B

First combine the number of responses in the extreme categories, and using a $p = \frac{1}{2}$, determine whether this number is significantly different from the number of responses in the "just-about-right" category. State whether the "just-about-right" responses are significantly larger (i.e. more) than the combined data from the extreme categories. Next, compare (again using $p = \frac{1}{2}$) the extreme categories with one another to determine whether a significant product defect exists (and if so, its direction). Once again, do not consider the "just-about-right" responses as tie scores, as this would be an unacceptable way to increase the N, thereby making it easier to obtain a significant product defect.

Other single-sample analyses may be attempted; however, they require assumptions about the estimated frequency of response in each category (e.g. χ^2). We have not found any acceptable criteria on which to base such estimated or expected frequencies.

The task of finding an appropriate analysis for determining statistical significance between related samples is even more difficult. In our opinion, the bipolar character of the "just-about-right" scale limits the value of standard two-sample analysis methods. Finally, analyses which compare the distributions between samples tell us little about which distribution is the more desirable.

3. Option C

This analysis is based on serial use of the Stuart–Maxwell and the McNemar tests as described by Fleiss (1981). The test is for matched products in which there are more than two scale categories. The Stuart–Maxwell test is used to determine whether

Table 3.1 Hypothetical data to illustrate the Stuart–Maxwell test[a]

Product B	Product A			
	Too sweet	**Not sweet enough**	**Just about right**	**Total**
Too sweet	20	10	20	50
Not sweet enough	7	20	3	30
Just about right	5	10	5	20
Total	32	40	28	100

[a] The entries are the responses to both products for each subject. For example, of the thirty-two subjects who indicated product A was too sweet, twenty indicated product B was too sweet, seven said it was not sweet enough, and five said it was just about right. Of the forty subjects who said product A was not sweet enough, ten said B was too sweet, twenty said B was not sweet enough, and ten said B was about right.

there is a significant difference in the distribution of responses for the products. Where a significant difference is obtained, the data matrix is collapsed into a series of matrices and the McNemar test is used to determine individual scale categories for which differences are significant.

Table 3.1 contains the appropriate sorting of data from 100 consumers who evaluated two products using the three-category just-about-right scale. To construct this table, it was necessary to determine the number of too sweet, not sweet enough, and just-about-right responses assigned to product A when product B was scored too sweet, not sweet enough, and just about right. Obviously, this categorization of responses should be planned in advance to minimize repetitive handling of the original database. The Stuart–Maxwell statistic, as described by Fleiss (1981) for a three-category classification, is as follows:

$$\chi^2 = \frac{\bar{n}_{23}d_1^2 + \bar{n}_{13}d_2^2 + \bar{n}_{12}d_3^2}{2(\bar{n}_{12}\bar{n}_{13} + \bar{n}_{12}\bar{n}_{23} + \bar{n}_{13}\bar{n}_{23})}$$

where

$$\bar{n}_{ij} = \frac{n_{ij} + n_{ji}}{2}$$

$$d_1 = (n_{1.} - n_{.1}),\ d_2 = (n_{2.} - n_{.2}), \ldots, d_k = (n_{k.} - n_{.k})$$

and $n_{..}$ is the total number of matched pairs, $n_{1.}$ the number of paired responses in row 1, and $n_{.1}$ the number of paired responses in column 1. Applying this formula to the data in Table 3.1 yields the following value for χ^2:

$$\chi^2 = \frac{\frac{3+10}{2}(50-32)^2 + \frac{20+5}{2}(30-40)^2 + \frac{10+7}{2}(20-28)^2}{2\left(\frac{10+7}{2} \times \frac{20+5}{2} + \frac{10+7}{2} \times \frac{3+10}{2} + \frac{20+5}{2} \times \frac{3+10}{2}\right)}$$

$$= \frac{3900}{485.50} = 8.03$$

Table 3.2 Two-by-two table for comparing ratings of "too sweet" for products A and B[a]

Product B	Product A		
	Too sweet	**Other**	**Total**
Too sweet	20	30	50
Other	12	38	50
Total	32	68	100

[a] Note that the entries were derived from Table 3.1 by combining categories.

which with two degrees of freedom is significant at the 0.02 level. We conclude that the distribution of responses for product A is different from that for product B.

Because the distributions have been found to be different, it is necessary to determine those categories or combinations of categories that are significantly different. Fleiss correctly warns us that a control is needed to minimize the chances of incorrectly declaring a difference as significant when a number of tests are applied to the same data. The suggested control is to use the table value of χ^2 with $k - 1$ degrees of freedom (where k is the number of scale categories).

Using the McNemar test where

$$\chi^2 = \frac{[(b - c) - 1]^2}{b + c}$$

with the data in Table 3.2, we obtain

$$\chi^2 = \frac{[(30 - 12) - 1]^2}{30 + 12} = \frac{17^2}{42} = 6.88$$

The critical value of χ^2 with two degrees of freedom is 5.99. Since the obtained value of McNemar's χ^2 is larger than the table value, we may conclude that product B has significantly more "too sweet" responses than does product A.

Recently, an additional method for analysis has been applied to jar responses, called TURF analysis, adapted from media research. The primary objectives are stated to include optimizing a line of products, whether they are colors, flavors, etc., to identify the combinations that will have the most appeal, and the incremental value of adding to a line of products (see Cohen, 1993).

D. Other Scales of Interest

In addition to these three scaling techniques, there is another family of scales that is of interest to the sensory professional. In particular, we refer to scales such as semantic differential, appropriateness measures, and Likert or summative scales. These scales are used primarily by market research to measure consumer behavior as it relates to product image, social issues, sentiments, beliefs, and attitudes. They impact sensory evaluation when results are used to direct product formulation efforts or

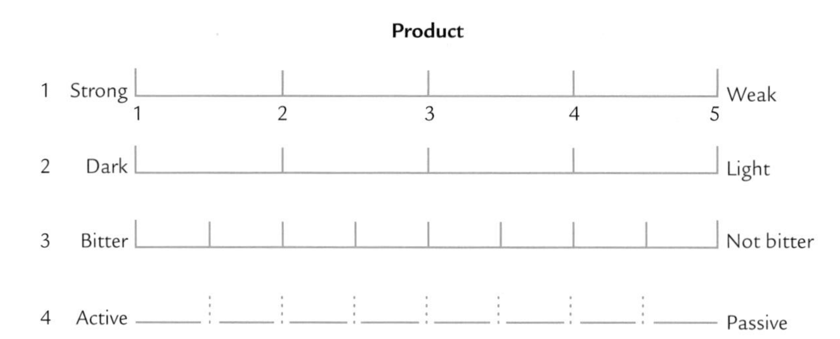

Figure 3.9 Examples of possible semantic differential scales. Note that the selection of word pairs and type of scale are the responsibility of the experimenter.

when results are compared with those from a sensory test. However, when combined with appropriate sensory analysis data, the relationships between the two types of information have major benefits for a company. Sensory professionals should be familiar with them and their relationship to sensory testing activities. They are not a substitute for sensory data; however, they extend the information base and lead to more informed product business decisions.

Semantic differential scales may be characterized as a series of bipolar scales with as many as thirty scales anchored at the extremes with word pairs that are antonyms. The scales are often referred to as summative because the scores can be summed across scales. Examples of some alternative formats for this scale are shown in Fig. 3.9, and as can be seen, there are numerous variations. As Hughes (1974) observed, there are five basic issues that are addressed in the preparation of semantic differential scales: balanced or unbalanced categories, types of categories (numerical, graphical, and verbal), number of categories, forced choice or not, and selection of word pairs. In each instance, the experimenter has an option to establish which particular scale format will be used. While this can be considered advantageous, it also assigns some risk to the experimenter. For example, if the word pairs are inappropriate or are misinterpreted by the subjects or the experimenter, this will introduce problems in interpretation of the results.

Likert scales also are used regularly by market research, and like semantic differential scales can take different forms. Basically, the measurement is one of agreement (or disagreement) with a particular statement, as shown in the examples in Fig. 3.10.

There is no question that these scales provide useful information about products whether it is during concept development, when assessing the potential impact of advertising, or when linking the imagery and the sensory information. We will have more to say about this in Chapter 6. More discussion about these techniques can be found in Hughes (1974) and Nunnally (1978).

IV. Conclusions

In this chapter, we described the four basic types of measurement techniques; nominal, ordinal, interval, and ratio. We identified the properties of each scale type along

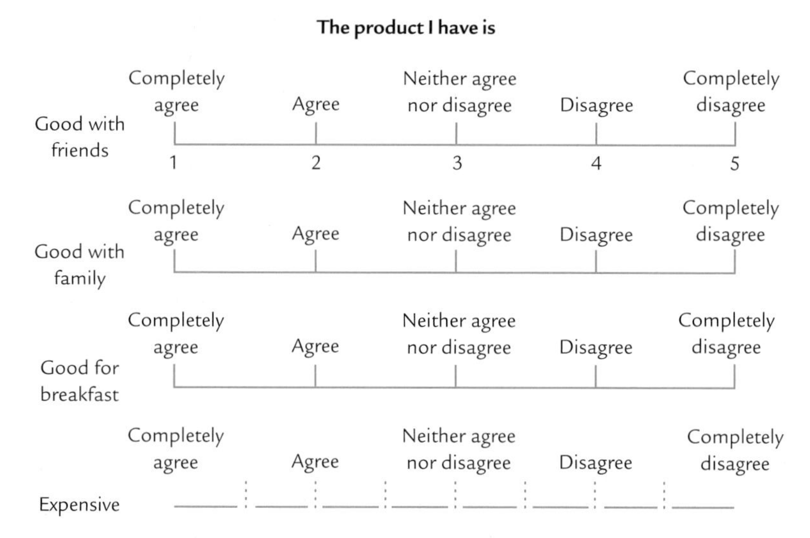

Figure 3.10 Example of Likert scale; the subject's task is to mark the scale at that point which reflects degree of agreement.

with examples of how they are applied to the sensory evaluation of products. There is no question that these measurement techniques are a necessary part of sensory evaluation. It is useful, at this point, if we give some consideration to the question of whether one of these scales is best. While having just one scale might appear to be most helpful, current evidence supports a position that is exactly the opposite. For any particular problem, more than one scale can be appropriate, just as more than one test method can be applicable.

It is reasonable to expect that behavioral research will result in the development of new measurement techniques and this will be of benefit to sensory evaluation. However, the sensory professional should not assume that what is new is necessarily better. In the past two decades since the first edition of this book, there have been numerous developments in sensory evaluation. Much of this has been associated with the ease of data capture and real-time analyses, the application of methods or adaptations rather than in enhanced methods of measurement. It must be kept in mind that selection of a scale should always occur after a problem has been defined and the objective stated. In proceeding from nominal to ratio scales, the instructional set becomes more complicated and demands on the subject increase in terms of the type of responses that they provide. Thus, each scale offers advantages and disadvantages, and it is only after the problem is defined that the sensory professional can make a decision as to which scale is best for that specific test.

Suggested methods for analysis according to the specific measurement technique also were listed. Additional details about these procedures will be found in Chapter 4 and in the three chapters on sensory test methods (Chapters 5–7). Those chapters will clarify the relationship between the test objective, experimental design and analysis, test method, and measurement technique is achieving reliable and valid product information.

Test Strategy and the Design of Experiments

4

I. Introduction

Every test, beginning with the request and ending with the recommendation(s), must reflect a strategy that addresses the key questions being asked; that is, the test's objective(s) and how the results will be used. Strategy is used here to mean a plan that enables the sensory professional to determine the basis for the request, how the test will be designed to answer the question(s), and how the results will be communicated. A test objective may have several parts and may not be entirely clear; that is, looks can be deceiving, nonetheless, it is essential that the sensory professional establish the primary

Sensory Evaluation Practices 3rd Edn
ISBN: 0-12-672690-6

purpose or purposes for the request before any test strategy can be formulated. Once the objective has been established and there is agreement as to the specific question(s) to be answered, the test strategy can be formulated. This includes selecting an appropriate test method, determining which qualified subjects are available, selecting an appropriate experimental design and method for analysis, determining when and where the products were prepared (i.e. pilot plant or production, etc.), and when and how they will arrive at the test site. While these activities will require additional time before the test is implemented, it is critical that the objective(s) be clearly understood. A test with one objective is often the exception; in many situations, there will be several questions needing answers and the professional must engage the requestor in a dialogue to be sure that all relevant information has been obtained. Otherwise, the sensory professional may have proceeded with a particular strategy that yields less useful results. For example, the discrimination test provides information as to whether there is a perceived difference between products but it cannot be used to determine the basis for the difference. Only through a dialog with the requestor can the sensory professional conclude that the discrimination model is appropriate. Further dialogue and bench screening of the products may make it clear that the product differences are easy to detect and a descriptive test is a more appropriate choice. In practice, requestors often want several kinds of product information of which preference is usually somewhere in their discussion. Obviously, a single test cannot satisfy both the difference and the preference question and some discussion is necessary to separate the issues and establish priorities. For example, establishing that preference information will not directly determine that products are different or the basis for a difference is a sensory responsibility; however, the sensory professional must make this point clear to the requestor before the test is initiated. These alternatives are discussed in more detail in the chapters on test methods (Chapters 5–7); however, our interest at this point is to emphasize their importance to the sensory professional in formulating an appropriate test strategy. From a sensory viewpoint, the issue is not a simple matter of selecting a "right or wrong test," but rather a matter of selecting a test plan that takes into account all reasonable alternatives and most important, the business objective. Test methods are not interchangeable nor should an attempt be made to answer different questions within the same test method. Not only is it wrong for that request, but it will have longer-term implications, particularly with regard to sensory's reputation of independence and professionalism. Thus, test strategy involves integration of several elements into a cohesive plan that is most likely to satisfy the objective(s) and the requestor, as well.

As a further complication, a strategy must take into account the impact of the product in relation to the psychological errors of testing and the product source, as well. With regard to the former, we refer to testing errors such as first-sample effects, contrast and convergence, and the error of central tendency (to name the most common), all of which will influence the outcome of a test (Guilford, 1954; Amerine *et al.*, 1965; Lawless and Heymann, 1999). Product source also impacts strategy, particularly with regard to recommendations. Results of a test with products prepared at the bench will not likely have the same effects as those prepared at a pilot plant or at a full-scale production facility. Furthermore, knowledge as to when and how products were prepared must be known otherwise recommendations need to be qualified. All too often, different results are obtained based solely on source of manufacture and this information is not generally shared with all parties to a project. As a result, decisions are made that are not supported in subsequent tests leading to credibility issues. Product source will be discussed further in the methods sections in subsequent chapters.

While sensory professionals generally are aware of testing errors, it is not clear that there is as much appreciation for their effects in the design of a test as there should be and this leads to confusion not only in test planning and design but also in interpreting results. To those not familiar with testing errors, the situation can be very confusing, if not troubling, in the sense that one can "manipulate" the serving order to achieve a particular result. For those unfamiliar with testing errors, this has the effect of clouding the scientific nature of the process. Nonetheless, it is important to share this information with a requestor when a particular array of products has the potential of causing such errors to occur. It is equally important to understand that not all testing errors occur in a test nor are biased responses easily identified, as such. It is not easy to demonstrate that using qualified subjects minimizes Type 2 decision errors, or that one- or two-digit codes are more susceptible to number biases than three-digit codes, and so forth. The effects of these errors are neither easily recognized nor do they occur all of the time and to the same extent, or are they easy to demonstrate to those who question their impact. Even the more obvious use of red lights (in an attempt to mask color differences not intended as part of the test) continues to create confusion in decision-making, yet many still do not grasp the implications of this atypical testing environment on response behavior. The problems caused by a disregard for these errors occurs much later when business decisions are found to result in no sales improvement or consumer complaints that products thought to not be perceived as different are, in fact, perceived and the consumers express their unhappiness with declining sales and/or complaints to the company.

This chapter focuses on test strategy in relation to experimental design, taking into account the request for assistance (and the requestor), product criteria, and the impact of psychological errors on response behavior. Experimental design also is considered with a sensory orientation. The reader is assumed to have a working knowledge of statistics, and to be seeking a guide to the design subtleties of a sensory test and thereby developing a greater appreciation for response behavior beyond their numerical representations. This latter issue is especially critical, for like the detective story, this behavior is an important clue. By and large, subjects are telling us something about products and we must be able to identify that "something" without hiding behind a screen of numbers.

II. Test Request and Objective

In Chapter 2, test strategy was discussed in the context of the overall positioning of a sensory program within the research and development structure. We now focus on strategy as it is applied to the individual request for assistance. The overall goal is essentially unchanged; that is, to formulate and implement a test plan that will satisfy the stated objective. Specific issues that need to be considered before a plan is completed, and the test implemented, are in addition to the more obvious considerations of test priority, objective, and product identification and availability. In particular, appropriateness of the products relative to the objective and how the results will be used, and the possible effects of psychological errors on response behavior must be taken into account before the sensory professional can proceed with preparation of the actual experimental design, the scorecard, and so on.

Although test objective was discussed previously (see Chapter 2), its importance to formulating a strategy demands that we include it in this discussion. As a preliminary step, the sensory professional has to ensure that all the necessary information is provided and that the request is reasonable should review a written or electronic request. Reasonable in the sense that what is being requested is consistent with sensory goals and objectives and with corporate goals and objectives, and warrants the expenditure of effort. For example, measuring purchase intent and/or attempting to represent unique population segments are unreasonable design variables in a sensory test involving only forty or fifty subjects. While the issue of what is reasonable can be a source of disagreement between the sensory professional and requestor, it must be addressed. Not only does it require direct discussion between the two, but further increases the likelihood that the best possible plan will be formulated. In most situations, products will be examined to ensure they are appropriate. To the extent possible, such meetings should provide for a thorough exchange of information regarding the products and possible methodological approaches. Questions about an objective also should be thorough to avoid problems after a test is completed. Occasionally, a requestor will withhold information unknowingly, or in the belief that this information is not relevant or will create experimenter bias. This is more likely to lead to an unsatisfactory test. For example, if the objective is to compare several competitive products with each other, the design strategy will be different from a test in which the objective is to compare products to a market leader but not to each other. Both tests will have some common design features, but there could be differences in the product serving order, in the analyses, and any conclusions drawn from the results. Failure to obtain a clear understanding of a test's objective increases the likelihood of dissatisfaction after that test is finished, and over the long term it will erode the mutual trust between the sensory program and the requestor. Questionable results are remembered long after confused objectives are forgotten. Over time requestors will become more sophisticated in the preparation of requests and discussions about objectives and consideration of reasonableness will be minimized, leading to a more efficient and productive evaluation process.

III. Product Criteria

Test strategy should include the possibility of an initial rejection of a request if the products are inappropriate or the basis for the request cannot be justified. Receipt of a request should not automatically result in a test or in rejection of the request.

Previous results or other product information may eliminate the need for a test. For example, product instability or variability may be greater than a contemplated ingredient change, and sensory evaluation's responsibility is to provide such an explanation with a rejection.

Rejecting products because they are not appropriate is a necessary part of test strategy and one that is likely to provoke considerable dialog, at least initially. Little is gained from a discrimination test that yields 90–100% correct decisions or from a test involving one or more easily recognized products. A test of very different products typically results in biased response patterns for some of the products. Later in this chapter, we will discuss contrast and convergence effects that can occur in such tests. Initially, requestors may consider this approach as a lack of cooperation or as an attempt to exert too much influence over their work. However, it is important that the sensory staff be very rigorous in considering product appropriateness. To an extent, the sensory professional is educating the requestor with regard to the many problems that can arise because of indiscriminate testing or testing products that are either not ready or a test is not warranted. It is not a question of a subject's ability to complete a scorecard but rather the difficulty in assessing response bias and the concomitant risk in the decision-making process. There are, of course, guidelines that can be used as an aid in reaching a decision about appropriateness; however, each product category will have its own unique characteristics, and the sensory professional must identify these to requestors to minimize conflict and enable them to be more selective in their product submissions. General guidelines include the following: (1) products obviously different from each other should not be tested in a discrimination test; (2) easily recognized product (e.g. branded on the product) will significantly alter response patterns to it and other products in a test; and (3) comparing experimental products with competitive products, especially during the early stages of development will yield atypical results (a variation of the theme – know the source(s) for all products).

Although assessing product appropriateness would appear to be time consuming and potentially disruptive, its importance far outweighs any additional time or delay in testing. Obviously not every request or every product will require such scrutiny. With experience, this increased vigilance is more than rewarded by a much greater level of awareness by all professionals involved with the sensory program. The reader should keep in mind that concern about product does not end with the initial review. In fact, vigilance is essential just prior to the actual test to be sure that the products are the same as what was observed when the request was first discussed. In some instances, the sensory staff are surprised when the products are prepared for the test and are found to be different from the original plan. This calls for immediate action; for example, contacting the requestor and determining whether the test will proceed as planned. In our experience, the product is often the single most critical element in a sensory test (besides subjects). The simple question of asking which product is control and where it was produced often yields a very interesting dialog that helps to explain unexpected results, hence our emphasis on product. We now turn our attention to an associated issue, psychological errors in testing.

IV. Psychological Errors

One of the more intriguing aspects of a sensory test is the extent to which psychological errors influence individual responses. What Guilford (1954) has referred to as "peculiarities of human judgment, particularly as they affect the operation of certain methods of measurement," is the topic of interest. With an awareness of the peculiarities, we need not be puzzled by atypical response patterns; and in many instances, we can organize and design a test to minimize the impact of these errors or at least to enable them to affect all products equally. For example, the first product in a multiproduct preference test typically is assigned a higher score compared with the score it will receive in subsequent serving positions. This phenomenon is referred to as a first-sample effect, which falls within the much broader classification of a time-order error. To minimize the impact of this error and ensure that it has an equal opportunity to affect all products, the products must be served equally often in the first position. In addition, data analysis must include provision for examination of response patterns by serving order. Of course, it is also true that some individuals will purposely request a single product or monadic test, knowing that it could result in a higher score. In effect, one is taking advantage of specific knowledge about human behavior. Single product tests are very popular when a company has established action standards for a product to move into a larger-scale market test that includes, among other criteria, a specific preference score such as a 6.5 on a nine-point hedonic scale. By moving to a larger test, the appearance of progress has been realized and there always is the hope (mistaken) that product acceptance will improve!

A more comprehensive discussion about the various types of errors is provided in the psychological literature (see Guilford, 1954, for an example). Our intention is to discuss these errors in relation to their impact on the product evaluation process. In general, many of these errors are more noticeable when subjects are naive and unfamiliar with the test method and/or the particular product or product category. Obviously, the impact of these errors can be reduced if one works with experienced and trained subjects, following the recommended procedures and practices described in Chapter 2. However, there are psychological errors that are more directly related to the specific products being tested; for example, contrast and convergence, and other context effects that can be minimized but never totally eliminated, through appropriate experimental design considerations. The key issues for the sensory professional are awareness of these errors and the importance of designing each study to minimize their effects, and to ensure that their effects will have equal opportunity to occur to all products.

A. Error of Central Tendency

This error is characterized by subjects scoring products in the mid-range of a scale, avoiding the extremes (or extreme numbers) and having the effect of making products seem more similar. This scoring error is more likely to occur if subjects are unfamiliar with a test method or with the products, or are relatively naive with regard to the testing process. The more experienced (and qualified) subject is less likely to exhibit this scoring error.

Avoidance of scale extremes is a particularly interesting issue. For example, it is occasionally suggested that the nine-point hedonic scale (Jones *et al.*, 1955; Peryam and Pilgrim, 1957) and similar category-type scales are in effect more restricted; that is, the extremes are avoided, and in the case of the nine-point scale one actually has a seven-point scale. Guilford (1954) and Amerine *et al.* (1965) recommended that this avoidance of extremes could be offset by changing the words or their meaning or by spacing the terms further apart. This approach is more applicable to scales other than the nine-point hedonic scale, which does not produce this error when product serving order is balanced and subjects are familiarized with the scale and the products prior to a test. Schutz and Cardello (2001) introduced a "labeled affective magnitude scale" to improve spacing between scale categories. More research will be needed using this latter scale before it can be assessed as helpful. One of the more illogical extensions to the avoidance of the extremes is to propose dropping two of the nine-point scale categories and using a seven-point scale. Unfortunately, this does not alter the error and therefore one now has a five-point scale that is significantly less sensitive than a nine-point scale. Avoidance of extremes also will occur with subjects who have been trained (directly or indirectly) to think that there are correct responses for perceived attribute intensities. This is likely to occur when using references (or standards) and subjects are advised to always assign specified value(s) for those standards (e.g. the scale mid-point in difference from reference judgments). The problem here is the inherent variability in standards and in the subjects themselves, a topic discussed more extensively in Chapter 3. Nevertheless, this error of central tendency can be minimized through standard sensory procedures and practices. In tests with naive consumers, demonstrating scale use before the test has a very beneficial effect and minimizes this error.

B. Time-Order Error

This error is referred to as an order effect, first-sample, or position error. This error in scoring results in the first product (of a set of products) being scored higher than expected, regardless of the product. The error can create difficulties in interpretation of results if the serving order is not balanced and results are not discussed as a function of serving order. Although it is possible to statistically measure the effect of order through the use of a Latin-square design (Winer, 1971), these designs are seldom used in sensory evaluation, primarily because of the unlikely assumption that interaction will be negligible. Interactions between subjects and products are not unusual, nor are interactions resulting solely from various treatment combinations. However, examination of response patterns by order of presentation as a means of assessing the error will provide very useful information about product similarities and differences.

The series of examples shown in Table 4.1 is intended to demonstrate this point as well as to illustrate the close relationship between the impact of a psychological error and product differences as perceived by a panel (when is the difference attributable to the order error and when to the products?) Example A (in Table 4.1) demonstrates the typical product served first effect; both products were scored higher by an average of 0.3 scale units. The conclusion derived from these results is that both products were liked equally and the time-order error affected both products equally. Example B

Table 4.1 Examples of scoring patterns from a series of two-product tests displayed by serving order as a demonstration of order effects

Example	Serving order	Product		
		X	Y	
A	First	6.4[a]	6.3	6.3
	Second	6.1	6.0	6.1
	Pooled	6.3	6.1	
B	First	6.5	6.4	6.5
	Second	6.7	6.1	6.4
	Pooled	6.6	6.2	
C	First	6.3	6.5	6.4
	Second	6.2	5.9	6.1
	Pooled	6.3	6.2	
D	First	6.4	6.5	6.5
	Second	7.0	6.5	6.7
	Pooled	6.7	6.5	

[a] Entries are mean values based on the use of the nine-point hedonic scale (1, dislike extremely; 9, like extremely), $N = 50$ in each case except for pooled values, with a monadic-sequential serving order. See text for further explanation.

provides a more complicated possibility; product X was liked more when evaluated after product Y. When served first, product X obtained a score of 6.5 and this score increased to 6.7 when it was served second. The reverse was obtained for product Y; when served first the score was 6.4 and it decreased to 6.1 when it was served second. The net result of this would be a recommendation that product X was preferred over product Y. It is possible that the 6.6 versus the 6.2 pooled result was sufficient to reach statistical significance at the 95% confidence level; nonetheless, the more telling issue was the 0.6 scale units of difference between products in the second position. If my product were Y and I were interested in attracting consumers of product X, these results would let me know that I would not be very successful from a product perspective!

Example C provides another possible outcome, except both products show the decline as occurred in example A; however, the magnitude of change was greater with Y (suggesting possible vulnerability of Y or opportunity for X). Example D provides another outcome in which X increased and Y remained essentially unchanged. Once again, a possible explanation for the increased preference for X over Y (7.0 compared with 6.5) in the second position would be that Y has a sensory deficiency that was only apparent after first evaluating Y (and then X).

Obviously, the sensory professional cannot afford to look at these scoring patterns solely in the context of the time-order error, but must consider the product scoring changes relative to each other and relative to the test objective. Simply assigning the change in a mean score to a time-order error is quite risky at best, as is the reporting of only results from the first position. Besides the issue of selective reporting, the loss of comparative information about the products should be a very significant concern to the sensory professional and to the test requestor.

C. Error of Expectation

This error arises from a subject's knowledge about the product and is manifested in the expectation for specific attributes or differences based on that knowledge. For example, in a discrimination test, the subject is likely to report differences at much smaller concentrations than expected. Conversely, the subject may overlook differences that are not expected in that type of product. In effect, the subject may have too much knowledge about products and should not have been selected to participate in the test. In descriptive testing, procedures that expose subjects to a broad array of irrelevant references will produce an error of expectation observed as a "phantom attribute" representing an attribute not in, or not at a perceptible level in, the test products. Such phantom perceptions represent "false hits" for the presence of that attribute. It is reasonable for subjects to expect an attribute if the panel leader has *a priori* provided them a reference for that attribute.

D. Error of Habituation and of Anticipation

These errors arise from the subject providing the same response to a series of products or questions. For example, in threshold tests where products are systematically changed in small increments by increasing or decreasing stimulus concentration, the subject may report "not perceived" beyond the concentration where the stimulus actually is perceived (habituation). An example of anticipation error is when the subject reports perception of the stimulus before a threshold concentration is actually achieved, but is anticipated at any time because there has been a series of "not perceived" responses. To some extent, these errors are similar to the error of expectation.

E. Stimulus Error

This error occurs when subjects have (or think they have) prior knowledge about products (i.e. stimuli) in a test, and as a result will assign scores based on knowledge of the physical stimulus rather than based on their perception of the stimulus or will find differences that are unexpected. Of course, this latter situation can be especially difficult to address, since non-product variables may arise from the normal production cycle or if the product was formulated in a way that was non-representative. To reduce this risk, the sensory professional must be very thorough in examining products before a test and make sure that there is sufficient product available to avoid using one or two containers of product and assume they are representative. If one follows test procedures as described in this book, then this particular error should not be of major concern. It also is one of the reasons why individuals who are directly involved in formulation of a product should not be subjects in a test of that product.

F. Logical Error and Leniency Error

These errors are likely to occur with naive subjects who are not given precise instructions as to their task. The logical error occurs when subjects are unfamiliar with the specific task and follow a logical but self-determined process in deciding how the products will be rated. The leniency error occurs when subjects rate products based on their feelings about the experimenter, and in effect, ignore product differences. These errors can be minimized by giving subjects specific test instructions and by using experienced subjects; the use of qualified and trained subjects is required for analytical tests.

G. Halo Effect

The effect of one response on succeeding responses has been associated by Guilford (1954) with stimulus error in the sense that it involves criteria not of direct interest to the particular experiment. One example of a halo effect is a test in which consumers provide responses to product preference followed by responses to a series of related product attributes. In this situation, the initial response sets the stage and all subsequent responses justify it; alternatively, asking preference last will not change or eliminate the effect. Halo effects are more observed in tests involving consumers and particularly in those situations in which there are many questions to be answered. With many questions, product re-tasting becomes necessary, which, in turn, leads to physiological fatigue, further exacerbating the situation and leading to errors of central tendency. To gain insight into this problem, one can examine response patterns and variance measures within and across scorecards. To overcome or circumvent halo effects, some investigators will require test participants to start (their evaluations) at a different place on a scorecard or to change the order in which the questions are listed. While such approaches have surface appeal, the problem still remains but now it affects responses to different questions. In addition, there is an increase in the amount of time required to complete a scorecard and an increase in the number of incomplete scorecards. While it is not our intent, at this point, to analyze the relative merits of lengthy consumer scorecards (this will be discussed in Chapter 7), it is necessary to make the reader aware of this particular effect, because it will have direct implications insofar as scorecard preparation and business decisions based on results from such tests are concerned. Also, it is unreasonable to expect that one can design out of a study the halo effect, which is behavioral in origin. Either one is prepared to accept its presence and apply reasonable caution when interpreting results or, to minimize the number of questions asked and thus minimize the impact of the effect.

H. Proximity Error

In this error, adjacent characteristics tend to be rated more similar than those that are farther apart. Thus, the correlations between adjacent pairs may be higher than if they were separated by other attributes, and as Guilford (1954) has suggested, this would be one reason not to put great emphasis on these correlations. It has been suggested that this error could be minimized by separating similar attributes, by rating attributes on repeated sets of products, or by randomizing the attributes on the scorecard. Unfortunately, each of these suggestions raises questions as to their practicality and usefulness in a business environment. Perhaps more important is the question of whether this error can be demonstrated in most consumer products (foods, beverages, cosmetics, and so forth). Research on the error appears to be associated with social studies, that is, personality traits, and not with consumer products. Nonetheless, some problems associated with the proposed solutions warrant consideration.

In descriptive tests, the subjects decide on the sequence in which the attributes are perceived and scored (usually in the order of their perceived occurrence) and efforts to randomize the sequence creates confusion (and variability). For example, subjects allowed to score attributes on a random basis demonstrate three effects that do not appear to lessen with time; an increase in variability, an increase in test time (by as much as 50%), and a tendency to miss some attributes entirely! We are not aware of situations in which the proximity error has been demonstrated in sensory tests.

I. Contrast and Convergence Errors

Probably the most difficult errors to deal with are those of contrast and convergence. Their impact on evaluation of foods was described in detail by Kamenetzky (1959). These errors are product related, and often occur together. The contrast error is characterized by two products scored as being very different from each other and the magnitude of the difference being much greater than expected. This could occur when a product of "poorer" quality was followed by a product of "higher" quality. The difference was exaggerated, and the higher quality product was scored much higher than if it were preceded by a product closer in quality. Convergence is the opposite effect, usually brought about by contrast between two (or more) products masking or overshadowing smaller differences between one of these and other products in the test. In tests involving three or more products the existence of one effect most often is accompanied by the other. These two effects are depicted in Fig. 4.1; the upper examples represent the impact on intensity measurement and the lower examples are for preference. Obviously, this exaggeration of the difference for some products and compression of the difference for other products can have serious consequences. While it is reasonable to acknowledge that this problem can be minimized through proper product selection, it is quite another matter to delineate "proper product selection." In the first instance, the two errors are more likely to be encountered when one or more of the products are recognizable, or several of the products are experimental and one is commercially available (such as a "gold standard"). Of course, one may still find it necessary to include such products, in which case experimental design and examination of responses by serving sequence become particularly important. For example, with a balanced design in which every product appears in every serving position, results can be examined when a particular product is served last and, therefore, has no effect on the preceding products. In this way,

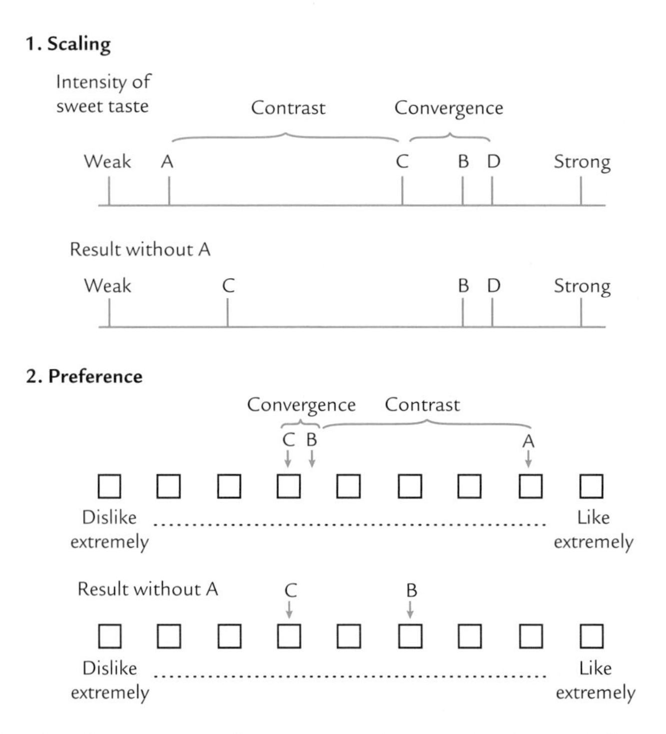

Figure 4.1 Examples of scoring and preference patterns demonstrating contrast and convergence effects. For purposes of display only, the products appear to be scored on a single scale. In actual tests, each product would have its own scorecard.

estimates can be obtained for the effects of contrast and convergence. There also can be situations in which a product is always served in the last position so as to eliminate at least one of these two effects. To the extent possible, the sensory specialist must be able to assess products, well in advance of a test, to be able to determine the potential for contrast and convergence before deciding on a test design.

However, the question of reporting these results remains. One cannot ignore the errors and report the results, or simply state that the particular testing errors had a significant effect on responses and, therefore, no conclusion can be reached. Somewhere between these two extremes exists a reasonable approach to reporting. The most reasonable approach is to describe the results in relation to the product(s) serving order. Consider the preference data in Fig. 4.1 (lower portion of the figure), where product B was more preferred than product C (when A was not a factor in the decision). This approach serves two purposes: first, it satisfies the requestor's objective; second, it makes the requestor aware of the consequences of including products in a test that are predisposed to these errors.

In this discussion about psychological errors, the intent has been to alert the sensory professional about the potential impact of these errors on response behavior. For the most part, careful product selection and the use of qualified subjects will minimize the impact of many of these errors, but will not eliminate them entirely. Results must always be reviewed for the presence of these errors, particularly when there is a concern based on a pretest examination of the products.

V. Statistical Considerations

Sensory evaluation uses statistics to determine whether the responses from a group of subjects are sufficiently similar or represent a random occurrence. Knowing that there is this degree of similarity enables the sensory professional to make a decision about the products being tested with some stated measure of confidence in the context of that population of subjects and where appropriate to subjects, in general. The remainder of this chapter focuses on statistical issues that sensory professionals consider (or should consider) when determining the most appropriate experimental design and analysis for a particular problem. The reader is assumed to have a reasonable knowledge of statistics and be familiar with commonly used summary statistical procedures, including the analysis of variance (AOV). (For a review of these methods as they relate to sensory evaluation, see Sidel and Stone, 1976; Korth, 1982; O'Mahony, 1982; Gacula and Singh, 1984; Gacula, 1993.) While we do not provide detailed mathematical steps for the various methods, some attention is given to methods of particular value to sensory evaluation, for example, the analysis of data derived from split-plot designs and other related designs. The latter provides the means by which one can analyze results from different groups of subjects who have evaluated a set of products at different locations and/or at different times. The chapters on specific sensory test methods (Chapters 5–7) also include recommended designs and analyses appropriate for those methods. However, a more thorough exposition on statistics can be found in Alder and Roessler (1977), Bock and Jones (1968), Box *et al.* (1978), Box and Draper (1987), Bruning and Kintz (1977), Cochran and Cox (1957), Cohen and Cohen (1983), Cohen (1977), Guilford (1954), Hays (1973), Krzanowski (1988), McCall (1975), McNemar (1969), Morrison (1990), Phillips (1973), Smith (1988), Winer (1971), and Yandell (1997).

The design of a test, the selection of a statistical method for analysis, and the interpretation of results are responsibilities of the sensory professional. Delegating this responsibility to a statistician or to some other individual is not recommended. A statistician cannot be expected to be cognizant of the subtleties of sensory evaluation, to be aware of the kinds of subject-by-product interrelationships described earlier in this chapter, or to easily accept some of the trade-offs that occur when the sensory requirements of a problem take precedence over the mathematical and statistical requirements. This should not be misconstrued as a recommendation to avoid statisticians, but rather it is an acknowledgment that the experienced sensory professional must have sufficient knowledge about statistics to recognize when and what type of assistance is required.

In many sensory tests, the statistical design requirements cannot be completely satisfied and compromises must be made. For example, one uses a pre-screened number of subjects who meet specific sensory requirements (i.e. they are not a random selection of people), who will most likely evaluate each product on a repeated basis, and will use a scale that may not be linear throughout its entire continuum. The products are not selected randomly. The subject's responses will most likely be dependent, not independent, and in most instances the number of subjects will be about twenty. For many statistical methods, it is easy to cite examples of a "failure to meet" one or more of the requirements based on these criteria; however, this should not constitute a basis for modifying a test plan or for not using a particular statistical analysis. It must be kept in mind that statistical models are based on stated assumptions about the response behavior of the individuals in a test; however, these assumptions are not absolute, they are not laws. In fact, the average score will likely not represent any one subject's score! When one or two assumptions are violated, there is a potential risk of reaching an incorrect conclusion. As noted by Hays (1973),

> *... statistics is limited in its ability to legislate experimental practice. Statistical assumptions must not be turned into prohibitions against particular kinds of experiments, although these assumptions must be borne in mind by the experimenter exercising thought and care in matching the particular experimental situation with an appropriate form of analysis.*

For some tests, statistical risk can be determined in relatively precise terms; for example, in the case of multiple *t*-test comparisons. When one is deciding that differences between products are significant, the error rate increases very rapidly in direct relation to the number of comparisons. As discussed by Ryan (1959, 1960), if one were comparing 10 means at the 0.01 level of statistical significance, the error rate per experiment would be equal to 0.45. In fact, multiple *t*-tests should be avoided because of this problem. There also are examples where a precise statement of risk is less clear. For a discrimination test, a precise computation of risk is difficult because assumptions must be made as to the true magnitude of difference between products, the actual sensitivity of the subjects, and the use of replication, which is a necessary part of the discrimination test. These issues are discussed in more detail in Chapter 5, as they relate to the discrimination process. However, it should be mentioned that one of the consequences of repeated trials testing is thought to be an increased potential for finding differences. Since we want to minimize unanticipated changes (i.e. minimize β risk), this particular risk would seem to have a positive effect. It would be foolish not to obtain replicate responses within a test just because there is a risk that the responses may be dependent. The mathematical, and particularly, the behavioral implications of this risk need more study. Our purpose here is to provide a frame of reference for the role of statistics in the overall scheme of sensory evaluation. After all, statistics, in itself, is not perfect in its analysis of responses, and new procedures continue to be developed. Sensory evaluation uses statistics as one of several tools in helping to solve a problem. This tool may not be entirely satisfactory, primarily because it was not designed exclusively for that purpose (sensory evaluation); nonetheless, we use it just as we make use of scales and subjects that are not perfect. They are perfect enough to enable actionable product decisions to be made with minimal risk.

In the discussion that follows, attention is given primarily to parametric, as compared with non-parametric, statistical methods. By parametric, we refer to methods that assume data that are normally distributed; while non-parametric methods are distribution free; that is, no assumptions are made about the distribution from which the responses were obtained. Interest in non-parametric methods was very strong in their early development (during the mid-1940s) because the methods were quite easy to use (e.g. Wilcoxon Signed Rank Test, Mann–Whitney, etc.) and enabled the experimenter to utilize proportions or other similar kinds of data that could be categorized in contingency tables. It should be clear that non-parametric tests provide the sensory professional with additional tools for data analysis, when there are reasons to justify their use. As O'Mahony (1982) noted, parametric methods are preferred because they use scaled data as they were obtained from the subjects. Using scaled data directly as obtained from the subjects is very important because it provides an unobstructed view of the responses with no modifications or transformations that are mathematically correct but destroy individual differences. It is the latter that often provides important clues as to the nature of product similarities and differences. However, there can be situations where a few subjects may score a product very different from all the other subjects, and those results would be sufficient to change a difference, for example, from significant to non-significant. In this situation, converting to ranks eliminates the magnitude effect, and an appropriate non-parametric procedure can be used. For more details on non-parametric methods, the reader is referred to Hollander and Wolfe (1973) and Daniel (1978).

Before describing some statistical tests, it is useful if we briefly discuss issues of a more general nature: for example, reliability and validity, replication, independence versus dependence of judgments, the concept of random selection of subjects, and Type 1 and Type 2 errors and risk in the decision-making process. Some of these issues also will be considered in the discussions about the analysis of data obtained using specific test methods.

A. Reliability and Validity

These two related elements (reliability and validity) should be of concern to every sensory professional, as they have a direct effect on each test and on program credibility. By reliability we mean the extent to which subjects will provide similar responses to similar products on repeated occasions. The closer this agreement, the higher the degree of reliability and, therefore, the greater confidence there will be in the potential validity of the results. However, a high degree of reliability is no guarantee of validity, and with low reliability there can be no consideration of measuring validity. For example, if a group of subjects replicate their judgments but are assigning responses opposite to the known or expected direction, there would be a high degree of reliability but no validity. This could occur if subjects were scoring a series of products containing known amounts of some ingredient such as an added flavor. If the subjects were confused about what they were measuring or how to use the particular scale, one could achieve a high degree of reliability and equally high variability but with no guarantee of validity. In the discussion on analysis of descriptive data (Chapter 6), a method is described for establishing a numerical measure of reliability for each subject. There are other procedures for estimating reliability and these can be found in the sensory literature (see, e.g. Sawyer *et al.*, 1962; Bressan and Behling, 1977; Zook and Wessman, 1977).

For analytical tests (discrimination and descriptive), the need for reliability cannot be underestimated. These tests typically rely on about ten to twenty subjects, which is a relatively small number of people on which to make an actionable recommendation. If the recommendations and the results are to be accepted as valid, then the experimenter must have a high degree of confidence in those subjects, and such confidence is derived in part from the data; that is, from the repeated measures, which provide the basis for computing a reliability estimate. Even if one were to increase the number of subjects in these tests, the trade-off would not be equivalent. For example, results from a discrimination test using fifty subjects would not carry the same "weight" as the results from twenty-five subjects with a replicate (in both instances, the $N = 50$). Just as any physical or chemical test would be done more than once, so too would a sensory analytical test. What is surprising is how little attention is given to this issue yet is fundamental to minimizing risk in decision-making.

Validity is more difficult to deal with because it is not directly measured and there are several kinds of validity (for which researchers disagree on the types and definitions). In its broadest sense, it may be considered as the degree to which results are consistent with the facts. Of the different kinds of validity, we are most interested in face validity and external validity. We state there is face validity when we measure what we intended to measure and results are consistent with expectation. For example, if we know that product A was formulated to contain more sweetener and the results show that this product was scored as more sweet than other products in a test, then we can conclude with confidence that the results have face validity. However, this observation by itself would not necessarily be sufficient to conclude that the results are therefore generalizable. External validity would need to be considered. By external validity we mean that given a different and/or larger group of respondents, will the same conclusion be reached? How confident are we that the conclusion reached in test A will be repeated in test B? For many sensory problems, determining that there is face validity, or external validity, in particular, is usually more difficult than the relatively simple sweetener example. The effects of ingredient or processing changes are not always known or easily measured and they are not usually very direct as stated in the sweetener example. That is, the addition of any ingredient is likely to alter sensory properties in an indirect manner. A process variable might alter product appearance or the change may be too small to be detected. Therefore, one's expectations about the validity of results will require more investigation.

Dialog with the requestor may provide further information about product formulation that would explain observed response patterns and, in turn, this might be sufficient to substantiate the face validity. However, the question of external validity cannot be completely and directly addressed through technology but rather through testing in the marketplace. Are consistent results obtained when the same products are evaluated by two groups of consumers? Note that we talk in terms of consistency, rather than in terms of an exact agreement of the numerical values. In any comparative study, one expects the results for two (or more) tests to be consistent; however, the expectation that the numerical values will be exactly the same is quite unrealistic. When considering the external validity of test results, it is important to remember that the basis for determining that this validity exists is whether the conclusions we reach are the same and, therefore, can be generalized.

From a purely sensory perspective, a concerted effort should be made to develop evidence for the validity of sensory test results. Since there is usually a bias associated with the use of employees for sensory tests, in general, the issue of validity, and especially external validity, becomes very important (see Chapter 2 for more discussion on this problem of use of employees versus non-employees in a test). More dialog about measuring validity is needed and a stronger case should be made for the importance of validity in the long-term development of a sensory program's credibility.

B. Replication

In the previous section, the importance of replication in assessing subject and panel reliability was noted as input for the determination of validity of the results. It is useful if we also consider replication in the context of the test itself and the trade-off between subjects, products, and the practicalities of repeated testing in a single session and over a period of several days.

Replication is absolutely essential for all sensory analytical tests; that is, for discrimination and descriptive tests, because of the very nature of the tests and the limited number of subjects in each test. In the first instance, analytical tests provide precise information about product differences and the specific attributes that form the basis for those differences. Like physical and chemical analyses, there must be more than a single analysis and the analysis is done using more than a single sample of a product. As described in Chapter 2, subjects are selected based on their sensory abilities as determined from a series of screening tests. By eliminating individuals who are insensitive or are inconsistent, and selecting those who are most sensitive, a more precise sensory instrument is created. This enables one to rely on fewer (and more precise) subjects. However, one must obtain replicate judgments from each subject to be sure that they are consistent in detecting differences. In addition, because there are a limited number of subjects, each one's contribution to the database is relatively large and a few atypical responses could shift a result from significance to non-significance or the reverse. The use of replication provides insight into individual response behavior. Given several opportunities to score products or to select the one most similar to an identified reference, how similar are the responses? If they are not similar, then one must determine their impact on test conclusions and decide whether a qualified recommendation is appropriate. Such attention to detail is critical to the successful use of sensory evaluation small-panel testing, which probably represents as much as 75% of the activity of most sensory evaluation programs in business today.

Thus far, no attempt has been made to state how much replication is necessary. Obviously, a replicate is superior to none, but at what point does it no longer become useful and additional responses have no impact on the conclusions. In addition, as the total number of judgments increases, the greater the likelihood of finding statistically significant differences of no practical value. For discrimination testing, we have observed that a single replicate (each subject evaluates each product twice) has proven to be sufficient, providing the experimenter with sufficient information to monitor discrimination ability and to allow a conclusion about the products with minimal risk. With a replicate, each subject will have sampled six products within a 20–30-minute time period, which usually is sufficient without experiencing any sensory fatigue. For descriptive tests, three to four replicates are usually sufficient to assess subject reliability and again, to reach conclusions about the products. Empirically, we have observed that variability decreases somewhat as one proceeds from the first to the second replicate and levels at the third replicate but subsequent replications do not exhibit any further decrease in variability. Of course, having a measure of within-subject variability improves the sensitivity of a statistical test and increases the likelihood of finding a difference. A more detailed discussion about the use of replication within the context of specific test methods is provided in Chapters 5 and 6.

There are practical as well as statistical considerations involved in the planning of an experiment and a decision as to the extent of the replication necessary. Practical considerations include product availability, preparation requirements, subject availability in terms of numbers and frequency, and the nature of the request (early stages of a project or just prior to test market). If insufficient product is available or the preparation procedures are so demanding as to cause concern for product stability, then a design which includes testing on successive days may not be realistic without finding larger than expected variability. Replication, in this instance, would have to be achieved within a single day by having several sessions.

To some extent, additional subjects can be used in place of replication; however, it should be approached with an appreciation for the risks involved – as noted above, the exchange is not equivalent. With replication, a subject has additional opportunity to score products, which, in turn, provides a measure of within-subject variability and leading to an increased likelihood of finding significant differences (i.e. statistical power is increased). The expectation that increasing the number of subjects will compensate for any advantage gained through replication is not necessarily true in every instance. Empirically, it can be shown that variability in scoring decreases with replication and the largest decreases occur from first to second, and from second to third replicates, respectively. Of course, if a project is in its early stages and several experimental versions of a product are under consideration, then a single replicate may be sufficient. On the other hand, as a project progresses and there are fewer experimental products and differences are smaller, the need for more replication becomes greater. The sensory professional must consider these issues when planning a test. However, it is important to keep in mind that without replication, risk in decision-making increases, and no amount of additional subjects can compensate for it.

A statistical approach to the problem of replication also is possible. By selecting appropriate mean and variability (e.g. standard deviation) values and the probability value for accepting or rejecting the null hypothesis, one can compute the number of judgments and then divide by the number of subjects to determine the extent of replication that is necessary. Obviously, this assumes a database about the products and/or the subjects is available.

In affective testing, replication is atypical, because of the more subjective nature of the judgmental process and because of the manner in which the results are used; that is, to estimate market potential, purchase intent, etc. Such broadly based objectives require larger numbers of respondents, particularly if one is dealing with, and representing, unique population segments. With a larger number of qualified (demographic and product usage) consumers, the various statistical measures become better estimates of the target population and thus the generalizations have greater validity. A broad representation of potential consumers is desirable for determining if there are any product deficiencies evident to a subset of the population and the extent to which those deficiencies represent business problems (or opportunities). If one intends to segment results based on typical demographic criteria, such as age, sex, and income, or based on other criteria (such as preference clustering), then the importance of a large database is more meaningful. Affective testing is discussed in greater detail in Chapter 7.

The issue of how much replication is necessary, like many other aspects of sensory evaluation, is not and perhaps should not be mandated. Each problem has a unique set of requirements, just as each product has a unique set of properties, and therefore the exact amount of replication cannot always be stipulated.

C. Independence and Dependence of Judgments

For sensory evaluation, the concept of independent judgments is not realistic, at least not in a literal sense. All individuals participating in tests have experience as product users (a primary screening criterion), and to that extent, their responses will reflect this dependence along with prior test participation. From a sensory design viewpoint, the use of a balanced serving order and other design considerations enable the experimenter to minimize the impact of this dependence, or at least to more evenly distribute its effect across all products. As a further consideration, a monadic sequential serving order is most appropriate; that is, only one product and a scorecard are served and then both are removed before the next product and scorecard are served. In that sense, the evaluations are made independently; however, the responses still have some dependency. The impact of dependence on the results and conclusions of a test is not entirely clear. While some statistical models (e.g. one-way AOV and *t*-test for independent groups) assume independence of judgments as a requirement, the risk is not well defined. These models require more subjects than their respective dependent models (e.g. two-way AOV and dependent *t*-test), and this introduces risk of finding more differences.

D. Random Selection of Subjects

In sensory evaluation, the random selection of subjects is rarely achieved, or rarely if ever desired. Sensory tests involve a limited number of subjects who are selected from a larger group of screened and qualified individuals. Selection of those subjects will be based on immediate past performance and the frequency with which these individuals have participated in tests. Test design reflects this selection, as will be described in the section on Experimental Design.

E. Risk in the Decision-Making Process: Type 1 and Type 2 Errors

An important consideration in the statistical analysis of results is the probabilistic statement that is made about those results and the risk implicit in that statement. The question most frequently asked is whether there is a difference between the products, if the difference is statistically significant (discussed at length in Chapter 5) and the probability that the result is real and not due to chance. In sensory evaluation, it is accepted practice to consider a difference as statistically significant when the value for α is ≤ 0.05. In effect, when α is ≤ 0.05, we are concluding that there is a difference between products A and B, and we are confident enough to conclude that there is only one chance in twenty that this result was due to chance. If there is reluctance to accept this degree of risk, then the criteria for statistical significance can be changed; for example, setting $\alpha \leq 0.01$ decreases the probability of wrongly concluding there is a difference. From a practical point of view, however, changing the decision criteria has its own risk. Others may view this changing of the decision criteria as using statistics to suit the particular situation, and in particular to demonstrate that statistical significance was obtained. On the other hand, marketing and marketing research may be using an α of 0.20 (or some other level), which also creates the potential for conflict. The magnitude of difference necessary to achieve significance at an α of 0.20 is smaller than that for an α of 0.05, and marketing research could easily conclude that their test found differences missed by sensory evaluation. Of course, the choice of α in this instance could be based on knowledge that consumers are less sensitive and/or the product is inherently variable, so a less restrictive significance criterion might be appropriate. This particular problem is reconsidered in Chapter 7, as part of a larger discussion on consumer testing, and is mentioned here as it relates to the need of the sensory professional to have a clear understanding of the level of statistical significance being used by others and its associated risk in the decision-making process. It is not a matter of one level being more or less correct or of everyone necessarily operating at the same level, rather the decision criteria and risk should be defined to prevent misunderstandings between the different business units. It is very possible that the significance level necessary to initiate the next action could be different for different product categories and this would not be wrong.

Taking risk into account acknowledges that the possibility of an incorrect decision still exists. For example, if we were to reject the null hypothesis when it is true, we will have committed an error referred to as a Type 1 error; this has a probability equal to α (which is the significance level). In practical terms, we might have a situation in which we are comparing an experimental product with a target product, and the hypothesis is that there is "no difference" between the products (referred to as the null hypothesis and expressed mathematically as H_0: $\bar{x}_1 = \bar{x}_2$). If we concluded from the results that there was a difference when in fact it was not true, then a Type 1 error was committed; the probability of such an error is equal to α. On the other hand, if we concluded that there was no difference when in fact there was a difference, then a Type 2 error was committed, and the probability of this error is equal to β. There is a mathematical relationship between α and β; when one decreases, the other increases; however, this relationship is determined by the number of judgments, the magnitude of the difference between products, and the sensitivity and reliability of the subjects.

This particular relationship is discussed in some detail in Chapter 5 on discrimination testing along with worked examples. However, its importance obviously extends to all sensory tests as well as to decisions about the selection of particular statistical tests for use after the AOV when there is a significant difference among the means. For example, the Newman–Keuls and Duncan multiple range tests are more protective with regard to Type 2 error compared with the Scheffé and Tukey tests, which are more protective with regard to Type 1 error. In tests after the AOV, these alternatives present the sensory professional with additional considerations as to which approach to use. Some worked examples are presented in Chapter 6, and are intended to demonstrate these risks and their effects.

As an additional consideration, the statistical power of the test also should be taken into account (see Cohen, 1977; Thorngate, 1995; Lawless and Heyman, 1999). Cohen (1977) described statistical power as follows:

> *The power of a statistical test of a null hypothesis is the probability that it will lead to the rejection of the null hypothesis, i.e., the probability that it will result in the conclusion that the phenomenon exists.*

Thus, by setting α, both β and the power are determined; however, the problem is somewhat more complicated. For example, if α is set very small, statistical power will be small and β risk will be high. As Cohen (1977) noted, the issue of statistical significance involves a series of trade-offs between the three factors. For example, with α set at 0.001, the statistical power might be equal to 0.10 and β to 0.90 (where $\beta = 1 - \text{power}$), which would be risky if one were attempting to minimize the prospects of committing a Type 2 error. This is a particularly important issue inasmuch as most product testing is focused on making changes that are least likely to be detected by the fewest people. We wish to minimize the risk of saying the products are the same when they are not.

As previously noted, there are several elements of a test that influence risk and statistical power. These are the number of subjects and/or responses, their sensitivity and reliability, the magnitude of the difference between products (the effect size), and the testing process itself. Obviously, a very large number of responses (e.g. several hundred or more) increases the likelihood that a given difference will be detected and β risk minimized. However, the use of large numbers of responses in a test as a means of minimizing β risk and of decreasing statistical risk carries with it the problem of obtaining differences that have no practical value.

Products also are a source of differences independent of the variable being tested. In practice, one often discovers that products are a greater source of variability than are subjects. Whether one is obtaining products from a production line or from a pilot plant, it is not unusual to discover that there are easily discernable differences among products within a production run or comparing production products to those from a pilot plant. Unfortunately, many of those differences are not controllable and the sensory professional must take this into account when designing each test. It should be kept in mind that the use of replication in a sensory test is essential to obtaining a measure of product variability; that is, by using more products, the responses represent the range of variability within the variable being tested. In addition, as Cohen noted, any procedures and/or controls that can be applied to eliminate non-test variables will increase power. This means strict adherence to test protocol (proper preparation and serving), use of an appropriate test site with environmental controls, and so on. Finally, it must be re-emphasized that the use of qualified subjects is, in all likelihood, the single most important element in minimizing risk.

In recent years, some researchers have taken another look at the Type 1 and 2 errors; however, no significant changes in thinking have occurred, other than to note the availability tables for calculating the β risk (Schlich, 1993) and further speculation about the process (Smith, 1981). Additional study will be useful because most sensory tests involve limited numbers of subjects and a database of not more than fifty responses while acceptance tests and market research tests use much larger numbers of participants. We would be remiss if we did not emphasize that these small panel tests are done with qualified subjects experienced with the test procedure, and each provide repeated responses, so there are some clear benefits to sensory tests that use replication as a integral part of every test.

F. Statistical Measures

We now direct our attention to a discussion about some statistical measures that may be considered basic to all sensory tests. Many of these measures should be obtained regardless of other analyses contemplated. First is the examination of responses by product and by order of presentation for each product and independent of product. Frequency distributions such as these provide for an assessment of any skewed response patterns, as well as an overall judgment as to the quality of the database. Second is the examination of means and standard deviations for the products, also by order of presentation. These latter measures provide for an assessment of order effects. It should always be kept in mind that these are summary statistics measures; that is, information is being summarized and the question of representativeness is addressed by observation of the frequency distributions.

In Fig. 4.2, results are presented from a group of forty subjects, each of whom scored each product on one occasion (i.e. no replication). The products were served in a balanced order, one at a time. For each product, the responses were plotted as a series of histograms; responses were pooled independent of serving order and whether served first or second. Also included were the means, SDs, N, and measures of the shapes of the distributions and the signs (+,−) of these latter measures which provides the direction and magnitude relative to a bell-shaped or normal distribution. A distribution is considered skewed when the value for skewness (Sk) exceeds ± 1. In the current example, none of the values approached this, ranging from +0.0314 to −0.6377. The measurement of kertosis (K) would yield a value of 3 for a normal distribution; the current results provide evidence for the more normal distribution for the responses to product B and the flatter distribution for product A. For more discussion about the measures of skewness and kertosis, the reader is referred to Duncan (1974). Whether one makes the decision to assess these measures or whether a simple perusal of the histograms is satisfactory, is judgmental. However, the important issue is that such an assessment is made because all subsequent tests will reflect the nature of the database. Considering the ease with which such analyses can be

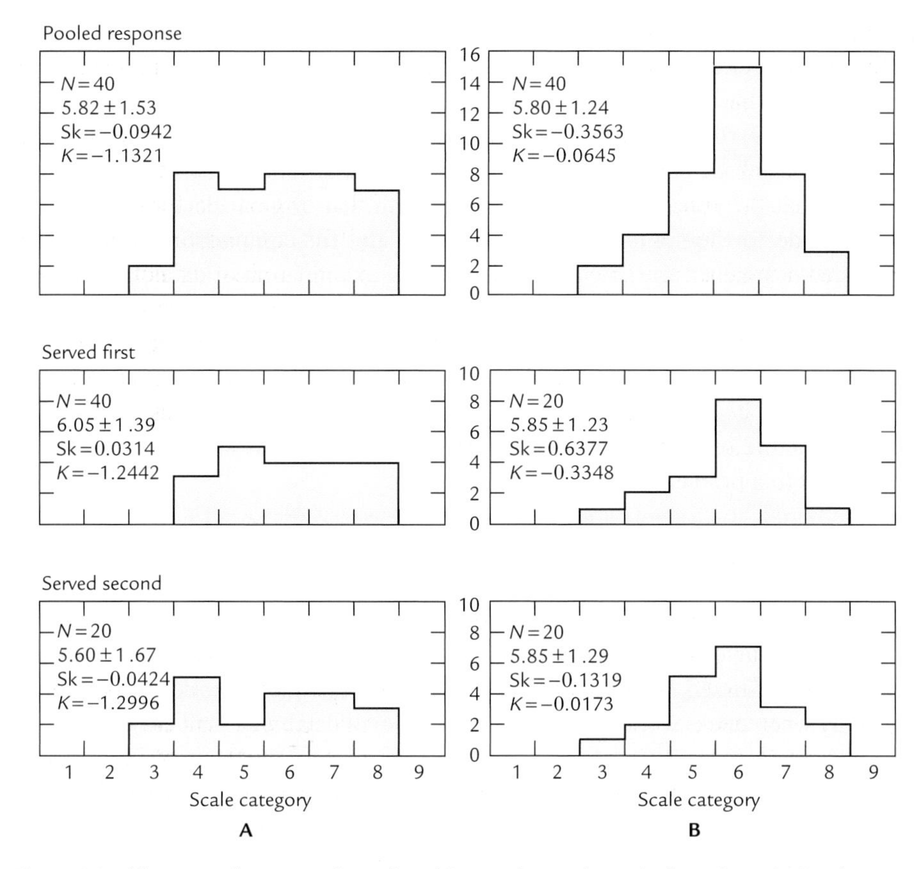

Figure 4.2 Histograms for two products, A and B, scored on a nine-point intensity scale. Results are tabulated for both serving orders and combined for each product. Also presented are the number of responses (*N*), mean ± SD, skewness (Sk), and kertosis (*K*). See test for additional explanation.

done with a laptop, it should be routine to subject all data to these and other summary displays of the responses. First, it should be noted that the histograms for each product are quite similar (served first and second compared with pooled), and, therefore, they provide no more information than can be gained from the pooled results. The relatively flat distribution for A means that about the same number of subjects scored it as 4, 5, 6, 7, or 8, while the distribution for B has a peak at the scale value of 6 and is more bell shaped with fewer judgments on either side.

In effect, this result could be interpreted as a reflection of greater agreement by these subjects concerning the score for product B and more disagreement concerning the score for product A. In this situation, the similarity in the means and standard deviations would be less informative or misleading. For the formulation specialist, such a similarity could be most frustrating, if there are no other clues as to product change. Of course, the usefulness of these measures is dependent on the total number of responses (N). When N is relatively small, for example, thirty or fewer judgments per product, then segmentation will yield smaller numbers for each subset and one must use caution when reaching any generalized conclusions. This would also be true if results were compared from different studies using different scales of measurement and the responses were standardized. Scales can be transformed on some common basis and appropriately tested for agreement (see McCall, 1975, or McNemar, 1969, for more detail). In each instance, however, it is very important that the original database be reviewed not only before but also after any transformations to ensure that the conclusions are consistent with that original database. Tests can also be made for homogeneity of the variance and for comparisons of variances (correlated or independent) as further steps in the examination of data.

The most important concern is for the sensory professional to recognize the need to assess the quality of each data set. The assessment should be more than just a perusal of a computer printout; it should be sufficiently extensive to determine its quality. Finally, it should be noted that no one measure can be expected to provide a complete picture of a database, just as no one statistical analysis can provide all of the answers to a problem.

1. The *t*-test

The *t*-test (or Student's *t* distribution) has been a very useful statistical procedure, although its popularity appears to have declined with the increase in multi-product tests (i.e. tests involving three or more products) and accessibility to AOV models using computer-based statistical packages. Nonetheless, the *t*-test does have utility, especially when one is working with a relatively small database (such as $N \leq 30$) and only two products are being tested. If more than two products are being tested, a single comparison of any two products is possible; however, the reader is cautioned that such a test is easily misused. In fact, an inappropriate and common error occurs when multiple *t*-tests are made from the same database. This incorrect use of the *t* statistic will result in a substantial and changing Type 1 error, an issue that is described by Alder and Roessler (1977) and Ryan (1959, 1960). Similarly, if large-sample statistical procedures are used for analysis of data that are appropriately analyzed by the *t*-test, the risk of a Type 1 error is increased. Additional discussion on this issue can be found in Alder and Roessler.

Selection of the appropriate *t* statistic and degrees of freedom for a two-product analysis will depend on a number of factors. These include paired or unpaired variates, equal or unequal numbers of judgments per cell, and equality or inequality of variances. Each alternative entails some computational differences and the sensory professional should be familiar with them.

Most sensory tests use the dependent *t* formula (paired-variate procedure) because the same subjects evaluated both products. However, if there is interest in determining whether there was a significant order effect for a product, then an independent *t*-statistic would be used in an unreplicated design, as shown in the following scenario. For this computation, responses from those subjects who evaluated product A in the first position would be compared with responses to product A served in the second position (obtained from the other subjects). If comparing product A with B in the first position only is of interest, then an independent *t*-statistic is appropriate. Similarly, a comparison of the products in the second position also would be made with the independent *t*-statistic.

Obviously, the t-statistic can be used in a number of ways to analyze results from a test. It is necessary that the researcher be clear as to the alternative(s) to be used, and care is taken that the data are consistent with the model. The relative ease with which the computations are made has made the method popular, and it should continue to be used.

2. Analysis of Variance

Of the many summary statistical procedures, the AOV is probably the most useful as well as the most frequently used method for data analysis in sensory evaluation. It is especially useful in analyzing multi-product tests and it can utilize data from a variety of experimental situations without serious compromise or risk in decision-making.

The analysis, as its name implies, is a statistical procedure designed to partition all the sources of variability in a test, thus providing a more precise estimate of the variable being studied. It might be considered an extension of the t-test, which is a two-product test (or a procedure that provides for the comparison of two means). The relationship between the two procedures can be shown in the one-way AOV and the independent t-test, in which the F value is equal to the t value squared. For a detailed discussion and description of these computations, the reader is referred to McCall (1975), Alder and Roessler (1977), and Bruning and Kintz (1987).

There are many different types of AOVs, depending on the nature of the problem, whether the variable is expected to have more than a single effect, and whether the subjects might be expected to respond differently to the different products, whether subjects evaluate each product on more than a single occasion, or whether different subjects evaluate each product on more than a single occasion, or whether different subjects evaluate the products at different times. For each experimental design, the particular AOV model will have certain distinguishing features. In most instances, these features are associated with partitioning the sources of variability and in determining appropriate error terms to derive the F value (the ratio of variances) for estimating statistical significance.

Before proceeding with a discussion about the different AOV designs, some of the common features of the AOV will be considered. As noted at the outset, the analysis involves a series of computations (in which scores are summed and squared or vice versa) to yield total sums of squares, treatment sums of squares, and error sums of squares. With unequal numbers of subjects, it is necessary that the sensory professional account for the missing observations. One possible alternative is to use a general linear model (GLM) hypothesis. With replication, decisions also will need to be made before any computations, regarding the most useful way to partition or group the treatment and error sums of squares. Replication is extremely important not only because it provides a measure of subject reliability, but also because it increases the statistical power of the test; that is, it increases the likelihood for finding a difference. The expectation is that within-subject variability will be smaller than the between-subject variability. For a trained panel test, how else can one directly demonstrate within-subject and panel reliability? The next computational step is the comparison of the various sums of squares (after dividing each value by its associated degrees of freedom), the assumption being that if the responses (to all the products) are from the same population, then the ratio will be unity. However, the more this ratio deviates from unity (and is greater than unity), the more likely we are to consider the responses as due to a true treatment effect. The ratio, referred to as the *F* ratio, is then compared with tabular values for determining statistical significance. It is common practice to summarize the computations using a source of variance table and listing the sources of variation, degrees of freedom, sums of squares, mean squares, *F* values, and associated probability values. A description of these computations with worked examples can be found in McCall (1975), Alder and Roessler (1977), Gacula and Singh (1984), O'Mahony (1986), and Bruning and Kintz (1987). Most statistical packages also provide the user with details regarding the output as well, and the sensory professional should read the information carefully.

The sensory professional must be familiar with the various types of AOV designs and how to read and understand results. As we will demonstrate in the next section, with studies involving more than a single treatment, the proper partitioning of the sources of variability becomes a critical issue in terms of identifying and isolating sources such as interaction that could mask a true treatment effect. Finally, the increasing reliance on statistical packages available on a PC is both an advantage and a disadvantage. The use of statistical packages is advantageous in that analyses are completed on a real time basis using one's PC; however, this can be a disadvantage if the statistical procedures are not clearly stated, or the package default analysis is not appropriate for the sensory test. For example, only one type of AOV model may be available (fixed effects) and this will lead to erroneous conclusions about differences if, for example, the particular design used was a mixed design; that is, fixed and random effects. Split-plot designs and other more complex designs require even more specific information from the sensory professional to ensure that the computations and the error terms selected for tests for significance will be appropriate. Attention to details is important, and one can never assume that the PC has done the thinking for you.

A brief comment about tests after the *F* test also is in order. The AOV provides evidence that there is a statistically significant treatment effect, but does not indicate specifically how the treatments differ. The answer requires the use of one of several tests that are referred to as range tests or tests after the *F* test. The seven most frequently used tests after the *F* test are Fisher's least significant difference (LSD) or *t*-test, Duncan's, Newman–Keuls, Tukey (a), Tukey (b), and the Scheffé and Bonferroni tests. An eighth test, the Dunnett test, also can be used, specifically when one is comparing products not to each other, but only to a control. In the discussion on descriptive analysis, the use of these tests and especially the former seven, is described in conjunction with several worked examples. Briefly, these tests provide more or less protection against a decision error (Type 1 and Type 2 errors) and depending on the problem, one test or another would be selected. The reader should be aware that the tests are not interchangeable, and also that these tests are applicable only if there is a statistically significant *F* value. Failure to observe this rule can lead to embarrassing consequences, such as reporting significant differences between certain products, when an *F* test would yield no significant difference.

3. Multiple-factor designs and analyses

The treatments-by-subjects (T × S) design is one of the most frequently used designs in sensory evaluation. It is a straightforward design with each product evaluated once by each subject. For example, if scoring four competitive products by forty subjects and determining whether there is a significant difference between any of the products is of interest, then a T × S design is appropriate. The products will be served in a balanced monadic sequential order one at a time to each subject, until all four products are scored. This design provides an assessment of each product relative to the others, and a basis for determining the effect of one product on (the score for) another. Typically, these effects are product dependent, hence the need to separate the effect from the variable of primary interest. This design is different from a completely randomized block design in which each subject evaluates only one product (forty responses per product in a four-product test will require 160 subjects). The former is preferred because it provides a more effective use of subjects and yields a separate subject term that can be partitioned from the error. It also can be expected to increase the likelihood for finding a difference because the extracting the variance for subject differences reduces the residual error term, hence the value of the T × S design.

Table 4.2 is a source of variance table for the T × S design. In this design, the error term is represented by the T × S interaction value (AS), which might be considered unsatisfactory even though it is appropriate. It is unsatisfactory in the sense that this source of variability contains more than interaction (variability that cannot be assigned elsewhere); however, the data cannot be partitioned any further. Keep in mind that the mean square interaction value (MS_{AS}) is used in the computation for F as the denominator, and the smaller this value, the more likely that F will be significant.

As shown in the source of variance table (Table 4.3), this error term can be improved with the addition of replication. If interaction is non-significant, it need not be used as the error term for testing treatment effects. Testing the treatment effect may be achieved by using the residual, or in the situation of a non-significant

Table 4.2 Source of variance table for a treatments × subjects design[a]

Source of variation	df	Sum of squares	Mean square	F
Treatments (A)	$a-1$	$ss_A = \frac{\sum^{a}\left(\sum^{s}x\right)^2}{s} - \frac{\left(\sum^{as}x\right)^2}{as}$	$ms_A = ss_A/(a-1)$	ms_A/ms_{AS}
Subjects (S)	$s-1$	$ss_S = \frac{\sum^{s}\left(\sum^{a}x\right)^2}{a} - \frac{\left(\sum^{as}x\right)^2}{as}$	$ms_S = ss_S/(s-1)$	ms_S/ms_{AS}
Residual (AS)	$(a-1)(s-1)$	$ss_{AS} = ss_T - ss_A - ss_S$	$ms_{AS} = ss_{AS}/(a-1)(s-1)$	
Total	$as-1$	$ss_T = \sum^{as}x^2 - \frac{\left(\sum^{as}x\right)^2}{as}$		

[a] Design plan: all subjects evaluate all products.

Table 4.3 Source of variance table for a treatments × subjects design with replications[a]

Source of variation	df	Sums of squares	Mean square	F
Treatments (A)	$a - 1$	$ss_A = \frac{\sum^{a}\left(\sum^{sr} x\right)^2}{sr} - \frac{\left(\sum^{asr} x\right)^2}{asr}$	$ss_A/(a-1)$	
Subjects (S)	$s - 1$	$ss_S = \frac{\sum^{s}\left(\sum^{ar} x\right)^2}{ar} - \frac{\left(\sum^{asr} x\right)^2}{asr}$	$ss_S/(s-1)$	
Treatment × subjects (AS)	$(a-1)(s-1)$	$ss_{AS} = \frac{\sum^{as}\left(\sum^{r} x\right)^2}{r} - \frac{\sum^{a}\left(\sum^{sr} x\right)^2}{sr} - \frac{\sum^{s}\left(\sum^{ar} x\right)^2}{ar} + \frac{\left(\sum^{asr} x\right)^2}{asr}$	$ss_{AS}/(a-1)(s-1)$	ms_{AS}/ms_R
Residual (R)	$as(r-1)$	$ss_R = ss_T - ss_A - ss_S - ss_{AS}$	$ss_R/as(r-1)$	
Total	$asr - 1$	$ss_T = \sum^{asr} x^2 - \frac{\left(\sum^{asr} x\right)^2}{asr}$		

[a] Design plan: all subjects evaluate all products.

interaction, by pooling the residual with the interaction sum of squares and the degrees of freedom (df) and using the resulting error term. However, it should be kept in mind that when the interaction is significant, it is the appropriate term for testing the treatment effect. Also, a significant subject effect is neither unusual nor of much consequence. It indicates that the subjects used different parts of the scale when scoring the products and should not be misconstrued as a problem with the subjects. Individual differences in scoring are to be expected, as was noted in Chapter 3.

When the research problem must accommodate two treatment conditions – for example, in evaluating a carbonated beverage product in which there are levels of carbonation and levels of flavor – then a treatment-by-treatment-by subject (T × T × S) design will be most appropriate. In this situation, the requestor may be seeking direction in formulation of a new product. Not only is it more test efficient to include an array of products that bear a relationship to each other, but the effect of one variable on another also can be measured. When each subject evaluates each product, further partitioning is possible using the various treatment interaction effects. As shown in the source of variance table (Table 4.4), the partitioning of the sources of variability is considerably more extensive, thus providing for more precise estimates for *F*. Although it would be possible to analyze this test as a treatment-by-subject design, the interaction between the two treatments is best analyzed with the T × T × S design. Similar to the unreplicated T × S design, each main treatment effect must be tested using its respective interaction value as the appropriate error term; for example, MS_A/MS_{AS} and MS_B/MS_{BS}. (See Lindquist, 1953, pp. 237–239, for additional information on this particular use of the interaction terms.)

Table 4.4 Source of variance table for a treatments × treatments × subject design[a]

Source of variation	df	Sum of squares	Mean square	F
Flavor concentrations (A)	$a - 1$	$ss_A = \frac{\sum^{a}\left(\sum^{bs} x\right)^2}{bs} - \frac{\left(\sum^{abs} x\right)^2}{abs}$	$ss_A/(a - 1)$	ms_A/ms_{AS}
Carbonation levels (B)	$b - 1$	$ss_B = \frac{\sum^{b}\left(\sum^{as} x\right)^2}{as} - \frac{\left(\sum^{abs} x\right)^2}{abs}$	$ss_B/(b - 1)$	ms_B/ms_{BS}
Subjects (S)	$s - 1$	$ss_S = \frac{\sum^{s}\left(\sum^{ab} x\right)^2}{ab} - \frac{\left(\sum^{abs} x\right)^2}{abs}$	$ss_S/(s - 1)$	
A × B (AB)	$(a - 1)(b - 1)$	$ss_{AB} = \frac{\sum^{ab}\left(\sum^{s} x\right)^2}{s} - \frac{\sum^{a}\left(\sum^{bs} x\right)^2}{bs} - \frac{\sum^{b}\left(\sum^{as} x\right)^2}{as} + \frac{\left(\sum^{abs} x\right)^2}{abs}$	$ss_{AB}/(a - 1)(b - 1)$	ms_{AB}/ms_{ABS}
A × S (AS)	$(a - 1)(s - 1)$	$ss_{AS} = \frac{\sum^{as}\left(\sum^{b} x\right)^2}{b} - \frac{\sum^{a}\left(\sum^{bs} x\right)^2}{bs} - \frac{\sum^{s}\left(\sum^{ab} x\right)^2}{ab} + \frac{\left(\sum^{abs} x\right)^2}{abs}$	$ss_{AS}/(a - 1)(s - 1)$	
B × S (BS)	$(b - 1)(s - 1)$	$ss_{BS} = \frac{\sum^{bs}\left(\sum^{a} x\right)^2}{a} - \frac{\sum^{b}\left(\sum^{as} x\right)^2}{as} - \frac{\sum^{s}\left(\sum^{ab} x\right)^2}{ab} + \frac{\left(\sum^{abs} x\right)^2}{abs}$	$ss_{BS}/(b - 1)(s - 1)$	
Residual (ABS)	$(a - 1)(b - 1)(s - 1)$	$ss_{ABS} = ss_T - ss_A - ss_B - ss_S - ss_{AB} - ss_{AS} - ss_{BS}$	$ss_{ABS}/(a - 1)(b - 1)(s - 1)$	
Total	$abs - 1$	$ss_T = \sum^{abs} x^2 - \frac{\left(\sum^{abs} x\right)^2}{abs}$		

[a] Design plan: all subjects evaluate all levels of two treatment conditions.

The next three designs, sometimes referred to as "split-plot" or "mixed" designs, represent useful models for product evaluation that extend the study of treatment interactions, providing for evaluation of matrices of products (i.e. multi-product tests) and the use of different groups of subjects. The latter practice is typical in evaluating the stability of products in storage. The designation of "split-plot" or "mixed" refers to the subplots of other less complicated designs that make up each design; for example, T × S and randomized blocks.

Table 4.5 is a source of variance table for a "one-within and one-between" split-plot design. This particular design would be most appropriate in situations in which, for example, different groups of subjects at different locations evaluated the same set of products or where different groups of subjects evaluated a product set representing different plants. Another application would be a test in which different subjects are presented with only one of several alternative concepts but all subjects evaluate all products. The latter situation enables the sensory professional to measure the effect of the concept on scores for the products, in effect, to determine whether responses to one or all products are more strongly influenced by one concept than by another (concept). Storage tests are especially well suited to these designs because different subjects evaluate each test product (the "within" variable) and the products change over time (the "between" variable).

The particular example in Table 4.5 yields a separate error term for evaluating the two main treatment effects ($MS_{error(b)}$ and $MS_{error(w)}$). The products are the "within" variable and the production plants are the "between" variable. The interaction term (A × B) is treated as the "within" variable in this design. If there is a choice, the variable of most importance should be used as the "within" variable.

A "two-within and one-between" split-plot design is a T × T × S design achieved with different subjects segmented according to a third test variable. The third test variable might be a production facility, a concept, a treatment variable such as flavoring options, or a demographic classification such as age or sex. The source of variance table for this design is Table 4.6. As was noted in the T × T × S design, special attention must be given to testing each main effect and interaction with the appropriate error term for testing the "between" treatment main effect and the three separate error terms for testing the "within" treatments main effects and interactions. In this particular example, the "within" variable is the flavor concentration and the two "between" variables are carbonation and sucrose; that is, a set of products has been prepared using different levels of carbonation, with all other formulae variables held constant, and another set of products has been prepared using different levels of sucrose. Both sets of products would have two different levels of added flavor.

Finally, Table 4.7 is a source of variance table for a "one-within and two-between" design. Note that the variables are the same as those listed in the previous design. However, the analysis of these variables is determined by which variables were evaluated by all subjects and which variables were evaluated by different groups of subjects.

Numerous other multiple variable designs have application in sensory evaluation. Most of these require a reasonable effort on the part of the sensory professional to

Table 4.5 Source of variance table for a split-plot one-within and one-between design[a]

Source of variation	df	Sum of squares	Mean square	F
Between-subjects	$bn - 1$	Between $ss_T = \frac{\sum^{bn}\left(\sum^{a} x\right)^2}{a} - \frac{\left(\sum^{abn} x\right)^2}{abn}$		
Production plants (B)	$b - 1$	$ss_B = \frac{\sum^{b}\left(\sum^{an} x\right)^2}{an} - \frac{\left(\sum^{abn} x\right)^2}{abn}$	$ss_B/(b - 1)$	$ms_B/ms_{error(b)}$
Error (b)	$b(n - 1)$	$ss_{error(b)} = \frac{\sum^{bn}\left(\sum^{a} x\right)^2}{a} - \frac{\sum^{b}\left(\sum^{an} x\right)^2}{an}$	$ss_{error(b)}/b(n - 1)$	
Within-subjects	$bn(a - 1)$	Within $ss_T = \sum^{abn} x^2 - \frac{\sum^{bn}\left(\sum^{a} x\right)^2}{a}$		
Products (A)	$a - 1$	$ss_A = \frac{\sum^{a}\left(\sum^{bn} x\right)^2}{bn} - \frac{\left(\sum^{abn} x\right)^2}{abn}$	$ss_A/(a - 1)$	$ms_A/ms_{error(w)}$
A × B	$(a - 1)(b - 1)$	$ss_{AB} = \frac{\sum^{ab}\left(\sum^{n} x\right)^2}{n} - \frac{\sum^{a}\left(\sum^{bn} x\right)^2}{bn} - \frac{\sum^{b}\left(\sum^{an} x\right)^2}{an} + \frac{\left(\sum^{abn} x\right)^2}{abn}$	$ss_{AB}/(a - 1)(b - 1)$	$ms_{AB}/ms_{error(w)}$
Error (w)	$b(n - 1)(a - 1)$	$ss_{error(w)} = \sum^{abn} x^2 - \frac{\sum^{ab}\left(\sum^{n} x\right)^2}{n} - \frac{\sum^{bn}\left(\sum^{a} x\right)^2}{a} + \frac{\sum^{b}\left(\sum^{an} x\right)^2}{an}$	$ss_{error(w)}/b(n - 1)(a - 1)$	
Total	$abn - 1$	$ss_T = \sum^{abn} x^2 - \frac{\left(\sum^{abn} x\right)^2}{abn}$		

[a] Design plan: each different group of "B" subjects evaluate all "A" products.

Table 4.6 Source of variance table for a split-plot two-within and one-between design[a]

Source of variation	df	Sum of squares	Mean square	F
Between-subjects	$cn - 1$	Between $ss_T = \frac{\sum^{cn}\left(\sum^{ab} x\right)^2}{ab} - \frac{\left(\sum^{abcn} x\right)^2}{abcn}$		
Carbonation (C)	$c - 1$	$ss_C = \frac{\sum^{c}\left(\sum^{abn} x\right)^2}{abn} - \frac{\left(\sum^{abcn} x\right)^2}{abcn}$	$ss_c/(c - 1)$	$ms_c/ms_{error(b)}$
Error (b)	$c(n - 1)$	$ss_{error(b)} = \frac{\sum^{cn}\left(\sum^{ab} x\right)^2}{ab} - \frac{\sum^{c}\left(\sum^{abcn} x\right)^2}{abn}$	$ss_{error(b)}/c(n - 1)$	
Within-subjects	$cn(ab - 1)$	Within $ss_T = \sum^{abcn} x^2 - \frac{\sum^{cn}\left(\sum^{ab} x\right)^2}{ab}$		
Flavor concentration (A)	$a - 1$	$ss_A = \frac{\sum^{a}\left(\sum^{bcn} x\right)^2}{bcn} - \frac{\left(\sum^{abcn} x\right)^2}{abcn}$	$ss_A/(a - 1)$	$ms_A/ms_{error1(w)}$
Sucrose level (B)	$b - 1$	$ss_B = \frac{\sum^{b}\left(\sum^{acn} x\right)^2}{acn} - \frac{\left(\sum^{abcn} x\right)^2}{abcn}$	$ss_B/(b - 1)$	$ms_B/ms_{error2(w)}$
A × B	$(a - 1)(b - 1)$	$ss_{AB} = \frac{\sum^{ab}\left(\sum^{cn} x\right)^2}{cn} - \frac{\sum^{a}\left(\sum^{bcn} x\right)^2}{bcn} - \frac{\sum^{b}\left(\sum^{acn} x\right)^2}{acn} + \frac{\left(\sum^{abcn} x\right)^2}{abcn}$	$ss_{AB}/(a - 1)(b - 1)$	$ms_{AB}/ms_{error3(w)}$
A × C	$(a - 1)(c - 1)$	$ss_{AC} = \frac{\sum^{ac}\left(\sum^{bn} x\right)^2}{bn} - \frac{\sum^{a}\left(\sum^{bcn} x\right)^2}{bcn} - \frac{\sum^{c}\left(\sum^{abn} x\right)^2}{abn} + \frac{\left(\sum^{abcn} x\right)^2}{abcn}$	$ss_{AC}/(a - 1)(c - 1)$	$ms_{AC}/ms_{error1(w)}$
B × C	$(b - 1)(c - 1)$	$ss_{BC} = \frac{\sum^{bc}\left(\sum^{an} x\right)^2}{an} - \frac{\sum^{b}\left(\sum^{acn} x\right)^2}{acn} - \frac{\sum^{c}\left(\sum^{abn} x\right)^2}{abn} + \frac{\left(\sum^{abcn} x\right)^2}{abcn}$	$ss_{BC}/(b - 1)(c - 1)$	$ms_{BC}/ms_{error2(w)}$
A × B × C	$(a - 1)(b - 1)(c - 1)$	$ss_{ABC} = \frac{\sum^{abc}\left(\sum^{n} x\right)^2}{n} - \frac{\sum^{ab}\left(\sum^{cn} x\right)^2}{cn} - \frac{\sum^{ac}\left(\sum^{bn} x\right)^2}{bn} - \frac{bc\left(\sum^{an} x\right)^2}{an} + \frac{\sum^{a}\left(\sum^{bcn} x\right)^2}{bcn} + \frac{\sum^{b}\left(\sum^{acn} x\right)^2}{acn} + \frac{\sum^{c}\left(\sum^{abn} x\right)^2}{abn} - \frac{\left(\sum^{abcn} x\right)^2}{abcn}$	$ss_{ABC}/(a - 1)(b - 1)(c - 1)$	$ms_{ABC}/ms_{error3(w)}$

Table 4.6 *(continued)*

Source of variation	df	Sum of squares	Mean square	F
$\text{Error}_1(\text{w})$	$c(a-1)(n-1)$	$ss_{\text{error}_1(\text{w})} = \frac{\sum^{acn}\left(\sum^{b} x\right)^2}{b} - \frac{\sum^{ac}\left(\sum^{bn} x\right)^2}{bn} - \frac{\sum^{cn}\left(\sum^{ab} x\right)^2}{ab} + \frac{\sum^{c}\left(\sum^{abn} x\right)^2}{abn}$	$ss_{\text{error1(w)}}/c(a-1)(n-1)$	
$\text{Error}_2(\text{w})$	$c(b-1)(n-1)$	$ss_{\text{error}_2(\text{w})} = \frac{\sum^{bcn}\left(\sum^{a} x\right)^2}{a} - \frac{\sum^{bc}\left(\sum^{an} x\right)^2}{an} - \frac{\sum^{cn}\left(\sum^{ab} x\right)^2}{ab} + \frac{\sum^{c}\left(\sum^{abn} x\right)^2}{abn}$	$ss_{\text{error2(w)}}/c(b-1)(n-1)$	
$\text{Error}_3(\text{w})$	$c(a-1)(b-1)(n-1)$	$ss_{\text{error}_3(\text{w})} = \sum^{abcn} x^2 - \frac{\sum^{abc}\left(\sum^{n} x\right)^2}{n} - \frac{\sum^{acn}\left(\sum^{b} x\right)^2}{b} - \frac{\sum^{bcn}\left(\sum^{a} x\right)^2}{a} + \frac{\sum^{ac}\left(\sum^{bn} x\right)^2}{bn} + \frac{\sum^{bc}\left(\sum^{an} x\right)^2}{an} + \frac{\sum^{cn}\left(\sum^{ab} x\right)^2}{ab} - \frac{\sum^{c}\left(\sum^{abn} x\right)^2}{abn}$	$ss_{\text{error3(w)}}/c(a-1)(b-1)(n-1)$	
Total	abcn − 1	$ss_T = \sum^{abcn} x^2 - \frac{\left(\sum^{abcn} x\right)^2}{abcn}$		

[a] Design plan: each different group of "c" subjects evaluate all levels of two treatment conditions.

delineate the sources of variability, selecting the appropriate error term for testing the different effects, and to decide which comparisons are most appropriate, but this should not be an impediment to their use. Their use allows for the evaluation of arrays of products that might not otherwise be considered feasible. The sensory professional must take the time to become familiar with the range of possibilities, and if needed, to seek assistance from the specialist in statistics. This is the only approach that offers hope for achieving maximum information from every test. In the section on Optimization, in Chapter 8, we discuss some additional experimental designs (e.g. Response Surface) that are used in sensory evaluation.

Table 4.7 Source of variance table for a split-plot one-within and two-between design[a]

Source of variation	df	Sum of squares	Mean square	F
Between-subjects	$bcn - 1$	Between $ss_T = \frac{\sum^{bcn}\left(\sum^{a} x\right)^2}{a} - \frac{\left(\sum^{abcn} x\right)^2}{abcn}$		
Carbonation level (B)	$b - 1$	$ss_B = \frac{\sum^{b}\left(\sum^{acn} x\right)^2}{acn} - \frac{\left(\sum^{abcn} x\right)^2}{abcn}$	$ss_B/(b-1)$	$ms_B/ms_{error(b)}$
Sucrose level (C)	$c - 1$	$ss_C = \frac{\sum^{c}\left(\sum^{abn} x\right)^2}{abn} - \frac{\left(\sum^{abcn} x\right)^2}{abcn}$	$ss_C/(c-1)$	$ms_C/ms_{error(b)}$
B × C	$(b-1)(c-1)$	$ss_{BC} = \frac{\sum^{bc}\left(\sum^{an} x\right)^2}{an} - \frac{\sum^{b}\left(\sum^{acn} x\right)^2}{acn} - \frac{\sum^{c}\left(\sum^{abn} x\right)^2}{abn} + \frac{\left(\sum^{abcn} x\right)^2}{abcn}$	$ss_{BC}/(b-1)(c-1)$	$ms_{BC}/ms_{error(b)}$
Error (b)	$bc(n-1)$	$ss_{error(b)} = \frac{\sum^{bcn}\left(\sum^{a} x\right)^2}{a} - \frac{\sum^{bc}\left(\sum^{an} x\right)^2}{an}$	$ss_{error\,(b)}/bc(n-1)$	
Within-subjects	$bcn(a-1)$	Within $ss_T = \sum^{abcn} x^2 - \frac{\sum^{bcn}\left(\sum^{a} x\right)^2}{a}$		
Flavor concentration (A)	$(a-1)$	$ss_A = \frac{\sum^{a}\left(\sum^{bcn} x\right)^2}{bcn} - \frac{\left(\sum^{abcn} x\right)^2}{abcn}$	$ss_A/(a-1)$	$ms_A/ms_{error(w)}$

A × B	$(a-1)(b-1)$	$ss_{AB} = \frac{\sum^{ab}\left(\sum^{cn} x\right)^2}{cn} - \frac{\sum^{a}\left(\sum^{bcn} x\right)^2}{bcn} - \frac{\sum^{b}\left(\sum^{acn} x\right)^2}{acn} + \frac{\left(\sum^{abcn} x\right)^2}{abcn}$	$ss_{AB}/(a-1)(b-1)$	$ms_{AB}/ms_{error(w)}$
A × C	$(a-1)(c-1)$	$ss_{AC} = \frac{\sum^{ac}\left(\sum^{bn} x\right)^2}{bn} - \frac{\sum^{a}\left(\sum^{bcn} x\right)^2}{bcn} - \frac{\sum^{c}\left(\sum^{abn} x\right)^2}{abn} + \frac{\left(\sum^{abcn} x\right)^2}{abcn}$	$ss_{AC}/(a-1)(c-1)$	$ms_{AC}/ms_{error(w)}$
A × B × C	$(a-1)(b-1)(c-1)$	$ss_{ABC} = \frac{\sum^{abc}\left(\sum^{n} x\right)^2}{n} - \frac{\sum^{ab}\left(\sum^{cn} x\right)^2}{cn} - \frac{\sum^{ac}\left(\sum^{bn} x\right)^2}{bn} - \frac{\sum^{bc}\left(\sum^{an} x\right)^2}{an} + \frac{\sum^{a}\left(\sum^{bcn} x\right)^2}{bcn} + \frac{\sum^{b}\left(\sum^{acn} x\right)^2}{acn} + \frac{\sum^{c}\left(\sum^{abn} x\right)^2}{abn} - \frac{\left(\sum^{abcn} x\right)^2}{abcn}$	$ss_{ABC}/(a-1)(b-1)(c-1)$	$ms_{ABC}/ms_{error(w)}$
Error (w)	$bc(a-1)(n-1)$	$ss_{error(w)} = \sum^{abcn} x^2 - \frac{\sum^{abc}\left(\sum^{n} x\right)^2}{n} - \frac{\sum^{bcn}\left(\sum^{a} x\right)^2}{a} + \frac{\sum^{bc}\left(\sum^{an} x\right)^2}{an}$	$ss_{error(w)}/bc(a-1)(n-1)$	
Total	$abcn-1$	$ss_T = \sum^{abcn} x^2 - \frac{\left(\sum^{abcn} x\right)^2}{abcn}$		

[a] Design plan: each different group of "BC" subjects evaluate all "A" products.

VI. Experimental Design Considerations

In preparing an experimental design, that is, the written plan that designates product serving order, the sensory evaluation professional will have addressed all of the issues considered in the preceding sections (objective, product appropriateness, and so on). These latter issues may be considered as sensory input to test design as distinct from mathematical or statistical input. A considerable number of texts on experimental design exist (e.g. Cochran and Cox, 1957; McNemar, 1969; Winer 1971; Box *et al.*, 1978). Nevertheless, the unique requirements of sensory evaluation necessitate additional discussion and selected examples (of designs) to reflect these requirements.

Experimental design and statistical analysis act in concert to substantively influence the outcome of a test. The design dictates the serving order of the products as well as the most appropriate analysis to satisfy the specific test objective. One may still be able to analyze the results of a poorly designed study, but the variables of interest are likely to be confounded and therefore inseparable from other effects, so that any clear statement about the products may be quite risky. On the other hand, neither the experimental design nor the analysis can compensate for poor test execution or an ill-defined objective.

With these thoughts in mind, we direct our attention to consideration of the sensory requirements in experimental design, followed by selected examples of experimental designs and a discussion on the application of more sophisticated designs in sensory evaluation.

The following design guidelines reflect the aforementioned issues as well as the practicalities of the test as one of several sources of business information used to make a recommendation within the briefest possible time period.

1. Responses of a subject are easily influenced by familiarity with the products and by previous test experience. Use balanced-block designs that minimize, or evenly distribute, bias from the interactions of subject, products, and time.
2. When reasonable, all products should be evaluated equally often by each subject. By reasonable we mean tests involving four or fewer products. For tests involving five or more products, the number of permutations precludes strict subject adherence to this requirement. Alternatives are discussed in guidelines 5 and 6.
3. All products should be served equally often before and after every other product and in all positions equally.
4. With balanced-block designs, the complete permutation is served before repeating a serving order. This procedure helps to minimize any time-order effects.
5. Completely randomized designs are considerably less useful than balanced-block designs, because some serving orders will occur infrequently while others will occur too frequently. With large numbers of respondents, such as 100 or more, these deficiencies may be overcome. However, most sensory tests involve <50 subjects, which could introduce considerable order bias. Table 4.8 demonstrates such a problem with a four-product random plan (from Sidel and

Table 4.8 Serving order for a four-product random test plan (A) and the frequency of product serving by position (B) and the pairing sequence (C)

A.

Subject	Serving order	Subject	Serving order
A	4 3 1 2	M	1 3 2 4
B	1 2 4 3	N	4 3 2 1
C	2 1 3 4	O	2 1 4 3
D	3 2 1 4	P	3 2 1 4
E	4 3 2 1	Q	2 4 3 1
F	1 2 3 4	R	3 1 2 4
G	2 4 1 3	S	4 2 1 3
H	3 4 1 2	T	3 1 4 2
I	2 1 3 4	U	1 2 3 4
J	2 4 3 1	V	2 3 4 1
K	1 2 4 3	W	1 3 4 2
L	4 3 1 2	X	4 1 3 2

B.

	Serving position				
Product	First	Second	Third	Fourth	Total
1	6	6	7	5	24
2	7	7	4	6	24
3	5	7	7	5	24
4	6	4	6	8	24
Total	24	24	24	24	

C.

	Serving position			
Pairs	1–2	2–3	3–4	Total
1 2	4	1	3	8
1 3	2	3	3	8
1 4	0	2	2	4
2 1	3	3	2	8
2 3	1	2	0	3
2 4	3	3	2	7
3 1	2	2	2	6
3 2	2	3	1	6
3 4	1	2	3	6
4 1	1	2	1	4
4 2	1	0	2	3
4 3	4	2	3	9

Stone, 1976) for twenty-four subjects; Section II shows that each product is not served in each position equally often. The problem is further exacerbated if one considers the serving order based on adjacent pairs (see Section III). For example, the sequence of product 1 followed by product 2 is served a total of eight times; four in the first and second positions, once in the second and third positions, and three times in the third and fourth positions. On the other extreme, the sequence of product 2 followed by product 3 occurs only three times; once in the 1–2 serving position, twice in the 2–3 position, and not at all in the 3–4 position. Such an imbalance is avoided with the balanced-block designs.

6. If all products cannot be evaluated by each subject within a single session, the order is balanced across the panel within each session. Balanced-block designs are preferred to balanced-incomplete-block designs because they allow for all possible comparisons by each subject and also use the fewest number of subjects. With several sessions, it is possible for each subject to evaluate all products and avoid the use of an incomplete design. Incomplete block designs provide different product context and subtleties to the subjects. This recommendation should not be misconstrued to mean that incomplete-block designs should not be used, but rather that they should be considered only after a decision is reached that the balanced-block design approach is not possible. The literature contains numerous examples of incomplete designs (Cochran and Cox, 1957) and more continue to be published (see, e.g. Gacula, 1978). In defense of incomplete designs, however, it should be pointed out that their greatest value arises when one is looking at a large array of products requiring extensive time to evaluate. For example, one might be evaluating an array of twenty skin lotions and the test protocol requires a 2- or 3-day use. Data collection would be extended 60 days, which might be quite impractical to achieve and, therefore, an incomplete design might be preferred. "Mixed" designs (split-plot designs) might also be appropriate (see Lindquist, 1953); however, the sensory evaluation professional should consider the problem in detail before reaching a final decision. In our own work, we avoid incomplete block designs where each subject evaluates less than 65–70% of the product set.
7. If it is not feasible to have all subjects evaluate all products, serving order balance is maintained across the panel. For example, in tests involving five products, the number of serving order permutations is 120. The determination of the permutations is based on the formula $P_{n,n} = n!$ (from Alder and Roessler, 1977) where n,n refers to the number of products taken in n sets and $n!$ refers to n factorial; $(n)(n - 1)(n - 2)$ and so on. For five products taken in sets of five, $P_{5,5} = 5 \times 4 \times 3 \times 2 \times 1 = 120$ orders of presentation of the five products. In many situations, all 120 orders of presentation will not be served and it is the responsibility of the sensory professional to select serving orders that are within reasonable balance. Examples are given in Section VII of this chapter.
8. A monadic sequential serving order provides for greater control of the time interval between products, hence control of sensory interaction and sensory fatique, and provides for a more independent response to each product.

While it may be argued that these guidelines are obvious to the experienced sensory professional and the statistician, the evidence to date suggests that considerable confusion continues to exist concerning the concept of experimental design in relation to sensory evaluation test activities. The literature provides excellent references on the subject of experimental design, including Lindquist (1953), Cochran and Cox (1957), and Winer (1971). However, the more practical sensory issues remain relatively untouched. Although publications by Gacula (1978) and Mullen and Ennis (1979) represent efforts to correct this deficiency, much more work will be needed to improve the quality of sensory information that is so heavily dependent on design. This effort is especially important with the increased interest in systems for the optimization of products and the development of predictive models for product acceptance. These programs reflect the competitive forces of the marketplace where manufacturers seek to identify and develop products with unique characteristics. They are made more possible as a result of computer technology, statistical packages, and advances in sensory evaluation methodology. In Chapter 8, we discuss some of these optimization programs and the role of sensory evaluation in making them successful.

VII. Selected Product Designs

To supplement the guidelines, we have prepared a series of designs reflecting the sensory evaluation requirements of testing. These particular designs are presented here for illustrative purposes and should not be followed without consideration for the test objective. In large tests, those involving five or more products, the particular design presented here is one of many possible designs and is presented solely to demonstrate that each sensory professional must develop his or her personal file of experimental designs. The sensory professional will be able to handle test requests with minimal delay and will have one less source of error.

An experimental design for a three-product test is presented in Table 4.9. The six orders of presentation for the three products (3 factorial, 3!) are taken in sets of three,

Table 4.9 Balanced-block design for a three-product test[a]

	Product serving order				Product serving order		
Subject	First	Second	Third	Subject	First	Second	Third
1	1	2	3	19	1	3	2
2	2	3	1	20	2	1	3
3	3	1	2	21	3	2	1
4	1	3	2	22	1	2	3
5	2	1	3	23	2	3	1
6	3	2	1	24	3	1	2
7	2	3	1	25	2	1	3
8	3	1	2	26	3	2	1
9	1	3	2	27	1	2	3
10	2	1	3	28	2	3	1
11	3	2	1	29	3	1	2
12	1	2	3	30	1	3	2
13	3	1	2	31	3	2	1
14	1	3	2	32	1	2	3
15	2	1	3	33	2	3	1
16	3	2	1	34	3	1	2
17	1	2	3	35	1	3	2
18	2	3	1	36	2	1	3

[a] See text for an explanation of the entries.

so the number of subjects should be in multiples of 6; that is, 6, 12, 18, 24, and so on, if the balanced order is to be maintained. In this particular design, it can be seen that for every six subjects each product appears equally often (twice) in each serving position and precedes and follows every other product equally often. We refer to this as "unfolding" in the sense that the aforementioned balance is maintained as the test progresses. Thus, any effects that are time dependent will be more easily isolated, and any question regarding serving order can also be addressed. With thirty-six subjects, each product appears in each position twelve times, as do the pairings (1–2, 2–1, and so on). This particular design should not be construed as a recommendation for only doing three-product tests with thirty-six subjects; the only concern is that each product serving order is not compromised to an extreme.

A balanced-block design for a four-product test is presented in Table 4.10. There are twenty-four orders of presentation for the four products, so the number of subjects should be in multiples of 24 (6, 12, and so on). Of course, one can use fewer than twenty-four subjects and add replication as a means of achieving the desired balance. In this latter situation, one could use twelve subjects and have a single replicate; this would mean serving the thirteenth through twenty-fourth orders, shown in Table 4.10, as the replicate. There also will be test plans in which the number of

Table 4.10 Balanced-block design for a four-product test[a]

Subject	Serving order			
	First	Second	Third	Fourth
1	4	3	1	2
2	2	1	3	4
3	1	2	4	3
4	3	4	2	1
5	4	1	2	3
6	3	2	1	4
7	4	2	3	1
8	1	3	2	4
9	2	3	4	1
10	1	4	3	2
11	2	4	1	3
12	3	1	4	2
13	3	2	4	1
14	1	4	2	3
15	2	3	1	4
16	4	1	3	2
17	1	3	4	2
18	2	4	3	1
19	2	1	4	3
20	3	4	1	2
21	3	1	2	4
22	4	2	1	3
23	1	2	3	4
24	4	3	2	1

[a] See text for an explanation of the entries.

Table 4.11 Balanced-block design for a four-product test with replication[a]

Subject	Serving orders within and across the sessions			
	First session	Second session	Third session	Fourth session
1	1 2 3 4	3 2 4 1	2 3 1 4	4 2 1 3
2	2 4 1 3	2 1 3 4	3 4 2 1	1 4 3 2
3	3 1 4 2	4 3 1 2	1 2 4 3	3 4 1 2
4	4 3 2 1	1 4 2 3	4 1 3 2	4 2 3 1
5	2 3 4 1	3 2 1 4	1 2 3 4	1 3 2 4
6	3 1 2 4	2 4 3 1	2 4 1 3	2 1 4 3
7	4 2 1 3	1 3 4 2	3 1 4 2	4 1 2 3
8	1 4 3 2	4 1 2 3	4 3 2 1	1 3 4 2
9	3 4 1 2	2 1 4 3	2 3 4 1	2 4 3 1
10	4 2 3 1	1 3 2 4	3 1 2 4	3 2 1 4

[a] See text for an explanation of the entries.

subjects is not divisible by the serving orders. In Table 4.11, for example, is a design for ten subjects and four sessions, such that there is a reasonable balance. Each product appears equally often in each position; first, second, third, and fourth, but not in each session. All four sessions are necessary for this to be realized, and a similar case is made for adjacent pairings. Each of the adjacent pairs occurs on ten occasions across all four sessions and the ten subjects. When the balance is not possible within a reasonable number of sessions, some compromise must be made to minimize the imbalance that occurs. This particular issue is addressed in a design offered for a five-product test where the number of serving orders is 120 ($5! = 120$). Table 4.12 lists the serving orders for twenty subjects evaluating each product twice or forty subjects once, but with the serving order and the adjacent pairs kept in balance. However, as only forty of the possible 120 serving orders were used to construct the design and with larger panels, one can select serving orders that maintain the balance.

In the situation where the subjects are unable to evaluate all products in a single session but the desire is to stay with the balanced block, the serving orders can be prepared in the same way, as is shown in Table 4.11, and the products can be evaluated in separate sessions, as shown in Table 4.13. With twelve products, three sessions will be required for each subject to evaluate each product once. If replication is necessary, then the design will reflect this requirement and the sensory professional will verify the serving orders for individual products and adjacent pairs.

In the case of balanced-incomplete-block designs, the rules remain the same insofar as individual products and pairings are concerned. Incomplete-block designs require more subjects, and in situations involving products with very pronounced sensory interaction (chili, cigars, and so forth), these designs may be helpful. The number of permutations in an incomplete design is determined from the formula:

$$P_{n,r} = \frac{n!}{(n - r)!}$$

Table 4.12 Balanced-block design for a five-product test[a]

Subject	Serving order				
	First	Second	Third	Fourth	Fifth
1	4	5	1	2	3
2	5	2	4	3	1
3	1	4	3	5	2
4	2	3	5	1	4
5	3	1	2	4	5
6	3	2	1	5	4
7	1	3	4	2	5
8	2	5	3	4	1
9	4	1	5	3	2
10	5	4	2	1	3
11	1	3	5	4	2
12	5	1	2	3	4
13	2	5	4	1	3
14	3	4	1	2	5
15	4	2	3	5	1
16	2	4	5	3	1
17	4	3	2	1	5
18	3	1	4	5	2
19	5	2	1	4	3
20	1	5	3	2	4
21	1	2	3	4	5
22	2	4	1	5	3
23	3	1	5	2	4
24	4	5	2	3	1
25	5	3	4	1	2
26	5	4	3	2	1
27	3	5	1	4	2
28	4	2	5	1	3
29	1	3	2	5	4
30	2	1	4	3	5
31	2	3	4	5	1
32	3	5	2	1	4
33	4	2	1	3	5
34	5	1	3	4	2
35	1	4	5	2	3
36	1	5	4	3	2
37	4	1	2	5	3
38	5	3	1	2	4
39	2	4	3	1	5
40	3	2	5	4	1

[a] See text for an explanation of the entries.

when n is the number of products and r the number of products in a set. Thus, for a balanced-incomplete four-of-five design, there will be 120 orders; for a three-of-five design, there will be sixty orders. If all orders are not served, then every effort is made to maintain the balance of individual and adjacent pairs. Table 4.14 is a four-of-five design for forty subjects that meets these criteria.

Table 4.13 Example from a balanced-block design for a twelve-product test

Subject	Orders of presentation within and across sessions[a]		
	First session	Second session	Third session
1	7 8 9 10	11 12 1 2	3 4 5 6
2	8 10 12 2	4 6 7 9	11 1 3 5
3	9 12 3 6	8 11 2 5	7 10 1 4
4	10 2 6 9	1 5 8 12	4 7 11 3
5	11 4 8 1	6 10 3 7	12 5 9 2
6	12 6 11 5	10 4 9 3	8 2 7 1
7	1 7 2 8	3 9 4 10	5 11 6 12
8	2 9 5 12	7 3 10 6	1 8 4 11
9	3 11 7 4	12 8 5 1	9 6 2 10
10	4 1 10 7	5 2 11 8	6 3 12 9
11	5 3 1 11	9 7 6 4	2 12 10 8
12	6 5 4 3	2 1 12 11	10 9 8 7

[a] See text for an explanation of the entries.

In addition to these designs, there will be situations in which the emphasis is solely on a comparison of one product (a reference) to a series of other products (competitive, experimental, and so on) and there is no concern about how the competitive products compare with one another. The initial idea might be a design in which the subjects evaluate the products in pairs; for example, 1 versus 2, 1 versus 3, and 1 versus 4. However, this design is inefficient in the use of the subjects because of the need to include the reference as one of each pair. There will be more responses for the reference product resulting in an unequal number of judgments in one cell, and there is a risk that the subjects may recognize the reference resulting in some atypical response patterns. This particular approach is often used in the mistaken belief that including a reference with every evaluation increases test precision. Unfortunately, this approach also adds more variability to the testing process inasmuch as the reference product is variable and there also is an increase in adaptation – sensory fatigue. One solution to this problem is to not change the test design, but use a specific analysis of variance followed by Dunnett's test (intended for comparisons involving one product versus all the others).

This particular issue warrants further consideration because it can be troublesome for sensory evaluation. While the use of multiple paired comparisons is an acceptable design and there are appropriate statistical methods for analysis, the more basic issue is whether this is the most efficient use of the subjects' skills and the implication of always including a reference product in a test. From a strict sensory evaluation perspective, the use of multiple pairs is inefficient in the sense that for every test product response there will be a reference product response, which means that the database for the latter product will double that for the other products. This is not necessarily an undesirable situation; however, it will require an analysis that takes into account the unequal cell entries (if the data are pooled). The number of subjects

Table 4.14 Example of a balanced-incomplete-block design for a five-product test[a]

Subject	Serving order			
	First	Second	Third	Fourth
1	1	2	4	3
2	2	3	5	4
3	3	4	1	5
4	4	5	2	1
5	5	1	3	2
6	1	2	5	4
7	2	3	1	5
8	3	4	2	1
9	4	5	3	2
10	5	1	4	3
11	1	3	4	2
12	2	4	5	3
13	3	5	1	4
14	4	1	2	5
15	5	2	3	1
16	1	3	2	5
17	2	4	3	1
18	3	5	4	2
19	4	1	5	3
20	5	2	1	4
21	1	4	5	2
22	2	5	1	3
23	3	1	2	4
24	4	2	3	5
25	5	3	4	1
26	1	4	3	5
27	2	5	4	1
28	3	1	5	2
29	4	2	1	3
30	5	3	2	4
31	1	5	3	4
32	2	1	4	5
33	3	2	5	1
34	4	3	1	2
35	5	4	2	3
36	1	5	2	3
37	2	1	3	4
38	3	2	4	5
39	4	3	5	1
40	5	4	1	2

[a] See text for an explanation of the entries.

required for a test is increased substantially or if the same subjects are used, then the potential of product sensory interaction is concomitantly increased.

Products requiring extensive preparation may introduce additional variability, and the potential exists that the subjects recognize that one product in every pair is the same and this could alter their responses. Subjects might make comparative judgments, that is, the response would be a combination of response to the product coupled with the difference between the products. This is not to imply that a paired test should never be considered and implemented, but that alternatives should be thoroughly explored with the requestor before a final decision is reached. One final comment, the requestor should be aware that the multiple-paired test plan makes it very difficult for post-test comparisons between the experimental products. While there are procedures by which results from such a test can be converted to scaled values and thus enable such comparisons to be made, they must be planned in advance. In Chapter 3, we discussed paired versus scaled procedures and we will have more to say about the topic in Chapter 7.

The sensory professional is confronted with a vast array of options in terms of how best to design a test. There is no single best test method or ideal subject, just as there is no single test design or method of analysis that is applicable in every situation. Each request must be considered with care, to ensure that the test objective is consistent with the requestor's intent and that there is a clear understanding of how the results are expected to be used. The objective and the product will determine the specific method, the experimental design, and the method of analysis. Each element must be kept in perspective and only through a careful and logical process can the best plan be formulated for that particular problem.

Discrimination Testing

5

I. Introduction

Discrimination testing as a class of tests represents one of the two most useful analytical tools available to the sensory professional. It is on the basis of a perceived difference between two products that one can justify proceeding to a descriptive test in order to identify the basis for the difference, or the converse, products are not perceived as different, and appropriate action is taken; for example, the alternative ingredient can be used, etc.

Within this general class of discrimination methods are a variety of specific methods, some are well known, such as paired-comparison and triangle tests, while others are relatively unknown, such as the dual-standard test method. However, all the methods are intended to answer a seemingly simple question, "Are these products perceived as different?" Obviously the response to this question can have major consequences. If

Sensory Evaluation Practices 3rd Edn
ISBN: 0-12-672690-6

the two products are perceived as different (at a previously established level of risk) and the development objective is to not be different, then the objective has not been achieved and the planned sensory testing sequence will likely be changed. Knowledge of perceived product differences enables management to minimize testing where it is either unwarranted or premature, and to anticipate response to the products in the event of additional testing (e.g. products found to be different in a discrimination test will be described as different in a descriptive test). Reaching decisions about product differences based on carefully controlled tests, conducted in a manner that is well defined and unambiguous, leaves little room for error in the decision-making process. To attain this level of sophistication, it is first necessary to understand the behavioral aspects of the discrimination process, along with an appreciation for the nature of the products tested and then to combine that information with knowledge about the various test methods as part of the overall sensory testing scheme. As with any other testing, nothing can be done in isolation. In this chapter, we explore these issues in considerable detail in an effort to clarify what is possible when using discrimination testing.

In an early publication on difference testing, Peryam and Swartz (1950), in discussing flavor evaluation, observed that there existed a "tendency toward oversimplification in a complex field, this lack of appreciation of the true difficulties involved." It would seem that this lack of appreciation for the complexities of the discrimination test stems from the ease and simplicity with which the test is described and implemented. A typical instruction may be "Here are two products; which one has the stronger flavor?" or "Here are three products, which one is different from the other two?" The subject's task would initially appear to be relatively simple; however, this apparent simplicity has led many well-meaning individuals to devise a multitude of test variations without fully appreciating their consequences. In some instances, these variations were intended to increase the amount of information derived from the test; since the individual is there why not get more information! In other instances, the alternatives were proposed as providing a more precise measure of the difference or at the least, insight into the subject's decision-making process. As a result, the literature provides the investigator with an interesting array of options in test methods and analyses, many of which, it turns out, create more problems or do not, in fact, enhance the decision-making process. Whether Peryam and Swartz actually anticipated this outcome is difficult to say; nonetheless, their concern is still valid.

It is clear that the problem is due primarily to a lack of understanding of the basis for the discrimination test, lack of appreciation for subject qualification criteria, considerable confusion as to when the test is used, and the interpretation of the results (Roessler *et al.*, 1978; Stone and Sidel, 1978). At the same time, we need to be aware of the limitations of the discrimination model. After all, the response is a discrete judgment and as such, there are limitations as to what can be done with a result. As a consequence, ill-conceived practices prevail, such as combining difference with a preference question or with a series of descriptive questions, measuring the magnitude of the difference, or misinterpretation of results, such as equating the level of statistical significance with the magnitude of difference. While these efforts appear to have a research focus and/or an effort to extend or enhance the methodology, the sensory professional's failure to recognize the real likelihood for making a wrong decision as a consequence of the variations can have a far more significant and usually deleterious effect on test results and on the credibility of the sensory function within the company.

This problem of misinterpretation is exemplified in two modifications that involve the use of consumers in a discrimination test. It has been suggested that the difference test be used for screening consumers as a prelude to a preference test (Johnson, 1973). The objective of this procedure was to eliminate those individuals who were non-discriminatory and hence could not have a preference, and to obtain a truer measure of product preference. Unfortunately, this approach fails to take into account several basic issues about the discrimination test, not the least of which was the learning processes that all respondents go through when presented with a novel situation such as the discrimination test. This learning process requires many test trials, particularly when the evaluation process involves products that stimulate the chemical senses, and it would be impossible to determine after a single trial whether an individual succeeded or failed because of the novelty of the task, because of a failure to understand the task, or because of an inability to perceive the difference. Finally, consumers who participate in discrimination screening tests are no longer able to provide unbiased preference judgments. There also is a response bias toward the different product, a factor of some importance if one asks a preference question (Schutz, 1954) after the discrimination task. This proposed pre-screening of consumers had some early advocates; however, it appears to have been discarded based on the reasons listed here.

A second example of the misuse of the discrimination test, also involving consumers, is the use of large numbers of consumers. This action is typically proposed so that the results will be representative of the larger population. Testing several hundreds of consumers, a statistically significant difference could be found when the number of correct decisions is very close to chance. With 100 consumers, 59 (59%) correct matches would be significant at the 0.05 probability level; with 200 consumers, 112 (56%) correct matches would be needed for significance. The fundamental concern is not limited to discrimination but extends to any test in which large numbers of responses are obtained in the belief that "there is safety in numbers." While the results are statistically correct, the practical implications could be quite different (Roessler *et al.*, 1978; see also the discussion in Chapter 4 on Type 1 and Type 2 errors). Should one be prepared to state that two products are different in a test involving several consumers when that decision is based on a relatively small number of correct decisions above chance? One of the more ambiguous issues in sensory tests is the number of responses needed for a meaningful decision. In this particular example, the problem is also complicated by the use of consumers of unspecified skill. Consumers are not equally skilled, even at the most simplest of sensory tasks. It is not a question of the consumer's lack of ability to complete the task, but much more important, there is no way to know when the responses are valid. We will discuss this and other examples of misuse of the discrimination test later.

The sensory professional must recognize the inherent weakness and the risk associated with any approach based on faulty assumptions (whether these are subject related, method related, or product related). Failure to address these issues can only result in problems of credibility for a sensory program.

If the conclusions and recommended next steps from a discrimination test are to be accepted by management as reliable, valid, and believable, then it is important that each test be conducted with proper consideration for all aspects of the test – from design, to product preparation and handling and implementation, to data analysis and interpretation. Failure to appreciate all the subtleties of a test increases the risk of data misinterpretation. From a business viewpoint, the ultimate value of sensory evaluation, in general, and the discrimination test, in particular, derives from the reliability and validity of test results and in the manner in which decisions are made, based on the results. Finally, credibility is enhanced when recommended changes are made and subsequent consumer results confirm the decision.

The difference test, a special case of an ordinal scale, is a type of threshold test in which the task is to select the product that is different (Dember, 1963; Laming, 1986). In the classic threshold test, a series of products, some of which contain no stimulus, is presented to the subject one at a time. The subject's task is to indicate whether or not the stimulus was detected. The subject is not required to identify the stimulus, only to indicate that perception has occurred. When identification is required, this may be referred to as a recognition threshold test. Some types of directional difference tests involve recognition or at least differentiation according to a specific characteristic.

In product tests (food, beverage, tobacco, cosmetic, etc.), the problem for the subject is especially difficult because the variable being tested rarely has a one-to-one relationship with the output. That is, a change in the amount of an ingredient such as salt cannot be expected to only affect perceived saltiness, and, in fact, a change in saltiness may not be perceived at all. In addition, all the other sensory characteristics of the products are being perceived and the subject must sort all these sensory inputs to determine which product is different. These latter two issues are extremely important. The failure to appreciate the sensory complexities introduced by a product has caused considerable difficulty for sensory evaluation and for users of the service. For example, perception of salt differences in water would not be representative of the complexities entailed in evaluating salt differences in a prepared food. In spite of this, one continues to encounter use of salt thresholds as a basis for identifying individuals expected to perform above the average in evaluating products containing salt. The salt in a food will have numerous other flavor effects, and hence the direct extrapolation to model systems will be misleading. Finally, the method itself will contribute to task complexity. The methods are not equivalent; some methods involve only two products, while others involve three but require as many as three comparisons for a single decision. This latter issue will have a direct impact on the sensitivity of a subject. In the next section, we describe the most common test methods in preparation for addressing the more complex issues of test selection, data collection, and interpretation.

The subjects and their responses represent a third and equally important component. Difference testing involves choice behavior. The subject must either select one product as different from another, or according to specific criteria, select the one that has more of a specific characteristic; for example, sweetness, saltiness. From the subject's viewpoint, the situation involves problem solving behavior, a challenge in which there are correct and incorrect decisions; to be successful, one must make the correct choice, using all of the information and all of the clues that are available.

To a degree, choice behavior has been taken into account in the statistical analysis of the responses (Bradley, 1953; Roessler *et al.*, 1953; Gridgeman, 1955a). However, on closer examination, it appears that even here the situation is not totally clear. That is, the mathematical model on which the analyses are based does not completely satisfy all test possibilities such as replication. We will have more to say about this issue later in the chapter. In recent years, investigators have focused more attention on the decision criteria in an effort to devise mathematical models of the discrimination process (Ennis and Mullen, 1985, 1986; Bi and Ennis, 2001; Rousseau and Ennis, 2001). These investigators use an approach proposed by Thurstone (1927) and developed further in *signal detection theory* (Green and Swets, 1966). It is evident that the discriminal process continues to present investigators with many challenges not the least of which is a reaffirmation of the complexity of the process.

In view of the diversity of applications and the confusion that appears to exist about the various methods and their uses, it is useful if we first consider the methods in detail, followed by their applications. Only in this way can we hope to develop realistic guidelines for testing and for reaching meaningful decisions about product similarities and differences. While the early literature can provide us with insight into the development of specific methods as well as their modifications (Peryam and Swartz, 1950; Pfaffmann *et al.*, 1954; Gridgeman, 1959; Bradley, 1963), it remains for us to apply this information in the contemporary business environment without sacrificing quality, reliability, and validity. In so doing, we will discuss the discrimination tests used by sensory professionals to make product decisions, without digressing into a discussion about competing psychological theories or models attempting to explain the discrimination process itself.

II. Methods

Basically, the three types of discrimination tests that are used most often are paired comparison, duo–trio, and triangle. A number of other test types have been developed, but because of their lack of use in product evaluation, no more than a cursory examination is justified.

A. Paired-Comparison Test

The paired-comparison test is a two-product test, and the subject's task is to indicate, by circling or by some similar means, the one product that has more of a designated characteristic such as sweetness, tenderness, or shininess, with the designated characteristic having been identified before the test and stated on the scorecard. This method is also identified as a directional paired-comparison test, the "directional" component alerting the subject to a specific type of paired test. An example of the scorecard for the directional paired test is shown in Fig. 5.1, with the direction stated. Examples of test items provided to a subject are shown in Fig. 5.2.

Note that the instructions require the subject to make a decision; that is, the test is forced choice and the decision must be either one or the other of the two products (and not "neither"). This issue of forced-choice tests is discussed later in this chapter in connection with statistical considerations (see also Gridgeman, 1959).

Paired-comparison test

Name ______________________ Code ______________ Date __________

In front of you are two samples; starting with the sample on the left, evaluate each and circle the sample which is most sweet. You must make a choice, even it if is only a guess. You may retaste as often as you wish. Thank you.

847 566

Figure 5.1 An example of a scorecard for use with the directional paired-comparison test. The specific characteristic is stated on the scorecard, as shown here for illustrative purposes.

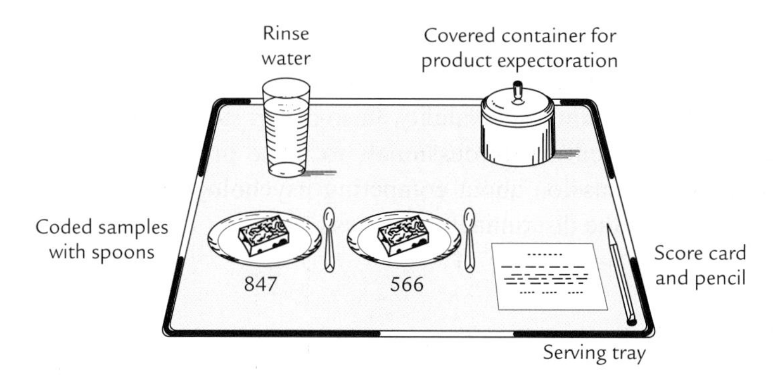

Figure 5.2 Display of samples, scorecard, and other supplies provided to the subject.

The paired-comparison test is relatively easy to organize and to implement; the two coded products are served simultaneously, and the subject, after sampling both products, makes a decision. However, it is often difficult to specify the difference or be confident that the subjects will understand or recognize that difference. By "understand," we mean that the subjects are able to perceive that characteristic in the product. The effect of a single variable such as sweetness or saltiness cannot be totally specified; that is, a single ingredient modification may affect many other product characteristics, and assuming the subjects have responded only to that one is risky. If we must take the time to qualify subjects and train them to recognize a specific characteristic, then the descriptive test should have been selected. In spite of this limitation of the directional, paired test, it still has many applications. For example, by changing the instructions and requiring the subject to indicate only whether the products are the same or different by circling the appropriate word on the scorecard, one can eliminate the issues of directionality and semantics. Of course, the subjects will require very precise instructions to remind them of the

Table 5.1 Number of correct decisions for the non-directional paired test according to serving order

Test	Serving order				Totals (correct/trials)
	AB	BA	AA	BB	
1	5[a]	5	4	5	19/40
2	7	7	0	1	15/40

[a] Entries are typical and used here for illustrative purposes.

change in the task. Almost all subjects have an expectation about product differences, that is, they expect the products to be different. If they are not informed of this change in instructions, their expectations will remain the same, and their responses could be atypical. The two orders of presentation in the directional paired test are AB and BA; however, the "same/different" form has four orders – AB, BA, AA, and BB. The latter two orders are necessary; otherwise, the subjects can state, and some will, that all of the product pairs are different and achieve 100% correct decision! This situation can be monitored if one tabulates responses according to the four orders of presentation. In Table 5.1 are two sets of responses; the first set of responses is consistent with expectation for the AA and BB series, while the latter set of responses is inconsistent and suggestive of misunderstood directions (or some similar problem).

Surprisingly, little use is made of this form of the paired test, yet it should have considerable application where product availability is limited and/or product characteristics (a strong-flavored product, spice mixes, tobacco, and so forth) suggest limiting subject exposure to the products.

Another version of the paired test is the A-not-A procedure. The subject is presented with and evaluates a single product that is then removed and is followed by a second product. The subject then makes a decision as to whether the products are the same (or different). This particular test procedure has considerable merit in those situations where non-test variables such as a color difference may influence results. Sensory evaluation professionals must recognize that a test method can be modified if the problem warrants it; however, these modifications have not changed the basic integrity of the task or the statistical probability.

The paired-comparison procedure is the earliest example of the application of discrimination testing to food and beverage evaluation. Cover, in 1936, described its use in the evaluation of meat (the paired-eating method). Additional attention was given to the discrimination procedure through the evaluation of beverages, as reported in a series of papers by the staff at the Carlsberg Breweries in Copenhagen by Helm and Trolle (1946) and as developed at the Seagram and Sons Quality Research Laboratory (Peryam and Swartz, 1950), and further utilized at the US Army Food and Container Institute. Statistical issues also were addressed by these workers; however, a more thorough discussion of these statistical issues can be found in the work of Harrison and Elder (1950), Bradley (1953, 1963), and Radkins (1957); it also is discussed later in this chapter.

B. Duo–Trio Test

The duo–trio test, developed by Peryam and Swartz (1950), during their work with the Quartermaster Food and Container Institute, represented an alternative to the very popular triangle test that, for some, was a more complex test psychologically; that is, grouping three unknowns.

The duo–trio test was found to be useful for products that had relatively intense taste, odor, and/or kinesthetic effects such that sensitivity was significantly reduced. In the duo–trio test, the subject is presented with three products; the first is identified as the reference (or control) and the other two are coded. The subject's task is to indicate which product is most similar to the reference. A suggested, but not recommended, option is to remove the reference before serving the two coded products. Removal of the reference alters the subject's ability to refer back to the reference, if necessary, before reaching a decision. The change may result in the test being more a test of memory.

The original description of the method also included the possibility for presentation of a warm-up product to minimize first-sample effects. In many tests, product availability may be limited or taste carry-over problems may be such that the use of the warm-up technique would not be feasible. First-sample effects should be minimized through the use of qualified subjects and balanced designs.

The scorecard for the duo–trio test, as shown in Fig. 5.3, is similar to that used in the paired-comparison test, except that there is an "R" to the left of the two coded products and instructions remind the subject to evaluate "R" before evaluating the other two products.

Examples of items provided to the subject are shown in Fig. 5.4. Two design options are available in the duo–trio test. The conventional approach is to balance the reference between the control and test products; however, in some situations, the reference may be kept constant, and the control is usually selected as the reference. As Peryam and Swartz observed, if one product is considered to be more familiar to the subjects, then it would be selected as the reference (this is usually a control or product currently being manufactured). The use of this latter technique is encouraged where changes are contemplated in a product currently available in the market place. This approach, referred to as the constant-reference duo–trio test method, is intended to reinforce the

Duo–trio test

Name ____________ Code ____________ Date ____________

In front of you are three samples, one marked **R** and the other two, coded; evaluate the samples starting from left to right, first **R** and then the other two. Circle the code of the sample different from **R**. You may retaste the samples. You must make a choice. Thank you.

R 132 691

Figure 5.3 Example of scorecard used in the duo–trio test. See text for additional explanation.

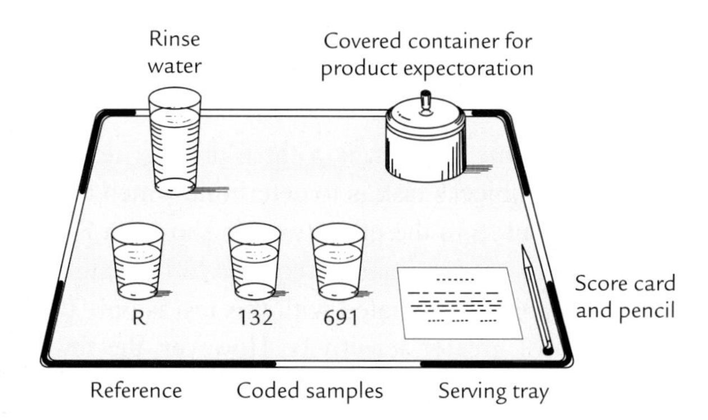

Figure 5.4 Example of items given to the subject for the duo–trio test.

sensory characteristics of the control and enhance detection of any product that is perceived as different. In situations where formulation changes are necessary for a product currently available in the marketplace (because of ingredient availability, cost, and so forth), it is important that the change be perceived by the fewest consumers possible. This objective stems from knowledge that the consumer, while not necessarily being aware, develops a sensory familiarity for a particular brand and would take a negative view of any perceived, unadvertised changes. As a result, changes in a branded product are not intended to be perceived; that is, we do not wish to modify or change the product in any way that might be detected by the consumer. The reader should not assume that the intention is to fool the consumer, but rather it is to ensure that the consumer's sensory reaction to the product remains unchanged! The use of the constant-reference design, by reinforcing the sensory properties of the current brand, increases the likelihood of perception of the difference, thus eliminating unwanted variables that might be perceived. This latter concern is given further consideration in the discussion on test strategy, risk, and the decision-making process.

The chance probability associated with the duo–trio test is identical with that of the other two product tests, $p = \frac{1}{2}$. There are four orders of presentation with the balanced reference versus two orders with the constant reference. A series of experimental designs for this and other discrimination tests is presented later in this chapter.

C. Triangle Test

The triangle test is the most well-known of the three methods. It has been used to a much greater extent because it was mistakenly believed to be more sensitive than other methods (i.e. based on the probability of $\frac{1}{3}$). In fact, the method often was equated with sensory evaluation; that is, individuals claimed they had an active sensory program because their products were "triangulated" (a rather sad fate). This was never anticipated by its developers. As previously mentioned, the method was developed at the Carlsberg Breweries by Bengtsson and co-workers (see Helm and Trolle, 1946) as part of an effort to use sensory tests for the evaluation of beer and to overcome difficulties associated with the directional paired method. The test was applied to a wide variety of products by other workers, most of whom found the method to be quite suitable.

The triangle test, as its name implies, is a three-product test in which all three products are coded and the subject's task is to determine which two are most similar or which one is most different from the other two. As shown in Figs 5.5 and 5.6, the subject is served three coded products and is required to indicate which one is most different. The chance probability associated with this test is only 0.33, which probably accounts for its claim of greater sensitivity. However, the fewer correct scores required for statistical significance should not be confused with the totally separate issue of sensitivity.

The triangle test also is a very difficult test because the subject must recall the sensory characteristics of two products before evaluating a third and then making a decision. In fact, the test can be viewed as a combination of three paired tests (A–B, A–C, and B–C). These issues of test complexity and of sensory interaction should not be ignored by the experimenter (yet often is) when organizing and fielding a triangle test.

After completing a series of olfaction studies comparing the triangle method with the three-alternative forced-choice (3-AFC) signal-detection procedure, Frijters

Triangle test

Name ______________________ Code ______________ Date ________

In front of you are three coded samples, two are the same and one is different; starting from the left evaluate the samples and circle the code that is different from the other two. You may reevaluate the samples. You must make a choice. Thank you.

624 801 199

Figure 5.5 Example of scorecard for the triangle test. See text for further explanation.

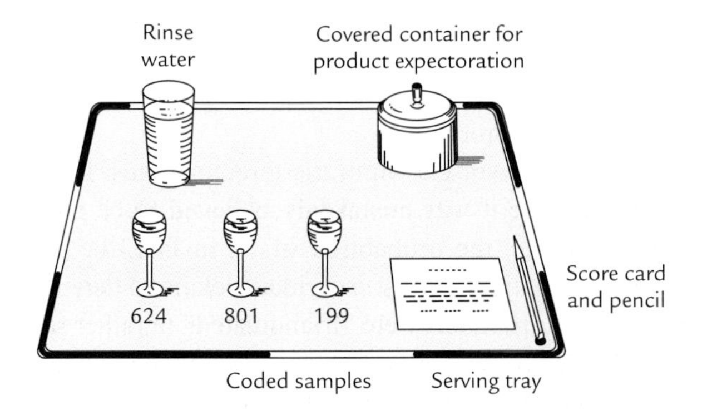

Figure 5.6 Example of items given to the subject for the triangle test.

(1980) concluded that the triangle procedure is improved by modifying the test instruction to read "which two of the three stimuli are most similar?" Intuitively, this instruction makes sense because products from a single production lot can be different thus presenting the subject with a real decision dilemma. This is not necessarily a new development so much as it is a reminder for the experimenter to be thorough in product screening before a test and to provide the subjects with less ambiguous instructions.

D. Other Test Methods

Other methods for discrimination testing, such as the dual-standard method, have been developed, but few have ever been used routinely for product evaluation. The dual-standard method was proposed for use in quality control situations (Peryam and Swartz, 1950). The subject is served four products; two are identified as references A and B and two are coded. The subject's task is to match the reference product with the coded product. The designation of the two references could reflect quality control limits or current production and product outside the limit. Other multi-product tests have been described and used by Mahoney *et al.* (1957) and Wiley *et al.* (1957). Both groups proposed comparing a series of treatments to a single reference; the hypothesis was that this would be relatively efficient and would enable the sensory professional to obtain more than just difference information. To this end, O'Mahony (1979, 1986) describes the *R-index*, a calculated probability value based on signal detection concepts, to provide a measure of the degree of difference between two products. The procedure requires more time and samples than the other methods and has not yet proven to be practical for routine business application. The *n-AFC* methods also provide a degree of difference measure, d' (see Bi *et al.*, 1997). The more complicated analysis, issues related to use of directional difference tests, and relevance of using numbers of correct responses to imply degree of product difference, have thus far resulted in limited used of these methods within the business environment. The availability of other methods, and especially descriptive methods, also make this latter use less viable, and there have been few publications of their application by other researchers. This does not mean that these test methods should be ignored, but rather that the experimenter should proceed with due consideration for all elements of the test; subjects, products, and handling procedure, before selecting a method. Or, at the least be able to differentiate between research and potential applicability of a new development.

Some other types of methods amounted to nothing more than sorting tasks, for example, separating the nine samples into two groups of five and four (Sawyer *et al.*, 1962). The idea is that very few correct choices would be required to achieve significance. Unfortunately, most products possess a multitude of sensations and these approaches, when combined with the human memory limitations, become much less feasible. Basically, one should be capable of handling any discrimination problem using the paired, duo–trio, or triangle test methods. However, the multiple standards method is finding some use in quality control situations.

III. Components of Testing

A. Organization and Test Management

Organization and management of discrimination test activities are essential to the success of any single test, as well as to the success of all testing independent of test type. In this section, we discuss the various issues that occur prior to, during, and after a test. Some are philosophical while others are easily identified as more practical in that they concern the number of subjects, the statistical significance, and so forth. For the sensory professional, however, these issues are interrelated and are discussed here as a practical guide.

Discrimination tests require thorough organization and planning to prevent confusion as to what will be done and how the results can be used. Being organized for testing assumes that there exists a system by which requests are documented, products are screened, objectives are defined, subjects and specific test method are selected, scheduled, and implemented, and, finally, results are reported in a way that is readily understood and actionable. Such organization initially takes time to develop but quickly pays for itself in terms of testing efficiencies, subject participation, and perhaps most important, credibility of the results.

As previously noted, the manner in which the sensory function is organized should reflect realistic industrial sensory practices. By realistic sensory practices we refer to rapid turnaround on requests and complete records concerning information requested, product handling, subjects used, and so forth. For discrimination testing, such records are relatively easy to maintain (e.g. using an Excel© file) once the resources are organized. Initially, this effort will result in a minor increase in record-keeping activities; however, the benefits far outweigh any initial time spent establishing the file. Of course, for those using direct data capture, the time requirements will be further minimized. The failure of sensory departments to maintain sufficient records on past experiences can and will result in duplication of effort. Companies frequently reintroduce technologies, ingredients, and/or products as a result of shifts in consumer behavior or changing economic conditions or as a result of changes in product managers. Duplication can also occur simply through a change in sensory personnel who are not familiar with work done several years earlier. The sensory professional must be able to quickly determine what has been done in the past and the extent to which the current request must be modified to reflect this past experience. For example, preparation procedures for a product may require special equipment or may preclude use of a particular method. A rapid search of the file could save considerable time and avoid a series of false starts.

Before discussing the management issues, it is useful to identify the elements of an organized effort. This information should be retained in a file such as the operations manual, and should comprise:

1. A clear statement of the objective of discrimination testing (this precludes misuse of the method).
2. A brief description of each of the methods; paired, duo–trio, triangle, and any other methods that might be used. Additional information should include

scorecards for each method and a detailed description of each procedure, including suggested containers and serving procedures.
3. A brief description of the test request sequence, including the interview with the requestor, if warranted, product review, test schedule, and report distribution.
4. Examples of the test request and report forms (paper and electronic).
5. A description of subject selection criteria, including screening procedures and performance monitoring.
6. Selected experimental designs with notes on their use.
7. Guidelines on test procedure, including product coding, amount of serving, timing, etc.
8. Methods for data analysis and their interpretation.
9. Suggested motivational efforts for subjects.

As other elements are identified and described, they should be added to the file. The current list is intended to serve only as a guide to those elements that have been found to be universally applicable. In the following sections these elements are discussed in detail to enable the reader to develop a greater appreciation for the specific recommendations.

Before discussing these elements, however, it is useful to address management issues, that is, approaches to making the system work to the best advantage of the company. It should be made clear that test management includes the determination as to whether products warrant a discrimination test, the test to be used, the products to be served, the subjects to be selected, and the reporting of results. Sensory evaluation cannot renege on its responsibility on any of these issues without seriously compromising its integrity. A common weakness is to allow the requestor to stipulate the test method or to consistently use one method for all requests. Basically, the specific objective (see Section IIC) and the characteristics of the product will determine which method is most appropriate. Failure to establish this qualification at the outset will cause some difficulties, as requestors will recognize your indecisiveness and/or your willingness to go along with their test preferences.

Sensory management must also be prepared to address unpopular issues such as rejecting a request because the products may not warrant discrimination testing. Other issues include the frequency of tests, the frequency of subject participation (e.g. once per day, once per week), and the basis for qualifying, selecting, or re-screening individuals. Firm control of what testing is being done must be demonstrated but without necessarily appearing to dictate what is needed. The sensory professional's role as manager is one of "controlled" flexibility; that is, applying sensory evaluation test guidelines in a very precise way while at the same time adapting test procedures to best satisfy unusual test requirements. After all, the science component cannot be compromised to any great extent before the validity of the results is destroyed.

The following sections describe the organization issues, and provide additional background information on the development of a management approach. The topics selected include those most frequently encountered as critical issues in discrimination testing.

B. Test Requests

The request for assistance (in this situation, the measurement of perceived differences) materializes in the form of a written or electronic test request. The use of a formal test request serves many purposes, as demonstrated in Table 5.2. The upper part of the form is completed by the requestor and the lower part is completed by a sensory professional or designate. The upper part includes the name of the requestor, date, priority, test objective, product identification (name, code, how, when, and where manufactured), amount of product available, location, preparation specifications if known, individuals to be excluded from the panel, and report distribution. Depending on sensory professional's experience with the product and the requestor, a meeting may be needed to complete the form. Once completed, the form becomes an essential document for all subsequent test activities for that product, including detailed instructions to the experimenter as well as for report preparation. It should also be noted that the form should be confined to a single page, making it relatively easy to handle and read.

In the following sections, items for the test request form are discussed in detail, in addition to other elements of the discrimination test.

C. Test Objectives

Identification and agreement on a specific test objective and, where appropriate, the overall project objective are essential for the success of a test, both in terms of design and in terms of conclusions and recommendations. In practice, there appears to be a reluctance and at times an inability to state a test objective on the part of the

Table 5.2 Example of a discrimination test request form[a]

To be completed by the requestor	
Experimenter:	Date:
Test objective:	Priority:
Product:	Project number:
Sample location, description, and history (storage, etc.):	
If storage, withdrawal date:	
Sample amounts and availability:	
People to be excluded from testing:	
Report distribution:	
To be completed by sensory evaluation	
Receipt date:	Serving conditions:
Type of test method:	Sample quantity:
Suggested test date:	Sample temperature:
Design:	Carrier:
Number and type of subject:	Serving container:
Methods of sample presentation:	Lighting conditions:
Number of replications:	Other:
Experimenter comments:	

[a] See text for additional explanation.

requestor. This confusion as to objective is especially noticeable during the early stages of program development or when working with an inexperienced requestor. Sensory professionals are often presented with requests in which the test objectives are stated as "do a triangle test between current production barbecue sauce and product code X47A" or some similarly vague statement. This request is neither informative nor a correct statement of an objective. Nonetheless, the sensory professional must proceed to develop, in cooperation with the requestor, an objective that reflects the purposes for the test and the project. For example, an appropriate test objective might be to determine whether there is a perceived difference in a barbecue sauce containing an alternative flavor versus a current flavor. The project objective may be to find a less costly flavor for barbecue sauce that is not perceived as different from that of current production. This information is especially helpful because it not only identifies the specific test objective but also alerts sensory staff to the potential of additional testing and to the fact that current production is the target (and if the duo–trio test were selected, the constant reference procedure would be used).

Alternatively, if the program objective was to screen new flavors, the test method might be the balanced duo–trio or the paired method followed by consumer acceptance tests. Some might choose to not conduct the discrimination test; however, the key here is having stated and documented an objective. It can be seen that test strategy will depend on the project and test objectives.

In those situations where the requestor is not clear as to the basis for the test or how the information will be used, the sensory professional may find it necessary to communicate directly with others who might have more information, for example, marketing research or with the brand manager. In addition to the objective statement, it also is important to determine action criteria and what action will be taken based on the results; for example, if a difference is reported, will products be reformulated or will there be a test to determine its effect on preference.

D. Test Procedures

Once the test objective is established, the sensory department must turn its attention to the other elements of the test. Some of these elements might be considered as cooperative aspects, in that they require assistance from the requestor, while others are strictly a sensory decision (e.g. test method selection).

1. Product screening

This issue precedes a decision that the test is warranted and most often arises during the initial (organization) stages of a sensory evaluation program or when requestors lack familiarity with sensory testing procedures. This does not mean that screening for all other situations can be assumed to be unwarranted, only that the timing (for screening) may be different.

Requestors, especially those who are inexperienced, often submit products that do not warrant testing because the difference is so obvious; that is, the likelihood of obtaining 90–100% correct decisions is very high and thus the test represents a considerable waste of experimenter and panel time and effort. At the time of the meeting, direct examination of the products with the requestor should enable that decision to be reached. In some situations, the sensory professional may still have to test products that have easily perceived differences. This effort can be considered in the context of an educational process, an opportunity for the sensory staff to demonstrate its professional judgment, for the requestor to gain experience in recognizing "easily perceived differences" and their impact on product formulation, and for both to benefit from pretest screening. Product screening may also reveal inherent variability in manufacturing that results in larger differences within a treatment variable than between treatment variables, making the discrimination test untenable, but leading to an alternative test method (e.g. a descriptive test).

Pretest screening also will enable the sensory professional to clarify any special requirements related to preparation and serving and to identify any additional background material required as it relates to the product or the test.

Occasionally, sensory evaluation may receive a test request but the product will not be available for preview until just before testing is scheduled to commence. This is obviously risky and the sensory staff will have to devise some means for dealing with this kind of situation. If previous work with the product or product class and with the developer has been successful, then one could proceed; however, there should be at least a last-minute check. It is not so much a matter of mistrust, but rather an issue of minimizing risk. Once data are collected, they cannot be disregarded (no matter what the requestor wishes) and the fact that the products were inappropriate may be forgotten. Product screening does not guarantee elimination of judgment errors; however, it will certainly minimize these kinds of risk.

2. Test selection

Selection of the specific test method can be a challenge for the sensory professional for several reasons. Requestors and sensory professionals often become attached to a particular method, and in the latter's situation, have organized their testing in such a way that is most convenient to use just that method. Unfortunately, this situation tends to feed on itself. Continued reliance on a single method causes one to develop a rationale for its continued use, and requestors also become "comfortable" with the method and express discomfort when it is not used. To avoid disagreements with requestors, sensory evaluation will continue to use the method and will receive reinforcement for this decision from test requestors, usually in the form of no disagreement.

The literature provides a somewhat conflicting selection of conclusions regarding the sensitivity of the various test methods; some sensory professionals suggest the triangle is more sensitive than the duo–trio and the paired tests, while others have arrived at the opposite conclusion (Dawson and Dochterman, 1951; Byer and Abrams, 1953; Hopkins, 1954; Schlosberg *et al.*, 1954; Gridgeman, 1955b; Hopkins and Gridgeman, 1955; Radkins, 1957; Buchanan *et al.*, 1987). Rousseau *et al.* (1998) reported that the same–different method is more powerful than the triangle and duo–trio; this will need to be confirmed further on an empirical basis with subjects screened for their discrimination ability and with a broad range of products and differences.

A careful examination of this literature provides useful insight concerning sensory evaluation methods research. Test method sensitivity appears to be more a matter of product, how the discrimination question is phrased, and the manner in which the investigator selected subjects than it is a matter of method (see, e.g. Buchanan *et al.*, 1987). The issue of subject qualification has not been given much consideration and will be discussed in the next section. On the other hand, the type of product is recognized as having an influence. However, there is no overwhelming database on sensitivity that could influence an investigator to select one discrimination test in preference to another. While the statistical literature does provide some evidence in support of the triangle test and the AFC methods, this conclusion must be considered solely within that context; that is, independent of behavioral issues such as subject skills, replication, and the products' sensory characteristics.

The reader is reminded that there also are conflicting conclusions with regard to this statistical conclusion (see Gridgeman, 1955b; Bradley, 1963). As stated at the outset of this discussion, on a practical application basis, we find no discrimination test method to be any more or less sensitive; all are equally sensitive. All discrimination methods have the same basic goal and all are essentially different forms of the two-sample choice situation. Differences between methods can and do arise as a result of the characteristics of the products and the use of qualified subjects. For example, products that have intense flavors and aromas, that are spicy and/or are difficult to remove from the palate, or that have physiological effects (cigarettes, distilled beverages) usually preclude the use of the triangle test. Subjects must smell and/or taste three coded products and make six comparisons – A versus B, A versus C, B versus C – before reaching a decision. While it might be argued that subjects do not always make the six comparisons, there is no question that there are more comparisons to be made in the triangle test than in the duo–trio; the fewest comparisons are made in the paired test. The point is that sensory evaluation must first consider product and objective before reaching a decision about the most appropriate method for that problem.

Whenever products are being compared with a current franchise (i.e. product now being manufactured), the duo–trio, constant-reference test method is most appropriate (Peryam and Swartz, 1950). As mentioned previously, this approach provides maximum sensory protection for the current franchise. Since there is one less comparison (R versus A, R versus B), there is a reduction in possible sensory interactions and there is maximum reinforcement of the sensory properties of the current product (it is evaluated twice versus once for the experimental product). Signal detection theory of perception indicates that the more familiar and focused one is with a signal (the stimulus) the more likely one will detect that stimulus which is different. Other factors also could reduce the choices to the paired procedure. The paired-comparison method remains the most widely used for strongly flavored products, those that have differences other than the variable being tested, and for many personal care products that require home use.

With simultaneously available products, visual difference as an unwanted influence on subjects is often treated in rather bizarre ways; for example, blindfolded subjects, darkened rooms, or a variety of colored lights. These extreme situations can arise when a researcher is inflexibly committed to one specific test method. In fact, visual differences can be more easily managed by using a paired method with a sequential serving procedure. This particular issue will be discussed further in the section on lighting.

Thus, test method selection is the result of a series of probing questions and answers by the sensory professional. The focus is on test objective, type and availability of product, preparation procedures, product sensory characteristics, test method capabilities, availability of qualified subjects, and the use of the results. Such an approach leads to a much higher quality database, and also provides more reliable and valid product information.

3. Subject selection

The importance of subject selection for a discrimination test has long been acknowledged (see Helm and Trolle, 1946; Giradot *et al.*, 1952), yet this has often been neglected in many sensory test operations. Current procedures vary widely, with the most common practice being the use of individuals who have previously participated and/or who are located close to the testing area. This approach appears to be based on the misconception that sensory skill and technical training/experience are equivalent; that one's knowledge about a project, such as direct participation in that project, automatically qualifies one to be a subject. While it is true that the more knowledge a subject has about product differences, the better he or she can focus attention, and their performance can be expected to improve (Engen, 1960). In fact, what happens is that these individuals (who work close to the test facility) base their judgments on what they think the response should not be what they actually perceive. Another approach makes use of large numbers of consumers, 100 or more; however, it is not clear as to the basis for this practice (Morrison, 1981; Buchanan *et al.*, 1987; Rousseau *et al.*, 2002). It has been suggested that use of unscreened consumers provides a more typical result of what can be expected in the marketplace. This approach overlooks several factors, including the fact that about 30% of the consumer population cannot discriminate differences and identifying these individuals takes as many as twenty or more trials. Using unqualified consumers results in a substantial amount of variability that will mask a difference, leading to a wrong decision. Alternatively, a significant difference could be obtained entirely by chance. Using large numbers of consumers increases the risk of finding statistical but not practical differences. We will have more to say about this latter issue in a subsequent discussion in this chapter. Finally, it should be kept in mind that the purpose for the test (in most instances) is to minimize the risk of concluding that there is no difference when, in fact, there is. Minimizing risk is achieved by using a homogeneous population of subjects qualified to participate based on their sensory skill. The issue of how one becomes qualified to participate is not a new or novel concept. For many years use of threshold tests have been advocated, and continues to be used especially for some descriptive tests, as a means of selecting subjects. Unfortunately, the evidence indicated that such threshold measures had no relationship to subsequent performance with more complex stimulus systems (see Giradot *et al.*, 1952). Mackey and Jones (1954) reported that the threshold measures did not serve as useful predictors of performance in product tests. Schlosberg *et al.* (1954), as part of a larger study on panel selection procedures, discovered only a weak relationship between selected life-history questions and results from a series of discrimination tests, or even between one test trial and another, although the latter trials were sufficiently promising to warrant additional study. As a footnote, the authors reported that "performance during the first two days of testing had a fair predictive value … during the following 20-day period."

In a related study, Sawyer *et al.* (1962) compared correct judgments from session to session, as well as performance within a session, and observed that it was possible "to predict the proportion of judges whose sensitivity can satisfy established specifications."

The literature clearly indicated that the selection process was critical to the quality (reliability and validity) of the results. Boggs and Hansen (1949), Peryam *et al.* (1954), Bennet *et al.* (1956), and Dawson *et al.* (1963a,b) all recommended that the subjects participating in a discrimination test be selected based on their skill. Later publications provided a reaffirmation of the positive impact of training on performance (see McBride and Laing, 1979; Frijters *et al.*, 1982; O'Mahony *et al.*, 1988). The former researchers emphasized experience, subject attitude, and past performance as factors that should be taken into consideration in selecting subjects. From a practical point of view, these requirements seemed reasonable and are consistent with our own experiences. It was clear from reviewing results from thousands of tests that screening individuals and excluding those who could not differentiate differences at greater than chance, yielded more consistent conclusions, results exhibited greater face and external validity, and from a practical point of view, there were no decision reversals based on other test results. This empirical evidence led us to develop a set of guidelines for discrimination testing that have proven to be extremely useful:

1. The recruited subjects must be "likers" of the product class or must be "willing to try" the product as determined from the product attitude survey (PAS). Since the subjects will be asked to participate on numerous occasions, product liking is important. Greater familiarity with product subtleties are another potential benefit of product users and likers. Dislike for a product eventually manifests itself in tardiness, greater variability in performance, and general disruption of the testing process.
2. All subjects must be qualified (based on sensory skill) and have participated in not less than two tests in the previous month. In general, the sensory forgetting curve is quite steep and an individual must maintain the skill through regular participation. For different types of products, the frequency of participation is empirically derived; however, it will probably not be less than once per month. This should not be construed to mean that practice tests should be created if no regular requests have been received. It is rare for a sensory program to not have tests scheduled every week. Similarly, one can overuse an individual subject; for example, testing several times per day for months at a time. This always results in poor motivation and poor performance. The major concerns here are absence of the subjects from their regular work and complaints from their management, along with test fatigue; that is, too much testing.

3. Each subject must have a composite performance record that is greater than chance probability (separate $p = \frac{1}{3}$ from $p = \frac{1}{2}$). No subject should be selected if his or her performance is poorer than chance based on at least the previous three or four tests where the panel result has declared that a difference is present. Including subjects that are non-discriminators increases the risk of incorrect decisions about product differences.
4. No subject should have specific technical knowledge about the products, test objective, and so on. A subject who has prior knowledge about the variables is likely to respond based on what the result is supposed to be rather than responding perceptually.
5. No more than one or two subjects from the same specific work area should be scheduled at the same time. While it may be highly desirable to complete a panel by scheduling everyone from a single location, this approach can have negative long-term consequences. Sensory evaluation should never empty a laboratory or work area, no matter how brief the test time; since participation is voluntary, it will alienate laboratory managers by causing undue disruption of their work.
6. Employee subjects should be rewarded (not monetarily) for their participation after each test and at other convenient times (e.g. holidays). Rewards for participation should never be taken for granted and subjects must be made welcome. Food and beverage rewards and acknowledging past performance all are examples of this welcome.
7. There is an upper limit to the frequency of testing for each subject. An individual could participate in several discrimination tests per week; however, situations may arise where there is need for two to three tests per day for several days. Such a situation should be agreed to in advance. From a skills point of view, testing more than once per day should lead to greater precision. From a practical point of view, this approach will be quite disruptive of that individual's regular work routine and will lead to conflict. Consider the manager who finds that his staff of ten is spending the equivalent of one or two man-days per week as test subjects!

These guidelines necessitate the development and maintenance of complete records for each subject. The importance of these records cannot be underestimated, for without them it would be difficult to make reasonable subject decisions. Once the decision is made to establish performance records, it then becomes a matter of determining how to organize the record such that it is accessible for both subject selection (monitoring performance) and adding new information (current results). The ideal system is one that has the stored information accessible with a PC and printer in the sensory facility. The performance records coupled with other subject records, including the PAS, will be of great value as the program develops.

One example of a performance record is given in Table 5.3. In this particular example, the first column is used for identification of product; all subsequent columns list the test date, test type, and rates of correct total decisions. Note that the $p = \frac{1}{2}$ and $p = \frac{1}{3}$ tests are separated to prevent errors in computation of performance. The actual layout of the record does not have to conform to Table 5.3 (i.e. the rows and columns

Table 5.3 Example of a performance record for an individual subject[a]

Name________________________ Location________________

	Test type			
	PC[b]	DT[b]	T[b]	DT
Date	25/11	28/11		
Dry cereal	1/2	2/2		0/2
Dry cereal			1/2	
Date	4/12	5/12		
Vanilla ice cream	2/2	1/2		

[a] Entries are the ratio of correct to total decisions. Note that $p = \frac{1}{2}$ and $p = \frac{1}{3}$ are separate. See text for additional explanation.
[b] PC, paired comparison; DT, duo-trio; T, triangle.

can be switched). The important point is that there be a record that is understandable to the sensory professional. The performance record is used with particular emphasis on the most recent 30 days, which is a realistic basis for selection. Earlier records provide a historical "perspective" on individual subjects and could be used for selection if an insufficient number of subjects were available for a test. This particular decision would be judgmental on the part of sensory evaluation.

In this discussion on subject selection, emphasis has been placed on the immediate past performance (e.g. the last eight to ten tests) of the subjects as a basis for selection. The expectation is that the individual subjects will maintain their proficiency; however, there should not be major concern if that does not occur in a single test. For example, if a subject is operating at 65% correct decisions, performance in a single test might diverge substantially, for example, 0 or 100% correct, without cause for concern. Obviously, criteria for not accepting a subject will need to be developed. One such criterion might be 50% or less correct decisions for four consecutive tests (with the panels in those tests finding a statistically significant difference and percent correct at ~65%).

Another aspect of subject performance-selection criteria is the change in performance over time. Considerable emphasis has been given to identifying and using subjects who are discriminators, that is, subjects whose performance is consistent and greater than chance. Following screening, the subjects participate in tests. Cumulative performance records are maintained and used as the primary basis for continued selection in testing. However, over time it may appear that the level of performance is decreasing, as if the subjects have "lost" some of their sensory skills. In fact, this movement toward chance performance should be viewed in more positive terms; the product differences are smaller (hence more difficult to perceive) because the formulation/development specialist is better able to prepare products as a result of information derived from previous tests. This is a dynamic system in which sensory skills that are improving with testing are being challenged by smaller and smaller product differences. This relationship, depicted graphically in Fig. 5.7, provides a visual display of the relationship between performance and product formulation.

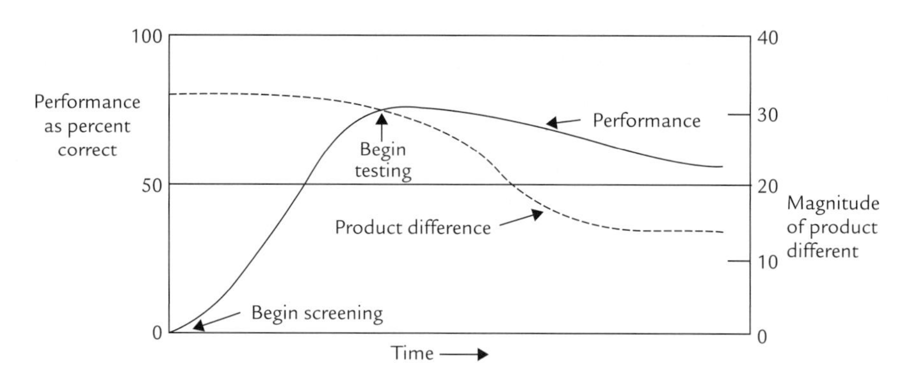

Figure 5.7 Visual representation of the changes that occur in the skill of the subjects over time as product formulation efforts yield products with smaller differences. See text for additional explanation.

There usually is a keen desire on the part of subjects to assess their own performance in comparison with that of their peers and this is particularly true for new subjects. Performance records permit graphing individual percent correct responses compared with the panel. The graphs can represent tests done on a chronological basis or a grouping of tests by product class. Each subject is given his or her own graph of correct matches or percentage compared with the panel. Confidentiality is easily maintained by sending individual graphs to each subject via the company's e-mail system, and the subjects can compare results with one another if they choose to do so. For some individuals, participation represents a mark of special significance relative to fellow workers, and to be more correct than other panel members can enhance this "special" identification. Annual awards recognizing best performances would further enhance their being special. Obviously, such an attitude is desirable for motivational purposes; however, it should not overwhelm the contribution of all other participants. From a sensory viewpoint, correctness of decision is important; but this must be placed within the context of the test itself because all responses are important, not just those that are correct.

Quite independent of these empirical approaches to subject selection, there also are statistical approaches, the most notable being the method described as sequential analysis. The method was adapted from the work of Wald and Rao (cited in Bradley, 1953) and a detailed description of the method can be found in reports by Bradley and others (Radkins, 1958; Steiner, 1966; Amerine and Roessler, 1983). Basically, the experimenter sets limits for the proportions of correct and incorrect decisions as well as the associated α and β risks. This information permits computation of two parallel lines, the distance between representing the area within which the subjects "remain" until their performance enables them to be accepted or rejected for a test. Depending on the levels of risk (and limits of sensitivity), these lines can be shifted. Radkins proposed using the technique as a basis for evaluating product differences, without depending on a fixed number of subjects. According to Radkins, this procedure has the "inherent advantage of smaller sample sizes ..." although the risks of such an approach compared with a fixed panel size were also recognized. However, all issues associated with subject participation must be kept in balance and assessed before any procedure that is used.

4. Product preparation and serving

The need for detailed attention to product preparation and serving conditions is often overlooked or understated. Earlier in this discussion, considerable emphasis was placed on product screening to be sure that the product and the test were suitably matched. The issue of product preparation also was considered. That particular problem should be resolved in advance so that preparation does not introduce another confounding variable. It must be clearly understood that all aspects of the test must be kept "constant" to ensure that the responses reflect only the variable being evaluated. After all, the subjects are well aware of the task and use all their senses to make a decision. In those situations where product differences are very small, any cues, conscious or subconscious, will influence the decision. Such minor issues as serving temperature, amount of serving, or the nature of that serving can have a substantial impact on some subjects. For example, in food evaluation, some samples of a salad dressing containing cheese could easily have more pieces of cheese than others, thus incorrectly cueing or confusing some subjects.

Product serving is especially important in the discrimination test because of the usual simultaneous serving, which provides for direct comparison. Since the subject's task is only to indicate whether there is a difference, any cue is used. It may be necessary to use a sequential serving procedure when product differences, other than the test variable, cannot be eliminated, such as a visual difference. This particular problem also is discussed in the section on lighting.

The serving procedure could be changed for some products. For example, evaluation of fragrance samples can be accomplished by having subjects move from station to station and then make their decisions. The distance between stations can be kept to a minimum, about 3–6 ft apart. The fact that the subjects move rather than the products does not affect the results. It is important for the sensory professional to make every effort to utilize existing methodology and to consider all the options.

Finally, we would be remiss if we did not comment on certain practices involving discrimination tests in which attempts were made to circumvent non-test variables by means of subject instructions. The most common practice is to tell subjects to ignore a known difference (e.g. visual or textural) and evaluate the flavor or feel, as if the perceptual and decision-making processes were independent. Subjects, no matter how well trained, will almost automatically focus on the variable that they are supposed to ignore. Such an approach can only lead to confusion and to questionable testing practices for sensory evaluation. The product's characteristics must be carefully considered to be sure that it can be served in a way that does not mask differences or provide cues. The responsibility for these decisions rests with the sensory staff.

5. Lighting

In discrimination testing, lighting will become an issue when visual differences occurred during product formulation that were unrelated to the variable being studied. Usually, the requestor cannot correct the difference without great inconvenience, so the test must be done in spite of the difference. In the discussion on booth lighting in Chapter 2, recommendations were made regarding the amount of light (controlled and up to 100 ft-candles illumination) and the type of light (incandescent for ease of handling). The problem encountered with lighting is the fascination with the use of red, yellow, or green lights, and especially the use of red lights to mask color differences (usually in foods). Although it is assumed that the light will mask the color difference, there is little evidence to support this assumption, and the use of colored lights for some products may even enhance a visual difference. Some facilities using colored lights are so designed that light from the preparation area comes through the pass-throughs and shines on the products during serving, allowing subjects to easily observe the differences. While it is possible to design a facility so as to provide complete control of the lights, the costs associated with such effort do not warrant the investment. In other procedures, subjects are blindfolded or rooms so darkened that vision is significantly impaired.

From a behavioral viewpoint, these procedures are quite risky, introducing additional variables, and are not recommended. To begin with, any conclusion about product differences (or lack thereof) must be stated in terms of the experimental condition; for example, a difference when served under red light (but is the difference due to the test variable, the effect of the lighting, or the combination of these). An aspect of this practice is the potentially negative impact on management. When management reviews results with products present, considerable doubt may develop concerning the test conclusion. For more discussion on this topic the reader is referred to Chapter 2. Test situations that are inherently weak or subject to misinterpretation must be avoided. Where differences unrelated to the test variable exist, sensory evaluation must make note in the record and then consider whether the discrimination test is appropriate. If so, the recommended procedure would be to use a monadic, sequential serving order; that is, serve the products one at a time, remove the first one before serving the second, and then request a decision (this is the non-directional paired comparison). This procedure minimizes the visual difference and provides a more realistic test of the variable.

It can be argued that this latter serving procedure does not overcome management's concern about obvious visual differences; however, the approach is more realistic in terms of the test conditions and more representative of the manner in which the product would typically be evaluated or is typically consumed.

Another approach is to use colored containers for the product. However, as with any other experimental modification, the sensory professional should ensure that such an approach does not contribute cues or serve as a confounding variable. It should be apparent that sensory evaluation must evaluate each situation with care, as there are no easy or simple solutions.

Despite all these arguments, one continues to encounter the use of lights and other atypical means for masking unintended product differences. It is unfortunate because it casts the science in a rather unscientific "light."

6. Carriers

The use of carriers in discrimination testing is a complex and at times emotional issue, especially for food and beverage evaluation. Carriers are defined as materials that accompany the product being tested. In food evaluation, a carrier could be milk served with a ready-to-eat breakfast cereal, cake with frosting, butter on bread, lettuce with salad dressing, and so forth. For other products, the use of carriers is generally less of a problem than the form of the product. For example, in evaluating different fabric treatments, the fabrics could be tested as swatches or as finished garments. On the other hand, evaluating differences in tobacco blends is best accomplished as a test of the finished product; cigar, cigarette, pipe tobacco, etc.

In general, carriers tend to dilute and/or mask differences and are not recommended. Nonetheless, they continue to be used and the issue must be examined in more detail. Probably the single most persuasive argument advanced by proponents of the use of the carrier is "that is how the product is consumed." While this observation is correct it should be kept in mind that not all of a product is consumed with a carrier. In addition, the use of a carrier should be viewed within the context of the discrimination test and its relationship to product consumption in the home. The discrimination test is not intended to duplicate product use at home. It is a unique test situation carried out in a controlled environment, using a selected and homogeneous group of subjects. The sole purpose of the test is to determine whether there is a perceived difference between two products, all other factors kept constant, and to determine the level of significance associated with that decision.

In most projects, the objective is to make a change (ingredient, process, and so on) that either is not detected or is detected by the fewest number of people. If the experienced subject cannot perceive the change under the most controlled of conditions, then we are confident that the difference will not be perceived by the consumer. Therefore, our test design incorporates many features that minimize the risk of an incorrect decision; that is, we use a group of qualified subjects (experienced, likers/users of product, known discriminators); we use a balanced serving order; and we take care to standardize product preparation and serving conditions. All of these "conditions" are intended to reduce the chances of the subject's decision being influenced by a non-test variable.

Carriers introduce the potential for problems in terms of testing procedure and in the interpretation of the result. Each carrier will have unique physical and chemical characteristics that will require standardization and that, in turn, may limit the extent to which results can be generalized. Use of a carrier does not allow us to state that the difference is perceived without a carrier.

Consider the following situation. The objective of the test is to determine whether there is a perceived difference between products A_1 and A_2 (the null hypothesis is that $A_1 = A_2$). If a statistically significant difference exists (without use of a carrier), variable A_2 is rejected; that is, the objective has not been met. Even if a second test with a carrier shows no significant difference, the sensory professional's response to the requestor must first emphasize that the variable does have an effect; that is, A_2 is perceived as different from A_1. It is especially risky to ignore a difference that can be masked by carriers; sensory evaluation is essentially reporting no difference when, in fact, there is a difference! Consumers do taste products without a carrier, as well as with a multitude of different carriers, so their use in testing will create additional problems.

This does not mean that carriers should be forbidden from discrimination testing. Rather, our intention is to call attention to one of the more perplexing aspects of testing.

If there is reason to believe that a particular carrier is essential due to specific flavor interactions, it might be appropriate to prescreen products, and if some doubt remains, to implement discrimination tests both with and without a carrier. Alternatively, some compromises are desirable in certain situations. For example, in the evaluation of a pizza sauce mix, it was agreed that flavor interactions with crust components resulted in a sauce flavor that could not be achieved by heating the sauce alone. However, owing to variability in pizza crust within a brand, it was determined that the pizza would be cooked and the sauce scraped from the crust and tested by itself. Thus, the chemical reactions were allowed to occur and the subjects' responses were not influenced by crust thickness or other non-test variables.

The sensory professional must evaluate each request in terms of the objective as well as the background of the request and the ultimate use of the information. In the case of carriers, all the options must be thoroughly explored before proceeding.

7. Coding

As noted in the previous chapter, products are coded using three-digit codes, and no two products should be assigned the same code in a test. It is naive to assume that subjects will not communicate with one another after a test, for example, when passing one another in the corridor. Perhaps more troublesome is the subject who assumes that a certain coding is always used. While one can never expect to eliminate this notion, adherence to three-digit coding, different for each product, will minimize these effects and reduce bias for a particular number or code.

8. Experimental design

The design of discrimination tests is reasonably well defined, with minimal opportunity for improvization. The primary concern is attention given to the balanced order of presentation and sufficient responses for confidence in the conclusions (Harries, 1956; Gridgeman, 1958).

The designs described herein are based on the use of replicate responses by each subject and a pooled database of approximately forty responses. The rationale for this approach is discussed in Section IIIE (see also Roessler *et al*., 1978).

For the paired comparison, the two orders of presentation are AB and BA; for the "same-or-different" form, the four orders of presentation are AA, AB, BA, and BB. Thus, one could easily develop appropriate experimental designs for any number of subjects. However, our desire to obtain replicate responses adds a degree of complexity, one that we will demonstrate is well worth the effort. Table 5.4 contains the serving orders for twenty subjects for the paired-comparison test, with direction specified (total N is forty for statistical analysis).

Several characteristics of this design warrant comment. First, some subjects are served the same order twice. This is recommended to minimize subjects' theorizing that if the first sample of the first pair is the "stronger" one, then it will have to be the second sample of the second pair. Remember that the experienced subject, used on a regular basis, will become especially aware of the entire testing process (consciously or subconsciously). The design in Table 5.4 results in four orders for the two pairs, presented one (pair) at a time, and in our experience minimizes subjects' belief that

Table 5.4 A serving order for the directional paired-comparison test[a]

Subject	Serving order	
	First set	**Second set**
1	AB	BA
2	BA	BA
3	BA	AB
4	AB	AB
5	BA	AB
6	AB	BA
7	AB	AB
8	BA	BA
9	BA	AB
10	BA	BA
11	AB	AB
12	AB	BA
13	AB	BA
14	BA	AB
15	AB	AB
16	BA	BA
17	AB	AB
18	BA	BA
19	BA	AB
20	AB	BA

[a] One replication per subject.

they "know" the answers (or have broken the code). Second, this particular serving order can and should be varied, so that the first subject does not always receive the same order, and so on.

For the non-directional paired test, same-or-different, the twelve orders of two pairs are presented one (pair) at a time as indicated in Table 5.5. Thus, the level of statistical significance can be computed on a total of forty-eight responses. As noted previously, these serving orders can be changed; however, the more critical issue is to remind subjects that a particular serving order is not related to previous orders and that their responses should reflect what they perceive in products they are evaluating at that moment.

For the duo–trio tests, balanced and constant-reference, the orders of presentation with replication are similarly organized. The layout for the balanced reference design for sixteen subjects is presented in Table 5.6. For the constant reference, the design layout for twenty subjects is presented in Table 5.7; there are two serving orders for each subject, presented one set at a time, yielding a total of 40 responses.

The six orders of presentation for the triangle test, as in the previous design layouts, offer additional orders of presentation with replication within the session. Table 5.8 provides the design layout for eighteen orders of presentation for two triads served one triad at a time, and yields a total $N = 36$.

In reviewing this layout, the reader should note that other orders of presentation are possible and that the different product is equally balanced between A and B for

Table 5.5 A serving order for the paired same-or-different test[a]

Subject	Serving order	
	First set	Second set
1	AB	AA
2	BB	BA
3	BA	AB
4	AB	BA
5	AA	BB
6	BB	AA
7	AB	BB
8	AA	AB
9	BB	AB
10	AA	BA
11	BA	AA
12	BA	BB
13	AA	BB
14	AB	BB
15	BB	AB
16	BA	AA
17	BB	BA
18	AB	BA
19	BB	AA
20	AA	AB
21	AA	BA
22	BA	BB
23	AB	AA
24	BA	AB

[a] One replication per subject.

Table 5.6 A serving order for the duo–trio test, balanced reference[a]

Subject	Serving order	
	First set	Second set
1	R_A AB	R_B BA
2	R_B BA	R_A BA
3	R_A BA	R_A BA
4	R_B BA	R_A AB
5	R_B BA	R_B AB
6	R_B AB	R_B BA
7	R_A AB	R_A BA
8	R_A AB	R_B AB
9	R_A AB	R_A AB
10	R_A BA	R_B BA
11	R_B AB	R_A BA
12	R_B AB	R_B AB
13	R_A BA	R_A AB
14	R_B BA	R_B BA
15	R_B AB	R_A AB
16	R_A BA	R_B AB

[a] One replication per subject.

Table 5.7 A serving order for the duo–trio test, constant reference[a]

Subject	Serving order: First set	Serving order: Second set
1	R AB[b]	R BA
2	R BA	R BA
3	R AB	R AB
4	R BA	R AB
5	R AB	R AB
6	R BA	R AB
7	R AB	R BA
8	R BA	R BA
9	R AB	R AB
10	R BA	R AB
11	R AB	R BA
12	R BA	R BA
13	R AB	R AB
14	R BA	R AB
15	R AB	R BA
16	R BA	R BA
17	R AB	R BA
18	R AB	R AB
19	R BA	R BA
20	R BA	R AB

[a] One replication per subject.
[b] In this series R is always the same, A or B.

Table 5.8 A serving order for the triangle test, balanced order[a]

Subject	Serving order: First set	Serving order: Second set
1	ABB	ABA
2	BAB	AAB
3	BBA	BAA
4	AAB	BAB
5	BBA	ABA
6	ABB	AAB
7	BAA	BAB
8	ABA	BBA
9	AAB	ABB
10	BAA	BBA
11	ABA	ABB
12	BAB	BAA
13	AAB	BBA
14	BBA	AAB
15	BAA	ABB
16	ABB	BAA
17	ABA	BAB
18	BAB	ABA

[a] One replication per subject.

each subject. One might also consider a triangle test design in which the different products in both triads could be the same for some subjects (e.g. AAB and BAA, or ABB and BAB). This latter approach would be appropriate when the triangle test is used on a regular basis (i.e. daily) and when concern exists about the subjects' guesses as to which product is not the different one based on the first test. The subject might conclude that if the first product was the different one in the first set, it will not be the different one in the second set. The extent to which this reasoning might apply is not known; however, one could speculate that if it were widely applicable, more significant differences could be expected to occur in the latter tests of a series (of tests). Nonetheless, it is an issue that the sensory professional must consider when monitoring test results on a long-term basis.

There is no question that additional design layouts should be developed for the various types of discrimination tests. Ideally, a series of these designs with explanatory notes should be available, so that the sensory staff does not have to recreate them before each test.

E. Data Analysis and Interpretation

Analysis of traditional paired, duo–trio, and triangle discrimination test responses is reasonably well defined, based on the binomial distribution or approximations of the binomial distribution derived from other types of distributions [e.g. chi-square (χ^2)], the normal probability curve (Bengtsson and Helm, 1946; Lockhart, 1951; Roessler *et al.*, 1953, 1978; Bradley, 1963, 1975; McNemar, 1969; Alder and Roessler, 1977). In this discussion, attention is focused on the determination of statistical significance, the interpretation of the statistical value, and some of the associated issues, such as one-tailed and two-tailed tests, and the importance of replication. In a subsequent section (and in Chapter 4), we discuss Type 1 and Type 2 errors and some of the options that are possible in terms of statistical power in the decision-making process. This discussion also covers the related topics of number of subjects per test and number of responses per subject per test.

Computing statistical significance was described by Roessler and co-workers in a series of publications (Roessler *et al.*, 1948, 1953, 1956; Baker *et al.*, 1954), such that one could refer to tables that would indicate whether a particular number of correct decisions was statistically significant at the 0.05, 0.01, and 0.001 significance levels. Formulae were also provided for computation of significance for values not included in the tables. The tables were well received because they were easy to use; there were no computations and a conclusion could be reached within minutes of obtaining the last scorecard. However, this simplicity had a disadvantage, which could not have been foreseen at the time. The popularity of the tables led to some misuse and to misunderstanding relative to the derivation of the tabular entries. It was felt that the basis for the tables should be clarified and additional tables prepared that would provide exact probability values for measuring statistical significance (Roessler *et al.*, 1978; Stone and Sidel, 1978). These tables are reproduced here (Tables 5.9–5.14) and one can quickly see their value in establishing whether a particular result is significant.

Table 5.9 Minimum numbers of correct judgments to establish significance at various probability levels for paired-difference and duo–trio tests (one-tailed, $p = \frac{1}{2}$)[a]

Number of trials (n)	Probability levels 0.05	0.04	0.03	0.02	0.01	0.005	0.001
7	7	7	7	7	7		
8	7	7	8	8	8	8	
9	8	8	8	8	9	9	
10	9	9	9	9	10	10	10
11	9	9	10	10	10	11	11
12	10	10	10	10	11	11	12
13	10	11	11	11	12	12	13
14	11	11	11	12	12	13	13
15	12	12	12	12	13	13	14
16	12	12	13	13	14	14	15
17	13	13	13	14	14	15	16
18	13	14	14	14	15	15	16
19	14	14	15	15	15	16	17
20	15	15	15	16	16	17	18
21	15	15	16	16	17	17	18
22	16	16	16	17	17	18	19
23	16	17	17	17	18	19	20
24	17	17	18	18	19	19	20
25	18	18	18	19	19	20	21
26	18	18	19	19	20	20	22
27	19	19	19	20	20	21	22
28	19	20	20	20	21	22	23
29	20	20	21	21	22	22	24
30	20	21	21	22	22	23	24
31	21	21	22	22	23	24	25
32	22	22	22	23	24	24	26
33	22	23	23	23	24	25	26
34	23	23	23	24	25	25	27
35	23	24	24	25	25	26	27
36	24	24	25	25	26	27	28
37	24	25	25	26	26	27	29
38	25	25	26	26	27	28	29
39	26	26	26	27	28	28	30
40	26	27	27	27	28	29	30
41	27	27	27	28	29	30	31
42	27	28	28	29	29	30	32
43	28	28	29	29	30	31	32
44	28	29	29	30	31	31	33
45	29	29	30	30	31	32	34
46	30	30	30	31	32	33	34
47	30	30	31	31	32	33	35
48	31	31	31	32	33	34	36
49	31	32	32	33	34	34	36
50	32	32	33	33	34	35	37
60	37	38	38	39	40	41	43
70	43	43	44	45	46	47	49
80	48	49	49	50	51	52	55
90	54	54	55	56	57	58	61
100	59	60	60	61	63	64	66

[a] Values (X) not appearing in table may be derived from $X = (z\sqrt{n} + n + 1) / 2$. See text. Reprinted from *J. Food Sci.* **43**, pp. 940–947, 1978. Copyright © by Institute of Food Technologists.

Table 5.10 Minimum numbers of correct judgments to establish significance at various probability levels for the triangle test (one-tailed, $p = \frac{1}{3}$)[a]

Number of trials (n)	Probability levels						
	0.05	0.04	0.03	0.02	0.01	0.005	0.001
5	4	5	5	5	5	5	
6	5	5	5	5	6	6	
7	5	6	6	6	6	7	7
8	6	6	6	6	7	7	8
9	6	7	7	7	7	8	8
10	7	7	7	7	8	8	9
11	7	7	8	8	8	9	10
12	8	8	8	8	9	9	10
13	8	8	9	9	9	10	11
14	9	9	9	9	10	10	11
15	9	9	10	10	10	11	12
16	9	10	10	10	11	11	12
17	10	10	10	11	11	12	13
18	10	11	11	11	12	12	13
19	11	11	11	12	12	13	14
20	11	11	12	12	13	13	14
21	12	12	12	13	13	14	15
22	12	12	13	13	14	14	15
23	12	13	13	13	14	15	16
24	13	13	13	14	15	15	16
25	13	14	14	14	15	16	17
26	14	14	14	15	15	16	17
27	14	14	15	15	16	17	18
28	15	15	15	16	16	17	18
29	15	15	16	16	17	17	19
30	15	16	16	16	17	18	19
31	16	16	16	17	18	18	20
32	16	16	17	17	18	19	20
33	17	17	17	18	18	19	21
34	17	17	18	18	19	20	21
35	17	18	18	19	19	20	22
36	18	18	18	19	20	20	22
37	18	18	19	19	20	21	22
38	19	19	19	20	21	21	23
39	19	19	20	20	21	22	23
40	19	20	20	21	21	22	24
41	20	20	20	21	22	23	24
42	20	20	21	21	22	23	25
43	20	21	21	22	23	24	25
44	21	21	22	22	23	24	26
45	21	22	22	23	24	24	26
46	22	22	22	23	24	25	27
47	22	22	23	23	24	25	27
48	22	23	23	24	25	26	27
49	23	23	24	24	25	26	28
50	23	24	24	25	26	26	28
60	27	27	28	29	30	31	33
70	31	31	32	33	34	35	37
80	35	35	36	36	38	39	41
90	38	39	40	40	42	43	45
100	42	43	43	44	45	47	49

[a]Values (X) not appearing in table may be derived from $X = 0.4714z\sqrt{n} + [(2n + 3)/6]$. See text.

Table 5.11 Minimum numbers of agreeing judgments necessary to establish significance at various probability levels for the paired-preference test (two-tailed, $p = \frac{1}{2}$)[a]

Number of trials (n)	Probability levels						
	0.05	0.04	0.03	0.02	0.01	0.005	0.001
7	7	7	7	7			
8	8	8	8	8	8		
9	8	8	9	9	9	9	
10	9	9	9	10	10	10	
11	10	10	10	10	11	11	11
12	10	10	11	11	11	12	12
13	11	11	11	12	12	12	13
14	12	12	12	12	13	13	14
15	12	12	13	13	13	14	14
16	13	13	13	14	14	14	15
17	13	14	14	14	15	15	16
18	14	14	15	15	15	16	17
19	15	15	15	15	16	16	17
20	15	16	16	16	17	17	18
21	16	16	16	17	17	18	19
22	17	17	17	17	18	18	19
23	17	17	18	18	19	19	20
24	18	18	18	19	19	20	21
25	18	19	19	19	20	20	21
26	19	19	19	20	20	21	22
27	20	20	20	20	21	22	23
28	20	20	21	21	22	22	23
29	21	21	21	22	22	23	24
30	21	22	22	22	23	24	25
31	22	22	22	23	24	24	25
32	23	23	23	23	24	25	26
33	23	23	24	24	25	25	27
34	24	24	24	25	25	26	27
35	24	25	25	25	26	27	28
36	25	25	25	26	27	27	29
37	25	26	26	26	27	28	29
38	26	26	27	27	28	29	30
39	27	27	27	28	28	29	31
40	27	27	28	28	29	30	31
41	28	28	28	29	30	30	32
42	28	29	29	29	30	31	32
43	29	29	30	30	31	32	33
44	29	30	30	30	31	32	34
45	30	30	31	31	32	33	34
46	31	31	31	32	33	33	35
47	31	31	32	32	33	34	36
48	32	32	32	33	34	35	36
49	32	33	33	34	34	35	37
50	33	33	34	34	35	36	37
60	39	39	39	40	41	42	44
70	44	45	45	46	47	48	50
80	50	50	51	51	52	53	56
90	55	56	56	57	58	59	61
100	61	61	62	63	64	65	67

[a] Values (X) not appearing in table may be derived from $X = (z\sqrt{n} + n + 1)/2$. See text. Reprinted from *J. Food Sci.* **43**, pp. 940–947, 1978. Copyright © by Institute of Food Technologists.

Table 5.12 Probability of X or more correct judgments in n trials (one-tailed, $p = \frac{1}{2}$)

n/*x*	0	1	2	3	4	5	6	7	8	9	10	11	12	13	14	15	16	17
5		0.969	0.812	0.500	0.188	0.031												
6		0.984	0.891	0.656	0.344	0.109	0.016											
7		0.992	0.938	0.773	0.500	0.227	0.062	0.008										
8		0.996	0.965	0.855	0.637	0.363	0.145	0.035	0.004									
9		0.998	0.980	0.910	0.746	0.500	0.254	0.090	0.020	0.002								
10		0.999	0.989	0.945	0.828	0.623	0.377	0.172	0.055	0.011	0.001							
11			0.994	0.967	0.887	0.726	0.500	0.274	0.113	0.033	0.006							
12			0.997	0.981	0.927	0.806	0.613	0.387	0.194	0.073	0.019	0.003						
13			0.998	0.989	0.954	0.867	0.709	0.500	0.291	0.133	0.046	0.011	0.002					
14			0.999	0.994	0.971	0.910	0.788	0.605	0.395	0.212	0.090	0.029	0.006	0.001				
15				0.996	0.982	0.941	0.849	0.696	0.500	0.304	0.151	0.059	0.018	0.004				
16				0.998	0.989	0.962	0.895	0.773	0.598	0.402	0.227	0.105	0.038	0.011	0.002			
17				0.999	0.994	0.975	0.928	0.834	0.685	0.500	0.315	0.166	0.072	0.025	0.006	0.001		
18				0.999	0.996	0.985	0.952	0.881	0.760	0.593	0.407	0.240	0.119	0.048	0.015	0.004	0.001	
19					0.998	0.990	0.968	0.916	0.820	0.676	0.500	0.324	0.180	0.084	0.032	0.010	0.002	
20					0.999	0.994	0.979	0.942	0.868	0.748	0.588	0.412	0.252	0.132	0.058	0.021	0.006	0.001
21					0.999	0.996	0.987	0.961	0.905	0.808	0.668	0.500	0.332	0.192	0.095	0.039	0.013	0.004
22						0.998	0.992	0.974	0.933	0.857	0.738	0.584	0.416	0.262	0.143	0.067	0.026	0.008
23						0.999	0.995	0.983	0.953	0.895	0.798	0.661	0.500	0.339	0.202	0.105	0.047	0.017
24						0.999	0.997	0.989	0.968	0.924	0.846	0.729	0.581	0.419	0.271	0.154	0.076	0.032
25							0.998	0.993	0.978	0.946	0.885	0.788	0.655	0.500	0.345	0.212	0.115	0.054
26							0.999	0.995	0.986	0.962	0.916	0.837	0.721	0.577	0.423	0.279	0.163	0.084
27							0.999	0.997	0.990	0.974	0.939	0.876	0.779	0.649	0.500	0.351	0.221	0.124
28								0.998	0.994	0.982	0.956	0.908	0.828	0.714	0.575	0.425	0.286	0.172
29								0.999	0.996	0.983	0.969	0.932	0.868	0.771	0.644	0.500	0.356	0.229
30								0.999	0.997	0.992	0.979	0.951	0.900	0.819	0.708	0.572	0.428	0.292
31									0.998	0.995	0.985	0.965	0.925	0.859	0.763	0.640	0.500	0.360
32									0.999	0.997	0.990	0.975	0.945	0.892	0.811	0.702	0.570	0.430
33									0.999	0.998	0.993	0.982	0.960	0.919	0.852	0.757	0.636	0.500
34										0.999	0.995	0.988	0.971	0.939	0.885	0.804	0.696	0.568
35										0.999	0.997	0.992	0.980	0.955	0.912	0.845	0.750	0.632
36										0.999	0.998	0.994	0.986	0.967	0.934	0.879	0.797	0.691
37											0.999	0.996	0.990	0.976	0.951	0.906	0.838	0.744
38											0.999	0.997	0.993	0.983	0.964	0.928	0.872	0.791
39											0.999	0.998	0.995	0.988	0.973	0.946	0.900	0.832
40												0.999	0.997	0.992	0.981	0.960	0.923	0.866
41												0.999	0.998	0.994	0.986	0.970	0.941	0.894
42													0.999	0.996	0.990	0.978	0.956	0.918
43													0.999	0.997	0.993	0.984	0.967	0.937
44													0.999	0.998	0.995	0.989	0.976	0.952
45														0.999	0.997	0.992	0.982	0.964
46														0.999	0.998	0.994	0.987	0.973
47														0.999	0.998	0.996	0.991	0.980
48															0.999	0.997	0.993	0.985
49															0.999	0.998	0.995	0.989
50																0.999	0.997	0.992

[a] Reprinted from *J. Food Sci.* **43**, pp. 940–947, 1978. Copyright © by Institute of Food Technologists.

18	19	20	21	22	23	24	25	26	27	28	29	30	31	32	33	34	35	36
0.001																		
0.002																		
0.005	0.001																	
0.011	0.003	0.001																
0.022	0.007	0.002																
0.038	0.014	0.005	0.001															
0.061	0.026	0.010	0.003	0.001														
0.092	0.044	0.018	0.006	0.002														
0.132	0.068	0.031	0.012	0.004	0.001													
0.181	0.100	0.049	0.021	0.008	0.003	0.001												
0.237	0.141	0.075	0.035	0.015	0.005	0.002												
0.298	0.189	0.108	0.055	0.025	0.010	0.004	0.001											
0.364	0.243	0.148	0.081	0.040	0.018	0.007	0.002											
0.432	0.304	0.196	0.115	0.061	0.029	0.012	0.005	0.002										
0.500	0.368	0.250	0.155	0.088	0.045	0.020	0.008	0.003	0.001									
0.566	0.434	0.309	0.203	0.121	0.066	0.033	0.014	0.006	0.002	0.001								
0.629	0.500	0.371	0.256	0.162	0.094	0.049	0.024	0.010	0.004	0.001								
0.686	0.564	0.436	0.314	0.209	0.128	0.072	0.036	0.017	0.007	0.003	0.001							
0.739	0.625	0.500	0.375	0.261	0.168	0.100	0.054	0.027	0.012	0.005	0.002	0.001						
0.785	0.682	0.563	0.437	0.318	0.215	0.134	0.077	0.040	0.019	0.008	0.003	0.001						
0.826	0.734	0.622	0.500	0.378	0.266	0.174	0.106	0.059	0.030	0.014	0.006	0.002	0.001					
0.860	0.780	0.678	0.561	0.439	0.322	0.220	0.140	0.082	0.044	0.022	0.010	0.004	0.001					
0.889	0.820	0.729	0.620	0.500	0.380	0.271	0.180	0.111	0.063	0.033	0.016	0.007	0.003	0.001				
0.913	0.854	0.774	0.674	0.560	0.440	0.326	0.226	0.146	0.087	0.048	0.024	0.011	0.005	0.002	0.001			
0.932	0.884	0.814	0.724	0.617	0.500	0.383	0.276	0.186	0.116	0.068	0.036	0.018	0.008	0.003	0.001			
0.948	0.908	0.849	0.769	0.671	0.558	0.442	0.329	0.231	0.151	0.092	0.052	0.027	0.013	0.006	0.002	0.001		
0.961	0.928	0.879	0.809	0.720	0.615	0.500	0.385	0.280	0.191	0.121	0.072	0.039	0.020	0.009	0.004	0.002	0.001	
0.970	0.944	0.903	0.844	0.765	0.667	0.557	0.443	0.333	0.235	0.156	0.097	0.056	0.030	0.015	0.007	0.003	0.001	
0.978	0.957	0.924	0.874	0.804	0.716	0.612	0.500	0.388	0.284	0.196	0.126	0.076	0.043	0.022	0.012	0.005	0.002	0.001
0.984	0.968	0.941	0.899	0.839	0.760	0.664	0.556	0.444	0.336	0.240	0.161	0.101	0.059	0.032	0.016	0.008	0.003	0.001

Table 5.13 Probability of X of more correct judgments in n trials (one-tailed, $p = \frac{1}{3}$)

n/x	0	1	2	3	4	5	6	7	8	9	10	11	12	13
5		0.868	0.539	0.210	0.045	0.004								
6		0.912	0.649	0.320	0.100	0.018	0.001							
7		0.941	0.737	0.429	0.173	0.045	0.007							
8		0.961	0.805	0.532	0.259	0.088	0.020	0.003						
9		0.974	0.857	0.623	0.350	0.145	0.042	0.008	0.001					
10		0.983	0.896	0.701	0.441	0.213	0.077	0.020	0.003					
11		0.988	0.925	0.766	0.527	0.289	0.122	0.039	0.009	0.001				
12		0.992	0.946	0.819	0.607	0.368	0.178	0.066	0.019	0.004	0.001			
13		0.995	0.961	0.861	0.678	0.448	0.241	0.104	0.035	0.009	0.002			
14		0.997	0.973	0.895	0.739	0.524	0.310	0.149	0.058	0.017	0.004	0.001		
15		0.998	0.981	0.921	0.791	0.596	0.382	0.203	0.088	0.031	0.008	0.002		
16		0.998	0.986	0.941	0.834	0.661	0.453	0.263	0.126	0.050	0.016	0.004	0.001	
17		0.999	0.990	0.956	0.870	0.719	0.522	0.326	0.172	0.075	0.027	0.008	0.002	
18		0.999	0.993	0.967	0.898	0.769	0.588	0.391	0.223	0.108	0.043	0.014	0.004	0.001
19			0.995	0.976	0.921	0.812	0.648	0.457	0.279	0.146	0.065	0.024	0.007	0.002
20			0.997	0.982	0.940	0.848	0.703	0.521	0.339	0.191	0.092	0.038	0.013	0.004
21			0.998	0.987	0.954	0.879	0.751	0.581	0.339	0.240	0.125	0.056	0.021	0.007
22			0.998	0.991	0.965	0.904	0.794	0.638	0.460	0.293	0.163	0.079	0.033	0.012
23			0.999	0.993	0.974	0.924	0.831	0.690	0.519	0.349	0.206	0.107	0.048	0.019
24			0.999	0.995	0.980	0.941	0.862	0.737	0.576	0.406	0.254	0.140	0.068	0.028
25			0.999	0.996	0.985	0.954	0.888	0.778	0.630	0.462	0.304	0.178	0.092	0.042
26				0.997	0.989	0.964	0.910	0.815	0.679	0.518	0.357	0.220	0.121	0.058
27				0.998	0.992	0.972	0.928	0.847	0.725	0.572	0.411	0.266	0.154	0.079
28				0.999	0.994	0.979	0.943	0.874	0.765	0.623	0.464	0.314	0.191	0.104
29				0.999	0.996	0.984	0.955	0.897	0.801	0.670	0.517	0.364	0.232	0.133
30				0.999	0.997	0.988	0.965	0.916	0.833	0.714	0.568	0.415	0.276	0.166
31					0.998	0.991	0.972	0.932	0.861	0.754	0.617	0.466	0.322	0.203
32					0.998	0.993	0.978	0.946	0.885	0.789	0.662	0.516	0.370	0.243
33					0.999	0.995	0.983	0.957	0.905	0.821	0.705	0.565	0.419	0.285
34					0.999	0.996	0.987	0.965	0.922	0.849	0.744	0.612	0.468	0.330
35					0.999	0.997	0.990	0.973	0.937	0.873	0.779	0.656	0.516	0.376
36						0.998	0.992	0.978	0.949	0.895	0.810	0.697	0.562	0.422
37						0.998	0.994	0.983	0.959	0.913	0.838	0.735	0.607	0.469
38						0.999	0.996	0.987	0.967	0.928	0.863	0.769	0.650	0.515
39						0.999	0.997	0.990	0.973	0.941	0.885	0.800	0.689	0.560
40						0.999	0.997	0.992	0.979	0.952	0.903	0.829	0.726	0.603
41							0.998	0.994	0.983	0.961	0.920	0.854	0 761	0.644
42							0.999	0.995	0.987	0.968	0.933	0.876	0.791	0.683
43							0.999	0.996	0.990	0.974	0.945	0.895	0.820	0.719
44							0.999	0.997	0.992	0.980	0.955	0.912	0.845	0.753
45							0.999	0.998	0.994	0.984	0.963	0.926	0.867	0.783
46								0.998	0.995	0.987	0.970	0.938	0.887	0.811
47								0.999	0.996	0.990	0.976	0.949	0.904	0.836
48								0.999	0.997	0.992	0.980	0.958	0.919	0.859
49								0.999	0.998	0.994	0.984	0.965	0.932	0.879
50								0.999	0.998	0.995	0.987	0.972	0.943	0.896

[a]Reprinted from *J. Food Sci.* **43**, pp. 940–947, 1978. Copyright © by Institute of Food Technologists.

14	15	16	17	18	19	20	21	22	23	24	25	26	27	28
0.001														
0.002														
0.003	0.001													
0.006	0.002													
0.010	0.003	0.001												
0.016	0.006	0.002												
0.025	0.009	0.003	0.001											
0.036	0.014	0.005	0.002											
0.050	0.022	0.008	0.003	0.001										
0.068	0.031	0.013	0.005	0.001										
0.090	0.043	0.019	0.007	0.002	0.001									
0.115	0.059	0.027	0.011	0.004	0.001									
0.144	0.078	0.038	0.016	0.006	0.002	0.001								
0.177	0.100	0.051	0.023	0.010	0.004	0.001								
0.213	0.126	0.067	0.033	0.014	0.006	0.002	0.001							
0.252	0.155	0.087	0.044	0.020	0.009	0.003	0.001							
0.293	0.187	0.109	0.058	0.028	0.012	0.005	0.002	0.001						
0.336	0.223	0.135	0.075	0.038	0.018	0.007	0.003	0.001						
0.381	0.261	0.164	0.095	0.051	0.025	0.011	0.004	0.002	0.001					
0.425	0.301	0.196	0.118	0.066	0.033	0.016	0.007	0.003	0.001					
0.470	0.342	0.231	0.144	0.083	0.044	0.021	0.010	0.004	0.001					
0.515	0.385	0.268	0.173	0.104	0.057	0.029	0.014	0.006	0.002	0.001				
0.558	0.428	0.307	0.205	0.127	0.073	0.038	0.019	0.008	0.003	0.001				
0.600	0.471	0.347	0.239	0.153	0.091	0.050	0.025	0.012	0.005	0.002	0.001			
0.639	0.514	0.389	0.275	0.182	0.111	0.063	0.033	0.016	0.007	0.003	0.001			
0.677	0.556	0.430	0.313	0.213	0.135	0.079	0.043	0.022	0.010	0.004	0.002	0.001		
0.713	0.596	0.472	0.352	0.246	0.161	0.098	0.055	0.029	0.014	0.006	0.003	0.001		
0.745	0.635	0.514	0.392	0.282	0.189	0.119	0.070	0.038	0.019	0.009	0.004	0.002	0.001	
0.776	0.672	0.554	0.433	0.318	0.220	0.142	0.086	0.048	0.025	0.012	0.006	0.002	0.001	
0.803	0.706	0.593	0.473	0.356	0.253	0.168	0.105	0.061	0.033	0.017	0.008	0.003	0.001	
0.829	0.739	0.631	0.513	0.395	0.287	0.196	0.126	0.076	0.042	0.022	0.011	0.005	0.001	0.001

Table 5.14 Probability of *X* or more agreeing judgments in *n* trials (two-tailed, $p = \frac{1}{2}$)[a]

n^x	3	4	5	6	7	8	9	10	11	12	13	14	15	16	17	18	19
5	0.625	0.312	0.062														
6		0.688	0.219	0.031													
7			0.453	0.125	0.016												
8			0.727	0.289	0.070	0.008											
9				0.508	0.180	0.039	0.004										
10				0.754	0.344	0.109	0.021	0.002									
11					0.549	0.227	0.065	0.011	0.001								
12					0.774	0.388	0.146	0.039	0.006								
13						0.581	0.267	0.092	0.022	0.003							
14						0.791	0.424	0.180	0.057	0.013	0.002						
15							0.607	0.302	0.118	0.035	0.007	0.001					
16							0.804	0.454	0.210	0.077	0.021	0.004	0.001				
17								0.629	0.332	0.143	0.049	0.013	0.002				
18								0.815	0.481	0.238	0.096	0.031	0.008	0.001			
19									0.648	0.359	0.167	0.064	0.019	0.004	0.001		
20									0.824	0.503	0.263	0.115	0.041	0.012	0.003		
21										0.664	0.383	0.189	0.078	0.027	0.007	0.001	
22										0.832	0.523	0.286	0.134	0.052	0.017	0.004	0.001
23											0.678	0.405	0.210	0.093	0.035	0.011	0.003
24											0.839	0.541	0.307	0.152	0.064	0.023	0.007
25												0.690	0.424	0.230	0.108	0.043	0.015
26												0.845	0.557	0.327	0.169	0.076	0.029
27													0.701	0.442	0.248	0.122	0.052
28													0.851	0.572	0.345	0.185	0.087
29														0.711	0.458	0.265	0.136
30														0.856	0.585	0.362	0.200
31															0.720	0.473	0.281
32															0.860	0.597	0.377
33																0.728	0.487
34																0.864	0.608
35																	0.739
36																	0.868
37																	
38																	
39																	
40																	
41																	
42																	
43																	
44																	
45																	
46																	
47																	
48																	
49																	
50																	

[a]Reprinted from *J. Food Sci.* **43**, pp. 940–947, 1978. Copyright © by Institute of Food Technologists.

Table 5.14 (*continued*)

20	21	22	23	24	25	26	27	28	29	30	31	32	33	34	35	36	37
0.002																	
0.004		0.001															
0.009	0.002	0.001															
0.019	0.006	0.002															
0.036	0.013	0.004	0.001														
0.061	0.024	0.008	0.002	0.001													
0.099	0.043	0.016	0.005	0.001													
0.150	0.071	0.030	0.011	0.003	0.001												
0.215	0.100	0.050	0.020	0.007	0.002	0.001											
0.296	0.163	0.080	0.035	0.014	0.005	0.001											
0.392	0.229	0.121	0.058	0.024	0.009	0.003	0.001										
0.500	0.310	0.175	0.900	0.041	0.017	0.006	0.002										
0.618	0.405	0.243	0.132	0.065	0.029	0.011	0.004	0.001									
0.743	0.511	0.324	0.188	0.099	0.047	0.020	0.008	0.003	0.001								
0.871	0.627	0.418	0.256	0.143	0.073	0.034	0.014	0.005	0.002								
	0.749	0.522	0.337	0.200	0.108	0.053	0.024	0.009	0.003	0.001							
	0.875	0.636	0.430	0.268	0.154	0.081	0.038	0.017	0.006	0.002	0.001						
		0.755	0.533	0.349	0.211	0.117	0.060	0.028	0.012	0.004	0.001						
		0.878	0.644	0.441	0.280	0.164	0.088	0.044	0.020	0.008	0.003	0.001					
			0.761	0.542	0.360	0.222	0.126	0.066	0.032	0.014	0.005	0.002	0.001				
			0.880	0.652	0.451	0.291	0.174	0.096	0.049	0.023	0.010	0.004	0.001				
				0.766	0.551	0.371	0.233	0.135	0.072	0.036	0.016	0.007	0.002	0.001			
				0.883	0.659	0.461	0.302	0.184	0.104	0.054	0.026	0.011	0.005	0.002	0.001		
					0.771	0.560	0.382	0.243	0.144	0.079	0.040	0.019	0.008	0.003	0.001		
					0.885	0.665	0.471	0.312	0.193	0.111	0.059	0.029	0.013	0.006	0.002	0.001	
						0.775	0.568	0.392	0.253	0.152	0.085	0.044	0.021	0.009	0.004	0.001	
						0.888	0.672	0.480	0.322	0.203	0.119	0.065	0.033	0.015	0.007	0.003	0.001

The exact probability tables are especially useful because they enable the sensory professional to assess risk in terms more precise than would be possible using Table 5.9 or 5.10, for example. In practice, most sensory decisions operate from statistical significance at the 0.05 probability level (also referred to as the α level); however, the final decision can involve other issues. The tables do not lead to any decision regarding the appropriate level of statistical significance, appropriate number of responses, or impact of replication on the final decision. The sensory professional must consider all of these issues before the test and then proceed with the interpretation.

Most discrimination tests are one tailed; the tail refers to a segment of the distribution curve (i.e. the tail end). Duo–trio, triangle, A-not-A, and same-or-different tests are one tailed because there is a single correct outcome. The directional paired-comparison test may be either one tailed or two tailed depending on the number of outcomes of interest to the experimenter. Because the discrimination test is a perceptual task rather than an instrument measure, it is not always correct to assume that the result must be in the same direction as the physical or chemical difference between two products. A product having less sweetener may be perceived as sweeter than, less sweet than, or equally as sweet as another product depending on the remaining sensory components of those products. If all possible outcomes in the directional paired comparison are of interest, the two-tailed table is recommended. More correct decisions are necessary to achieve statistical significance, which is a more conservative approach. For additional discussion about one-tailed versus two-tailed tests, see McNemar (1969).

Discrimination tests are forced-choice tests; the subject must make a decision and the issue should not be in doubt (see Gridgeman, 1959), yet one periodically encounters a sensory test operation where "no-decision" responses by subjects are permitted. This practice is not recommended because it is inconsistent with a basic principle of the discrimination test and the fact that guessing is accounted for in the design. From a practical viewpoint, when "no-decision" responses are permitted then the total database is reduced. As Gridgeman (1959) noted, the decision as to what to do with these "no-decision" responses poses a dilemma. One cannot ignore them, yet they are not included in the methods for analysis and they cannot legitimately be divided equally between correct and incorrect decisions. Finally, there is the problem of subjects using this option to avoid more difficult decisions; it becomes an "easy way out." This particular problem can be avoided by simply requiring subjects to make decisions and by not providing the "no-decision" option.

At the outset of any testing, sensory evaluation must be firm about certain aspects of the test, for example, promptness, following test instructions, including making a decision, and so on. Subjects will generally adhere to these requirements, and individuals who either cannot comply or believe they are exempt from rules, should be excused from testing. The fact that differences are relatively small is no reason for not making a decision; the subject must remember that the test is designed to account for small differences. It should also be kept in mind that in most operations, the differences are relatively small (remember that easily perceived differences are not worth testing) and if the "no-decision" option is included, more subjects will take that option. Finally, the developers of the methods did not recommend the "no-decision" option.

An attempt to work around this problem has come from developments in signal detection theory, although the authors did not have that purpose in mind at the outset. Nonetheless, signal detection theory has provided additional insight into the decision-making process. This application of signal detection also has led to some proposed practical applications that warrant consideration. O'Mahony (1979) and O'Mahony *et al.* (1979, 1980) devised a multiple-difference procedure that yielded measures of difference based on signal detection principles; it was suggested that the method would be especially useful as a means for assessing very small differences. The subject evaluates a set of products, one at a time, and indicates one of four response alternatives – yes, yes?, no?, no. Based on the number of products in the test, one then has a response matrix from which R values or $P(A)$ values (indices of difference) can be computed. The primary advantages one might gain from the use of the procedure is that it takes into account the subject's uncertainty in a decision and that it could be used to evaluate many samples within a brief time period. Whether knowledge of a subject's uncertainty results in a more meaningful decision about product differences remains to be demonstrated.

In industrial operations, the sensory professional is working with very skilled subjects and it is possible that uncertainty about a decision may provide no advantage and could reduce sensitivity by providing this option where none existed. Other factors that need to be taken into account in comparing this procedure and those used in traditional discrimination testing include the amount of product required for a test, number of evaluations per subject, and time required for a decision. O'Mahony (1979) noted that the method has potential for flavor measurement; however, more study will be required before the technique can be used effectively within the industrial environment. Developments such as these warrant consideration; however, they must be evaluated relative to current activities and in their entirety, including product preparation, subject test time, analysis, and interpretation.

Decisions as to number of subjects for a test and number of responses per subject are issues that are not well defined. A perusal of the current literature would lead one to assume that the decision is arbitrary, and that any number of subjects from ten to fifty (or more) would be adequate or that statistical power calculations dictate number of observations (Ennis, 1993; Schlich, 1993). Until recently (see Ennis and Bi, 1998; Bi and Ennis, 2001), less consideration appears to have been given to replication. By replication in this situation, we mean a subject evaluating more than one set of the test products in a single session. The actual procedure would be for one set of products and scorecard to be served, a decision made, followed by an appropriate interval of 1–3 minutes, and the procedure repeated (this would result in two responses from each subject within a single session).

Generally, most companies have not utilized replication effectively in test design. If subjects are allowed to consume the product rather than "sip and spit," it is easy to understand why replication is not successful. Sensory fatigue (decrease in sensitivity) causes the percentage of correct responses to decrease in the second trial. This problem is easily corrected, and the information obtained from the replicate responses substantially increases the power of the test and the confidence that the sensory professional has with the results. Response patterns can be extremely informative as shown in the following table:

Test	Serving order: First	Serving order: Second	Pooled results
A[a]	6/15[b]	12/15	18/30
B	12/15	6/15	18/30
C	8/15	10/15	18/30

[a] Each test was either paired comparison or duo-trio: $p = \frac{1}{2}$.
[b] Entries are the ratios of correct to total decisions.

Each of the three examples, A, B, and C, show the same total number of correct decisions; however, the response patterns are different. In test A, the number of correct decisions was twice as great for the second serving order, suggesting that some form of learning may have occurred. After completing the first set, the subjects were able to perceive the difference (more easily). It can be argued that such an occurrence reflects on sensory evaluation for having selected inexperienced subjects; however, a new variable could introduce flavor changes not familiar to the panelists and thus could account for the observed response pattern. This problem could be minimized through the use of "warm-up" samples; however, sensory fatigue, as described next, might occur.

In test B, the situation is reversed and performance has declined from the first set to the second set. This pattern suggests that some type of fatigue may have occurred; either the interval between sets was not sufficient and/or the subjects did not rinse sufficiently to recover. Finally, in test C, the number of correct decisions is similar in both orders, indicating none of the problems encountered in tests A and B. All three tests yielded a total of 18 correct decisions with a probability value of 0.181, which is not sufficient for rejecting the hypothesis that the products are perceived as similar.

However, there is a question as to whether these results are consistent. For tests A and B, we may be in error if we conclude that there is no significant difference between the products. While it is true that the total correct decision is not sufficient for statistical significance, sensory evaluation would be remiss if the results by serving order were not discussed. In fact, both patterns suggest the likelihood of a statistically significant difference, and depending on product and subject availability, the test might be repeated. Practically speaking, repeating a test usually is not possible, most often because of product supply, and a decision must be made using available information; hence, the conclusion that there is a perceived difference. In the non-directional test, the number of correct decisions can be monitored by order of presentation, as well as by the specific pair of products. As shown below, the four possible serving orders – AA, BB, AB, BA – are listed with their respective results:

Test	Same		Different		Pooled
	AA	BB	AB	BA	
D	2/10	2/10	9/10	9/10	18/30
E	5/10	4/10	9/10	7/10	18/30

Assuming subjects understood the task, the serving orders of AA and BB should yield approximately 50% correct decision. In test D, only four of the twenty decisions are correct, which suggests some subjects did not understand the task and circled "different" on every scorecard. Thus, the eighteen correct decisions for the AB and BA orders might be considered to be the result of a combination of true perception of a difference as well as a misunderstanding of the task. Examination on a subject-by-subject basis may also provide further insight into the source of the problem. For test E, the responses are more consistent with expectation. These examples serve as a reminder of the importance of examining response patterns on a subject basis as well as by serving order before preparing any conclusion and recommendation.

This discussion about replication has thus far focused on problems that are traced back to the experimenter and the subjects; however, it is also possible that the product can be at fault. Product changes can and do occur between test planning and the experiment, and the sensory professional must be vigilant to the prospect of this problem. Another aspect of this problem is product variation due to production variation and in some instances, this variability is as large as the variable being tested. This could result in a non-significant conclusion, which would be incorrect. One added benefit of replication is the use of more product so that the product variations do not have as great an effect. Of course, where it is known that typical production variation cannot be avoided and it always results in significant differences, then it is necessary to consider using an alternative methodology such as descriptive analysis (discussed in Chapter 6). Finally, one should not mix all the control product so as to blend the variability. Such an approach will yield a result that in of itself may be quite reliable, but have absolutely no practical value (or external validity). Of course, major concerns about the product are addressed before data collection; however, judgmental situations do arise and the solution becomes apparent only after a test is performed. Regardless of the problem, replication enables the sensory professional to identify problems to avoid in future tests with those products, and to reach a more realistic and meaningful decision.

It can be argued that replication within a test session violates the statistical rule of independence of judgments and therefore the standard tables for determining statistical significance are not appropriate (Ennis and Bi, 1998; Bi and Ennis, 2001). This particular issue warrants comment.

The χ^2-statistic can be used to determine if the proportions of correct decisions in the replicate are significantly different from those in the first trial and so on. When the proportions of correct decisions are not significantly different, they can be combined and the traditional tables (Roessler *et al.*, 1978) used for determining statistical significance.

Table 5.15 Number of testers and their performance in a duo–trio discrimination test with one replication

		Trial		
		Correct	Incorrect	Total
Replication	Correct	5[a]	$6_{(r_2)}$[b]	11
	Incorrect	$3_{(r_1)}$[c]	1[d]	4
	Total	8	7	15

[a] Entry is number of subjects (five) that were correct on both trails.
[b] Entry is number of subjects (six) that were correct only on the second trial (the replicate).
[c] Entry is number of subjects (three) that were correct only on the first trial.
[d] Entry is number of subjects (one) that were incorrect on both trials.
Note: $m = r_1 + r_2$; see text for explanation.

A quick method for determining if there is a significant difference between proportions of responses from the same subjects has been proposed by Smith (1981). In Smith's example, the same panel participates in two different tests. The total number of correct responses for the first test (r_1) is added to the total number of correct responses for the second test (r_2) to produce a value m (i.e. $r_1 + r_2 = m$). Using Table 1, 2, or 3 prepared by Roessler *et al.* (1978), Smith used m to represent the number of trials (n) and r_1 and r_2 are significant.

Smith's procedure may be expanded to the situation where the same subjects evaluate products on two trials. A worked example for a duo–trio test is presented in Table 5.15; of the nine subjects who were correct only once, three were correct on the first trial and six were correct on the replication. Using Smith's notation, we determine that $r_1 = 3$, $r_2 = 6$, and $m = 9$. Consulting Table 1 in Roessler *et al.* and substituting M for n, we note that neither r_1 nor r_2 is >8, which is the table value required for statistical significance with an n of 9. There is, therefore, no evidence to indicate that the proportions from these two replications are different, suggesting that it would then be reasonable to pool the responses.

Another statistical solution to the handling of replication would be to use only the data from subjects who were correct on both trials for analysis. The rationale is that these data may be considered as representative of discrimination. Exact probabilities may be obtained from the tables of the cumulative binomial probability distribution. When such tables are not available, a formula for computing a good approximation to the exact probability has been provided by Roessler *et al.* (1953, 1978) and is modified here as follows:

$$Z = \frac{(X - np) - 0.5}{\sqrt{npq}}$$

where X is the number of subjects correct on both trials, n the total number of subjects; p the probability of two correct decisions $[(p_1)(p_2) = p]$; in the triangle test $p = \frac{1}{3}$, in the duo–trio and paired comparison tests, $p_1 = \frac{1}{2}$, and $q = p - 1$. Tables 5.16 and 5.17 have been prepared to accommodate tests where twelve to eighteen subjects participate in a trial plus replicate session for either the duo–trio,

Table 5.16 Probability of X or more correct judgments on two successive trials [one-tailed, $p = (\frac{1}{2})(\frac{1}{2}) = \frac{1}{4}$]

n	1	2	3	4	5	6	7	8	9	10	11	12
12	0.968	0.842	0.609	0.351	0.158	0.054	0.014	0.003	0.000			
13	0.976	0.873	0.667	0.415	0.206	0.080	0.024	0.006	0.001	0.000		
14	0.982	0.899	0.719	0.479	0.258	0.112	0.038	0.010	0.002	0.000		
15	0.987	0.920	0.764	0.539	0.314	0.148	0.057	0.017	0.044	0.001	0.000	
16	0.990	0.937	0.803	0.595	0.370	0.190	0.080	0.027	0.007	0.002	0.000	
17	0.992	0.950	0.836	0.647	0.426	0.235	0.107	0.030	0.012	0.003	0.001	0.000
18	0.994	0.961	0.865	0.694	0.481	0.283	0.139	0.057	0.019	0.005	0.001	0.000

Table 5.17 Probability of X or more correct judgments on two successive trials [one-tailed, $p = (\frac{1}{3})(\frac{1}{3}) = (\frac{1}{9})$]

n	1	2	3	4	5	6	7	8
12	0.756	0.391	0.140	0.036	0.007	0.001	0.000	
13	0.783	0.432	0.168	0.048	0.010	0.002	0.000	
14	0.807	0.470	0.198	0.061	0.014	0.003	0.000	
15	0.829	0.508	0.228	0.076	0.019	0.004	0.001	0.000
16	0.848	0.544	0.259	0.093	0.026	0.006	0.001	0.000
17	0.865	0.577	0.291	0.111	0.033	0.008	0.001	0.000
18	0.880	0.609	0.322	0.131	0.042	0.011	0.002	0.000

Table 5.18 Probablities for data in Table 5.15

Trials	Duo–trio or paired comparison[a]	Triangle[b]
1	0.50	0.08
2	0.06	0.00
Combined	0.10	0.00

[a] Assumes results entered in Table 5.15 were derived from a duo–trio or paired-comparison test.
[b] Assumes results in Table 5.15 were derived from a triangle test.

paired-comparison, or triangle test. When the number of subjects exceeds these table values, the above Z formula is recommended.

Returning to the worked example in Table 5.15 and using Table 5.16 (if duo–trio or paired test) and Table 5.17 (if a triangle test), we obtain a p of 0.31 and 0.02, respectively, with five of fifteen subjects correct on both trials. Alternatively, analyzing the data in Table 5.15 for each trial separately and pooled, we obtain the results shown in Table 5.18. Although the analysis applied to the data in Table 5.15 allowed us to pool the responses, and the results from the discriminators (subjects who were correct on both trials) are in general agreement with the pooled data, observation of the different probabilities from the first and second trial reaffirm the value of separate trial-by-trial analysis prior to pooling or any other analysis. Equipped with this information, the sensory professional is in a better position to determine whether the products were found not to be different, or a learning effect occurred.

A second issue related to replication concerns the number of subjects participating in the test. As noted earlier in this section, the literature is not totally clear on this issue. The tables for estimating statistical significance do not differentiate between thirty responses derived from one, two, ten, or more subjects. Yet, as noted by Roessler *et al.* (1978), there can be a difference in the interpretation that would be applied to the results. Sensory evaluation might be reluctant to recommend, with confidence, a "no difference" (or a difference) based on responses from one subject tested thirty times. One reason for a panel of subjects is to move away from reliance on one or two individuals. Obviously, a panel size that ranges between more than one subject and some larger number of subjects will be a sensory decision.

From an operational point of view, the fewest subjects should be used for the least amount of time that will yield a result with minimal risk and maximal confidence. We find that sixteen to twenty subjects per test with a replicate is satisfactory, for the following reasons:

1. For routine tests, subjects will spend not more than ~15 minutes away from their regular work station, including travel time.
2. For most products, evaluating two sets is optimal relative to minimizing sensory interactions (for products with no chemoreceptor stimuli, the number of pairs could be increased).
3. A total of approximately forty responses is sufficient to minimize risk in the decision about product differences (quality control procedures will have a different set of conditions and fewer responses are needed).
4. This panel size minimizes product usage, product preparation and scheduling time, and total test time.
5. From an experimental design perspective, sixteen to twenty subjects is a practical panel size (most serving orders are multiples of two, four, or six).

Several practical issues associated with the number of subjects in a discrimination test have been identified, and we now approach the problem from a statistical point of view. In a discrimination test (as in any sensory test), a hypothesis about the products is established *a priori* the test; for example, there is no difference between product A and product B (or products A and B are perceived as the same), which is expressed as

$$H_0: A = B$$

and referred to as the null hypothesis. The alternative hypothesis is expressed as

$$H_a: A \neq B,$$

A is not the same as B. To reach a decision as to whether to accept or reject the hypothesis selected, a particular probability (or confidence) and a level of risk are assigned. The decision as to which probability level is most appropriate is quite arbitrary; for further discussion, see McNemar (1969), Winer (1971), or Hayes (1973). The traditional values used in sensory evaluation are 0.05, 0.01, and 0.001 (see Amerine *et al.*, 1965). By probability values of 0.05, 0.01, and 0.001, we mean that the probability of the difference occurring by chance is five times in 100 tests, once in 100 tests, and once in 1000 tests, respectively (on all other occasions, this was due to a perceived difference). The number of correct responses sufficient to achieve the statistical significance is not a measure of the magnitude of difference between two variables.

Whenever significance is considered, there is always risk, albeit a small one, that our decision may be wrong. Obviously, this possibility of making a wrong decision is one that we would like to minimize, but the cost of achieving no risk may be very high (e.g. testing all consumers of a particular product). One option is to increase N to some very large number, but this is not practical. In addition, it should be noted that as N increases, the number of correct decisions for statistical significance becomes proportionally smaller, such that one could have statistical significance with just one or two correct decisions above chance. How practical is this result? Obviously, compromises are made that allow testing within the controlled environment with a relatively small number of subjects, but with low risk and high external validity. This approach leads again to the problem of setting an acceptable level of risk. As noted previously (Chapter 4), when the probability is 0.05, there is a possibility of one error in twenty decisions when we say that the products are the same (H_0: A = B). This particular error is referred to as a Type 1 error, and the probability of it occurring is given by α (alpha). A second type of error that could occur when we say the products are the same, when in fact they are not, is a Type 2 error, and its probability is β (beta). These probabilities are also expressed as follows:

rejecting the null hypothesis when it is *true* is called an error of the first kind (Type 1) and its probability is α (alpha) or
accepting the null hypothesis when it is *false* is called an error of the second kind (Type 2) and its probability is β (beta).

It should be noted that the probability of α is the significance (or probability) value found in the aforementioned tables; that is, when we report that the number of correct decisions is statistically significant at the 0.05 level, we are stating the probability of a Type 1 error. These two errors are not of equal importance and as we will show, the decision about their relative importance requires an appreciation for all components of the test before a decision is reached. Historically, the emphasis has been on α and minimizing this error; inadequate attention has been given to the Type 2 error and its effect on the conclusion (Cohen, 1977). There is a relationship between the two errors in that once α is specified, β also is determined. The two errors also are inversely proportional; the smaller we set α (e.g. $\alpha = 0.01$ or 0.001), the larger β will be (which can be offset to some degree by increasing N). From a business perspective, it turns out that β often can be more important than α. In most discrimination tests, the objective is to minimize perception of difference by the consumer (any perceived change is considered negative). This particular situation is very common; for example, the availability, cost, and quality of raw materials change frequently, and it is important that their impact on product acceptance be evaluated.

The goal for most of these product modifications is to not have the change perceived by the consumer. To achieve this, we select our best subjects and possibly use the duo–trio test with a constant reference. We create a situation in which the likelihood of perceiving the difference is emphasized, and if the difference is not perceived at the appropriate level of significance, we are confident that the change can be made. There is minimal risk of detection by the consumer if our best discriminators under ideal conditions do not perceive the difference. We could also institute a statistical change: let $\alpha = 0.10$; thus fewer correct decisions will be necessary before there is statistical significance. This approach will result in β decreasing (all other factors being equal), and we are more likely (than if we operated at $\alpha = 0.05$) to reject some products that are not different. Since our objective is to protect the current franchise, we will "sacrifice" α for β. That is, we would rather reject some products that may not be different to ensure the acceptance of that "one" which we know is not perceived as different. When we make this tradeoff, we are reducing the risk of saying there is no difference when, in fact, there is. Of course, such a change in probability (from 0.05 to 0.10) may be cause for concern by the test requestor, who may wonder why the change is being made. In this case, it may be desirable to not change α.

It is interesting to note that the sensory literature contains very little information on computation of β risk. Two early publications (Blom, 1955; Radkins, 1957) and a subsequent discussion by Amerine *et al.* (1965; see especially pp. 439–440) provided procedures for the computation and additional insight into β risk. Using the equation provided in Amerine,

$$N = \left[\frac{z_{\alpha}\sqrt{P_0(1 - P_0)} + z_{\beta}\sqrt{P_a(1 - P_a)}}{P_a - P_0} \right]^2$$

where N is the number of judgments, z the z-value corresponding to α and β, respectively, P_0 the probability of the null hypothesis, and P_a the probability of the alternate hypothesis.

This formula enables one to determine β with a specific N or the N necessary for specific α and β values. However, the situation is not totally clear, because the experimenter must also specify the P_a and the P_0 values.

While it may be relatively easy to establish α, usually at 0.05, β may not be so easy to specify. If the desire is to minimize risk and we set β small, say $= 0.01$, the number of judgments required in the test may be quite large (e.g. >100). The problem is complicated by our inability to mathematically account for subject sensitivity and for replication in the statistical formula. In addition, the experimenter must decide on the values to be assigned to P_0 and P_a and how large or small a difference is reasonable between the null hypothesis, P_0, and the alternative hypothesis P_a. This difference is based on the true difference between the samples; however, it is not possible to know the value (which will vary from product to product). We usually set $P_0 = 50$; that is, the likelihood of A $=$ B is ~50%. But what probability can be assigned to P_a?

For discrimination testing, it may be necessary to approach this topic from our knowledge of the general sensory skills of the subject. That is, in most product situations, a qualified subject is expected to perceive product differences once the magnitude of the difference reaches ~20%. For some of the senses (vision and audition), the just-noticeable-difference is <20%, while for others it will be greater [e.g. olfaction (see Wenzel, 1949; Schutz and Pilgrim, 1957; Stone, 1963; Geldard, 1972)]. Because products stimulate many of the senses, we could arbitrarily set $P_a = 0.70$; the difference between P_0 and P_a is set at 0.20 (or 20%). In other words, we are substituting product difference for the subject's estimated ability to perceive the difference. With that as a guide, we compute N for a variety of test conditions as well as for several levels of sensory skill (Table 5.19).

It is obvious that the magnitude of the difference between products, P_a and P_0, will cause an increase or decrease in N, the number of judgments, as does the change in α and β. These data demonstrate that the greatest changes occur as the magnitude of difference decreases – the smaller the difference, the more responses required before this difference will be perceived. However, the reader should reflect carefully on the practical implications. By increasing N, one can expect to find statistical significance between two products from a production line selected within 1 minute of each other and the true difference could be 0.001 units or less. One will find significance but it will have no practical value!

Is it advantageous to shift the levels of α and β, which could mean using an unbalanced design or a large number of judgments? Before attempting to answer the question, we should establish the risk associated with the current procedure of limiting

Table 5.19 Number of judgments required in a discrimination test at specific α and β values[a]

	$\alpha = 0.05, \beta = 0.10$	$\alpha = 0.05, \beta = 0.05$	$\alpha = 0.05, \beta = 0.01$	$\alpha = 0.10, \beta = 0.05$
$P_a - P_0$	N	N	N	N
10	209	263	383	208
15	91	114	165	90
20	49	62	89	48
25	30	37	53	29
30	20	25	34	19

[a] Entries are total number of judgments per test for selected α and β values. Computed from Amerine *et al.* (1965). See text for additional explanation.

Table 5.20 Computed β-risk values for discrimination tests as determined from the number of judgments[a]

	Level of α	
N	0.05	0.10
44	0.1358[a]	0.0672
40	0.1671	0.0866
38	0.1853	0.0981
36	0.2050	0.1111
30	0.2757	0.1606
20	0.4377	0.3900

[a] Entries are β values computed using the formula from Amerine *et al.* (1965). See text for additional explanation.

judgments to ~30–40. In Table 5.20, computed β values are reported when $\alpha = 0.05$ and 0.10, at a fixed level of sensitivity of 20% ($P_a - P_0$). It is apparent that β risk almost doubled when α was decreased from 0.10 to 0.05. For $N = 40$, the risk of committing a Type 2 error is approximately 17% (0.1671), about one time in six, which may not be that serious.

Associated with this risk is the related issue of the statistical power of the test. Cohen (1977) defines power as "the probability that it will lead to the rejection of the null hypothesis ..." Or stated another way, power is equal to 1 minus the probability of a Type 2 error (Winer, 1971). McNemar (1969), Winer (1971), and Cohen (1977) all direct attention to the importance of power and the extent to which it is most often overlooked. In general, it can be stated that as α is reduced, for example, to 0.01 or smaller, the increase in β risk results in a decrease in statistical power. Furthermore, one can assess the relative importance (or seriousness) of the respective errors. Since power (P) is equal to $1 - \beta$ (and the greatest power is achieved when β is very small), then for $N = 40$ and $\alpha = 0.05$ and $\beta = 0.1671$, the statistical power is 0.8329.

We can also consider the situation in terms of its relative importance, that is, the ratio of Type 1 to Type 2 errors is 0.1671/0.05, or 3.4:1. We consider a Type 2 error as 3.4 times more likely to occur (or more serious) than a Type 1 error.

It should be kept in mind that these computations have not taken into account subject replication, a factor that further reduces β risk. A reasonably high degree of confidence in results can be obtained from twenty qualified experienced subjects with a test involving one replication. By maintaining subject performance records and using the appropriate test method, one should expect to further reduce β risk from that computed by as much as 50%. It remains for the researchers to develop the appropriate mathematical procedures to support this hypothesis.

F. The Just-Noticeable Difference

In Chapter 1, the importance of the just-noticeable difference (JND) was discussed in relation to the perceptual process and the discrimination test methodology. There also are situations in which it is useful to estimate JND as an element in establishing product manufacturing specifications. This practice is a step removed from the more typical applications of the discrimination model as described in this chapter. In effect, systematic changes made in a particular variable are used as a basis for estimating how much change is needed before it is perceived. Rather than determining whether or not ingredient "x" can be substituted without being perceived, the objective is to determine how much change can be tolerated! While this particular issue also is considered in the discussion on quality control in Chapter 8, it warrants some discussion here because of its unique discrimination methodology requirement.

To determine the JND for a particular variable and to express the relationship mathematically, the constant-stimulus method is most likely to be used (see Guilford, 1954; Schutz and Pilgrim, 1957; Stone, 1963; Perfetti and Gordin, 1985; Laming, 1986).

This procedure involves a series of paired comparisons, with the subject's task being to note which one of the pair is more intense. One of the pair is always the same (the constant) and the other is either weaker or stronger. A proper spacing of the latter products results in proportional judgments from which an equation for the line of best fit can be computed (Bock and Jones, 1968). An alternative single-stimulus method could also be used (see Schutz and Pilgrim, 1957); however, the result is identical in all other aspects.

For the test to be successful, it is necessary that the particular variable be controlled so that a set of test products can be prepared that bracket the "norm." While it is relatively easy to implement this control in model systems, it is often quite difficult in product manufacturing. Nonetheless, if a predictive equation is to be formulated with any degree of confidence, then it is essential that no evaluation be made unless the products are within the experimental limits. Obviously, if the products are too close together, the predictive equation will be based on too few points and be of less value!

However, once the JND is known, it can be used to gauge the impact of machine variability and the importance of such change on preference. The implications are far reaching and can be of considerable economic importance.

IV. Special Problems

Mention was made earlier in this chapter about the importance of utilizing the test procedures as they were developed, or at the least to carefully consider modifications within the context of the sensory task. For example, a monadic sequential serving procedure is a reasonable alternative to the use of lighting changes (e.g. red or yellow) which can introduce other undesired variables into the test. While such a modification is reasonable, many other modifications that have been described create considerably more problems than they propose to solve. Some modifications offer clearly demonstrated statistical advantages, but entail considerable disadvantage from a behavioral viewpoint and are often quite impractical in a typical business environment. In general, these modifications can be characterized as being of three main types; preference after difference, magnitude of difference, and description of difference (descriptive). In each case, it appears that the overall intent of the modification is to increase the amount of information obtained from the test. If one considers that a subject may take as much as 5–10 minutes to provide two responses (the usual number, but more responses are possible), it would seem to be a relatively small output compared with that of the descriptive test, for example, where the same amount of time might yield ten times the number of responses. Many of the modifications are supported by statistical computations (Radkins, 1959; Bradley and Harmon, 1964; Gridgeman, 1964; Steiner, 1966; Ferdinandus *et al.*, 1970); however, most modifications have limited behavioral support. In the discussion that follows, we take a behavioral approach to provide the sensory professional with a greater appreciation for the risks as well as the statistical advantages offered by each method.

A. Is there Preference after Difference?

This particular question is one that continues to plague the sensory professional, although there are many problems associated with it. In recent years, this approach of discrimination followed by preference has been used with consumers, providing still one more example of the misapplication of sensory methodology.

In the laboratory situation, the subject makes a discrimination decision followed by the preference task. An alternative has been to remove the products and scorecard after the discrimination task and then to serve the two products again and request the preference. Either approach leads to a high-risk situation. First, odd sample bias exists in discrimination tests (Schutz, 1954) and one cannot design away the bias. By odd sample bias, we mean avoiding the product that is different from the other two in a three-product test, and the product that is not "the same as …" in the paired situation. Some subjects will assume that the product that is different is not "as good."

A second weakness is inherent in the subjects themselves; they were selected based on discrimination skill and their attitudes about the products may be completely skewed. The panel size is small (about twenty subjects) and the database is equally small (thirty to forty responses), hardly sufficient for any meaningful preference information. Perhaps most important is the context of test tasks; there is no assurance that the subjects have made the psychological transition from perceiving a difference to stating a preference. The assignment may seem to be relatively simple, such as "tell me which product you prefer," and the subjects mark their scorecard; the fact is that two very different tasks are involved, and some subjects may not make the mental transition thus resulting in a response that is confounded.

A third objection concerns the preference responses by subjects who did not make correct decisions; that is, subjects who did not match the same pair or a panel that had an insufficient number of correct decisions to achieve statistical significance. If no statistically significant difference exists, then no difference in preference for the two products can be expressed. While this latter situation is clear, those situations where there is a difference between products still pose a problem. Does one only report preferences for the correct decisions, which means that one is selectively reporting results, or does one include results for subjects who do not perceive a difference! While it is true that there are statistical procedures for analysis of the results (e.g. Ferdinandus *et al.*, 1970; Woodward and Shucany, 1977), the basic issues we describe have been ignored.

The report by Ferdinandus and co-workers is especially troublesome for several reasons; the combining of difference with preference, the establishment of a new, combined probability of $\frac{1}{6}$ and the concept of non-recognition. In fact, the authors have chosen to discuss discrimination using the term "recognition." Behaviorally, one might be on rather tenuous ground with the term "recognition" versus "discrimination." A subject may be capable of perceiving a difference but may not recognize the sensation(s) responsible. The concept of non-recognition is also very confusing, especially in relation to accepting or rejecting a particular hypothesis. It is difficult to define non-recognition. Is it an inability to perceive a difference, a momentary loss of concentration, or a case of sensory fatigue? Could it be that the concentration difference was too small for that subject at that time? None of these options can be separated before, during, or after the test. Finally, what use is derived from knowledge that a subject did not "recognize" the difference on one particular occasion but did "recognize" the difference on another occasion? The problem with such approaches is the rationale; all products are "different," and given sufficient products and subjects, one can demonstrate that a statistically significant difference exists. Telling the requestor that a significant number of subjects did not recognize a difference might mislead that individual to assume that there was no perceived difference. Similarly, when there was a statistically significant difference, there could also be statistically significant non-recognition!

The discrimination–preference combination procedure has also been used in marketing research with consumers (see Morrison, 1981; Buchanan, *et al.*, 1987). It is assumed that if consumers cannot perceive product differences, they cannot have a valid preference. By eliminating the non-discriminators, one is left with individuals whose preferences are more precise. Unfortunately, the rationale, while possessing a certain appeal, is flawed. The idea that a single (or even two) discrimination test will identify a discriminator is inconsistent with the evidence. Screening subjects takes considerably more than a single trial; most individuals must first learn how to take a test. This does not mean that an individual cannot make a reliable judgment about which product is liked. As noted, the two tasks are quite different. Thus, one will have a group of consumers, some of whom are participating based on a chance decision and not based on actual perception.

The typical database used in these tests is derived from several hundred consumers. With such a large database, it is relatively easy to have statistical significance, leading the investigator to conclude that consumers can participate in discrimination tests, that one can observe differences not identified with laboratory panels, and by implication that the results are valid. The flaws in this approach have been described earlier in this discussion and elsewhere in this chapter. Sensory evaluation must address these issues directly and must delineate the characteristics of the discrimination test and ensure that it is not used as part of a consumer preference test.

B. Magnitude of the Difference

It has been suggested that one might also be interested in determining the magnitude of the difference between the products. In this procedure, the subject first makes a discrimination decision followed by a measure of the perceived magnitude. The measurement is usually achieved with a category-type scale – weak, moderate, strong, and so on – which is converted to numerical values for subsequent analysis. A detailed discussion about the method, including a procedure for data analysis that incorporates all responses from subjects, was given by Bradley and Harmon (1964). Although their approach utilized the triangle test, the authors noted that the procedure could be extended to the duo–trio test. It is emphasized that if one intends to collect magnitude of difference responses, then the approach described herein is certainly recommended. However, a more basic issue concerns the value of knowledge of the magnitude of the difference and whether such knowledge will be useful in product formulation.

Assume the test objective is to replace ingredient A with B such that the samples are not perceived as different (i.e. H_0: A = B). If no statistically significant difference exists, then we accept H_0 and any magnitude of difference information is of no value. If a statistically significant difference does exist, then we would turn our attention to the value of the magnitude. It must be kept in mind that the magnitude value is a sensory magnitude, and the relationship between the sensory response and a specific amount of ingredient is not established. For example, knowledge that the difference is two scale units may not be very helpful to sensory evaluation or to the test requestor, since these are sensory units. Sensory evaluation must still make a professional judgment in guiding the requestor.

Remember that prior to any test, products are screened by the sensory professional and obvious differences are eliminated. Gradually, formulation efforts result in submission of products whose differences are quite small, usually at or near the JND, and therefore warrant testing. The responses will be clustered around the lower end of the scale, but still it is a sensory magnitude. For sensory evaluation, the problem is considerably less complex in the sense that knowledge of JND provides general direction to the requestor. In the chemical senses, a JND of around 20% is typical (Schutz and Pilgrim, 1957; Stone and Bosley, 1965); for the other senses, a JND of approximately 15% (Geldard, 1972) is reasonable. Basically, the JND for the individual senses are smaller and larger than these values; however, one must take into account the complexity of products and the extent to which ingredients interact with one another, hence the guideline of approximately 20%. This approach is obviously less formal; however, the problem of sensory magnitude affords one little solace. Sensory evaluation must still establish the perceptual meaning of that value – one JND, two, and so on – to provide a meaningful course of action for the requestor. From a practical viewpoint, such effort provides no advantage for sensory evaluation, but does require further analysis and interpretation. On the other extreme of the spectrum, Meilgaard *et al.* (1999) describe a procedure to determine whether there is no perceivable difference between two products. This too has seen very little use in comparison to traditional discrimination approaches.

C. Description of Difference

Another modification to the discrimination test requires subjects to indicate the basis for their decisions. It is assumed that since the subjects perceive a difference they should also be able to specify that difference. The task can be made especially easy if one provides a checklist. Examples of these types of scorecards can be found throughout the literature (see especially Amerine *et al.*, 1965, p. 341), as well as in most company files on sensory testing. Historically, the methods appear to have been derived from production/quality control sources. The "cutting" session used in canning is one major source. Another source is the transfer from market research. The assumptions that have proven to be especially dangerous are "we have used it for years and it always worked" or "the subjects answered all the questions so it must be valid." These particular issues have been addressed previously (see Chapter 2) and are mentioned here to allow the reader to refer to the arguments associated with these issues.

Obviously, the procedures are filled with risk from beginning to end. Subjects will use different words to connote the same sensation (or the reverse). One cannot assume otherwise without some type of language training. Using a checklist will cue subjects to focus attention on product attributes that may not be perceived or that are not understood. If one makes a concerted effort to develop attributes that are meaningful to all subjects, then one has taken a major step toward creation of a descriptive analysis capability (see Chapter 6). This capability should not be combined with the discrimination task. All too often, the requestor will distort the results to meet personal expectations. The failure to appreciate the behavioral–product relationships results in considerable misinformation about product differences and ultimately erodes the credibility of sensory evaluation. To avoid these problems, one should use the discrimination test strictly as it was designed, to determine whether the products are perceived as different and to establish the level of significance for that difference.

V. Summary

The discrimination test is a powerful sensory evaluation method in terms of its sensitivity and providing reliable and valid results. The test method has evolved in response to a greater appreciation for the perceptual processes involved in the discrimination task. In this exposition of discrimination testing, considerable emphasis has been placed on the use of methods according to strict guidelines. Of paramount importance is the strict adherence to detection of a perceived difference. While the literature includes numerous references to modifications of the methods, most if not all modifications introduce problems, especially with regard to data analysis and interpretation. To a considerable degree, many of these problems arise from a lack of appreciation for the use of the method in relation to other test methods, and a failure to follow accepted testing guidelines. It is important that the sensory professional recognize the following innate qualities of discrimination tests:

1. In practice, all discrimination tests are equally sensitive.
2. The discrimination test is forced choice; subjects must make a choice.
3. The discrimination test usually precedes other testing (e.g. descriptive and preference).
4. Products not perceived as different cannot be assigned different preferences.
5. Products perceived as different can be equally liked for different reasons.
6. Not all products warrant testing.

To minimize problems and to develop a resource that is accepted, the following guidelines are recommended:

1. Use a discrimination test only to measure whether there is a perceived difference.
2. Base selection of a particular method on the test objective and the product's characteristics.

3. Subjects should be selected on the basis of specific performance criteria, including experience with the product or product category; a performance better than chance for at least the previous three or four tests.
4. Use "sip-and-spit" procedure for foods and beverages; for other products, use a standard procedure.
5. Replication is required.
6. Use a balanced serving order.
7. Do not use discrimination testing as part of a consumer acceptance test.
8. Design the test environment to minimize all non-product variables and do not attempt to simulate any other environment.
9. Avoid or minimize product carriers where possible.
10. Express results from a discrimination test in probabilistic terms.

Careful planning and attention to details are required to develop a capability that management can accept as reliable and valid. The results of discrimination testing have proven effective and have saved companies substantial amounts of time, money, and effort, for a relatively modest investment.

Descriptive Analysis

6

I. Introduction

Descriptive analysis is the most sophisticated of the methodologies available to the sensory professional (when compared with discrimination and acceptance methods). Results from a descriptive analysis test provide complete sensory descriptions of an array of products, provide the basis for mapping product similarities and differences, and provide a basis for determining those sensory attributes that are important to acceptance. The results enable one to relate specific ingredient or process variables to specific changes in some (or all) of the sensory attributes of a product. This latter application of the descriptive methodology will be discussed later in this chapter and in Chapter 8. From a product development viewpoint, descriptive information is essential in focusing efforts on those product variables that are identified as different among relative to a target, and also to establish causal relationships. For these and other reasons to be discussed, there continues to be much attention focused on the methodology and its applications as evidenced by an examination of the current sensory literature. Research continues on various methods, new as well as existing, along with proposed approaches to the screening and training of subjects, and the analyses of the responses. They reflect different sensory testing philosophies and approaches to the descriptive analysis process. Before describing these methods, it is

Sensory Evaluation Practices 3rd Edn
ISBN: 0-12-672690-6

useful to define descriptive analysis as discussed here as well as to provide a brief historical perspective to the development of the methodology.

> *Descriptive analysis is a sensory methodology that provides quantitative descriptions of products, based on the perceptions from a group of qualified subjects. It is a total sensory description, taking into account all sensations that are perceived – visual, auditory, olfactory, kinesthetic, etc. – when the product is evaluated. The word "product" is used here in the figurative sense; the products may be an idea or concept, an ingredient, or a finished product as purchased and used by the consumer. The evaluation also can be total, for example, as in the evaluation of a shaving cream before, during, and after use. Alternatively, the evaluation can focus on only one aspect, such as use. The evaluation is defined in part by the product characteristics as determined by the subjects, and in part by the nature of the problem.*

Considering the information obtained from a descriptive test, the substantial interest in the use of these methods is understandable. The value of descriptive analysis was appreciated by its earliest practitioners, the brewmasters, perfumers, flavorists, and others. Wine and food writers and reviewers also practise a form of descriptive analysis; however, it is a purely qualitative exposition and one should treat that information accordingly. The food industry's use of chefs for developing new and innovative flavors is an indirect example particularly when their descriptions become a part of the product message. The brewmasters, flavorists, etc. described products and made recommendations about the purchase of specific raw materials; they evaluated the effect of process variables on product quality (as they determined product quality), especially the determination that a particular product met their criteria (and that of their company) for manufacture and sale to the consumer. These activities served as the basis for the foundation of sensory evaluation as a science; although, it was not considered within that context. It was possible for the expert to be reasonably successful as long as the marketplace was less competitive. Limited choices were available to the consumer, as were the ingredient and technology options.

All this changed with the scientific and technological developments in most consumer products industries and especially in the food and beverage industry. The impact of technology, the use of more complex raw materials, and related developments made it increasingly difficult for experts to be as effective as in the past, and certainly not effective in a global sense. The expert's functions were further challenged by the increasingly competitive and international nature of the marketplace, the rapid introduction and proliferation of new products, and the sophistication of the consumer's palate. At this same time period, sensory evaluation began its development, providing specialized test methods, scales for measurement, and statistical procedures for the analysis of results. Formal descriptive analysis and the separation of the individual expert from sensory evaluation received its major impetus from the development of the Flavor Profile® method (Cairncross and Sjöstrom, 1950; Caul, 1957). These investigators demonstrated that it was possible to select and train a group of individuals to describe their perceptions of a product in some agreed sequence, leading to actionable results without dependence on the individual expert. The method was distinctive in that no direct judgment was made concerning consumer acceptance of the product; although most investigators assumed consumer acceptance based on the reporting process. The method attracted considerable interest as well as controversy (discussed later in this chapter); however, there is no question as to its "historical" importance to the field. Since then, other methods have been described and their applications have grown substantially (Stone *et al.*, 1974; Williams and Langron, 1984; Meilgaard *et al.*, 1999).

Before describing specific test methods, it is important to first review the more fundamental issues on which all descriptive methods are based. In particular, we refer to the subject selection process; the extent and duration of the training, including the development of the descriptive language (for the array of products being evaluated); the quantification of the judgments; and finally, the analysis of the data leading to actionable recommendations. Such a discussion is particularly important because there are numerous decisions made by the panel leader in the course of the organization, development and use of a descriptive panel. These decisions and actions derive from that person's knowledge and understanding of the perceptual process, in general, and the descriptive process, in particular. Unlike discrimination and acceptance tests, where subjects exhibit choice behavior in a global sense; that is, all perceptions are taken into account to yield a single judgment, the descriptive test requires the subject to provide numerous judgments for each product.

A descriptive test involves relatively few subjects (as few as ten to as many as twenty) and there must be good evidence that the specific differences obtained are reliable and valid, and not the result of spurious responses from one or two more sensitive subjects. In the case of Flavor Profile®, the number of subjects was limited to six; placing great reliance on the group achieving agreement before a decision could be reached about a product. Since the method, as originally developed, was qualitative, this agreement was important with regard to recommendations. Implicit in the use of a limited number of subjects is the knowledge that the subjects are qualified. However, as we will show, there is no unanimity with regard to what constitutes qualified. For example, subjects who have demonstrated their skill at perceiving differences at better than chance among products of the type that they will evaluate in the actual test serves as an excellent qualifying system. For Flavor Profile® this qualifying approach was tedious, taking more than 14+ weeks. Failure to adequately screen each individual raises serious questions as to that person's ability to describe differences or score the intensities with any degree of confidence and, of course, this increases the risk of a Type 2 error (β risk). It enables one to use the fewest number of subjects without loss of information. As was discussed in Chapters 2 and 5, not all people interested in participating in a sensory analytical test will meet minimal discrimination ability requirements, and that about 30% of those who volunteer will fail. In addition, it must be kept in mind that selecting individuals based on their sensitivity to particular chemicals (e.g. sweet, sour, salt, and bitter stimuli or a selection of odorants) or based on various personality tests will not substitute for demonstrated sensory ability with the products to be tested. That sensitivity to basic taste and odor stimuli continues to be recommended (see Powers, 1988; Meilgaard *et al.*, 1999) is surprising in view of earlier evidence that it provided no indication of a subject's subsequent performance (Mackey and Jones, 1954). We have observed that subjects qualified based on sensitivity to basic tastes and/or odorants (proposed as standards) usually repeat these experiences when they develop a language; that is, there appears to be an assumption on their part that these stimuli are expected to be present in the products. There is a clear lack of appreciation for the messages that are "communicated" to subjects without the experimenter appreciating this and its effects on their responses (for more on this topic, see Orne, 1981). Still another approach proposed no subject screening; anyone can participate as a subject (Williams and Langron, 1984; Williams and Arnold, 1985) and a type of factor analysis was used to identify meaningful results. Subsequent to its introduction, this method has been revised to include some training which appears to require more hours than required by QDA®, for example. While mathematical approaches to describing behavior are a topic of considerable interest and some successes, predicting perceptions appears to be a more complex and challenging issue. Clearly, there are very basic differences in the approaches that are used for the qualification of subjects and the panel leader must decide what procedure(s) they are willing to use in their descriptive testing.

In using the QDA methodology (Stone *et al.*, 1974), we observed that the discrimination methodology has been and continues to be the most effective procedure for identifying subjects who can and cannot perceive differences (after first determining that they are regular users of the specific product category). It takes relatively little time to identify individuals who can and cannot perceive differences. Using twenty to no more than thirty discrimination trials fielded over 2 or 3 days (sessions last about 90 minutes), one can select a pool of discriminators from amongst a group of totally naïve individuals. For more information on this procedure, the reader should review Chapters 2 and 5. The screening procedure, at this stage, has several purposes; to eliminate the insensitive non-discriminator, to identify the most sensitive and reliable, to familiarize all subjects with the sensory properties of the products. In effect, one wants to develop a panel that is representative of the discriminating segment of the population because these are the consumers who are likely to detect and respond to product differences. Only after data collection can one determine empirically the effectiveness of the screening and subsequent training activities.

Screening should be product category specific as is the subsequent training effort. For example, if one were testing coffee, then the screening would be done with various coffees and not fruit beverages. In this way, one minimizes the risk of including insensitive and/or unreliable subjects in a test for a particular category of products. This does not mean that one is confronted with the task of having to requalify subjects every time a different set of products is evaluated. Most subjects are very capable of meeting the qualifying criteria for many different categories of products, particularly after they participated in several tests. These are issues that a sensory professional must consider whenever a test is planned and reconsidered after a test, when examining subject performance records.

Screening subjects for more than one type of product (e.g. ice cream and frozen yogurt) could be efficient because it eliminates need for additional screening before each new product category. This neither guarantees that a subject will stay qualified for all the products nor does it eliminate the need for the other training activities, or assessing subject performance in anticipation of the next test. A potential problem with screening subjects on several products arises when the volume of testing is such that it impacts the subjects' regular work activities and their availability to test. A second concern is the assumption that the subject will want to participate that frequently and not lose interest, and a third is the likelihood that these other products will be tested within a reasonable time period (e.g. within the next 4–6 weeks). It may be better to develop a larger pool of qualified subjects and thus reduce reliance on a small subset of people for all testing (see Chapter 2 for more discussion on this topic). This is true whether one is using employees or non-employees.

In summary, it is necessary that subjects for a descriptive test demonstrate their ability to perceive differences at better than chance among the products that they will be testing; that for inexperienced individuals, this skill takes as many as twenty to thirty trials to demonstrate; and that about 30% of those who volunteer will fail to meet the chance probability requirement. Once subjects have participated in testing, the need for screening is removed and data analyses provide direct measures for each subject's performance in each test. This will be discussed in more detail later in this chapter.

The training process, which follows screening, also has a number of alternative approaches. It is primarily focused on developing or familiarizing subjects with a descriptive language that is used as a basis for scoring the products. There also are other equally important activities that are part of the training, and these include the grouping of attributes by modality (i.e. appearance attributes, aroma attributes, etc.), listing them by occurrence, developing a definition for each attribute, identifying helpful references for use during training, and familiarizing the subjects with the scoring procedure. Depending on the test method used, the training can be quite different. If the subjects are inexperienced and no terminology is available, then this training will take the maximum amount of time, about 7–10 hours (not continuous but within a limited time period of 5 days, for example). Inexperienced subjects presented with the task of learning to use an existing language also could require as much as 7 or more hours. If the subjects are experienced, the training time is reduced to about 5 hours. These times are presented solely as a guide inasmuch as the products and the skill of panel leader will have an impact on the entire training process. In all these situations, the subjects work individually and as a group to ensure that the attributes are fully understood and that all of the product's characteristics have been fully accounted for. In QDA®, all of this is done under the direction of a panel leader who does not participate in developing the language. The QDA® methodology was the first methodology and still is one of the few methods that excludes the panel leader from directly participating in the language development, contrary to the statement by Powers (1988). This is true whether one is working with an experienced group or one that has never participated before. The panel leader's primary responsibility is to facilitate communications among subjects. The panel leader who participates as a subject is a biased subject because they are aware of the product differences and the test objective. Not only does this action communicate the wrong message to the subjects (subjects will tend to defer to the panel leader whom they assume has the correct answer) but also, the end result is a group judgment rather than a group of judgments (see Jones, 1958 for more on this issue).

Developing a sensory language or using one that already exists is an interesting process and certainly one that is essential for the successful outcome of a test. For some, the language assumes almost mystical importance, such that a considerable body of literature has been developed in which lists of words are published for specific types of products (see, e.g. Johnson and Civille, 1986; Muñoz, 1986). It appears that most of these lists (or lexicons) were compiled from the literature by product technologists and collated and assigned some measure of credibility by being published. Unfortunately, this is not very different from the efforts of product specialists or experts of 50 or more years ago when they developed quality scales and corresponding descriptions for products as part of an effort to establish food quality standards. Besides their interest in evaluation of their respective company's products, their technical and trade associations often formed committees for the express purpose of developing a common language for describing the flavor (or odor) of the particular category of products. For purposes of this discussion we chose the publication by Clapperton *et al.* (1975) on beer flavor terminology as an example of the efforts (of the association of brewers) to develop an internationally agreed terminology. Another example of this approach to standardizing the sensory language is described by Noble *et al.* (1987). The former authors stated the purpose as "... to allow flavor impressions to be described objectively and in precise terms." Various literature and professional sources were screened for words (or descriptors) describing the flavor of beer, and after reviews, the committee arrived at an agreed-on list. As the authors noted, the issue of chemical names compared with general descriptive terms was resolved with the inclusion of both.

From a technical viewpoint, the use of chemical names was appealing because it was believed they could be related to specific chemicals in the beer. An example would be the term diacetyl, which could be ascribed to a specific chemical, as compared with buttery, a less precise term that might be ascribed to several chemicals. By including both, it was stated that the terminology would be of value to the flavor specialist (the expert) and the layman (the consumer). While the concept of an agreed, in advance, terminology should have appeal, careful consideration of this approach reveals significant limitations, especially in relation to its application in sensory evaluation. It is risky to decide *a priori* what words subjects should use to describe a particular sensation or group of sensations. The fact that product changes – for example, a formulation change, or a process change, – rarely change just one attribute, emphasizes the complex nature of the process. To restrict subjects to specific words assumes that language is unchanging in terms of these words and the meanings assigned to them. While the chemical terminology should have specific meaning to experts, it is unlikely to have the same meaning to the consumer or to trained subjects (see Chapter 8, Section III). From a behavioral viewpoint, this approach must, therefore, be viewed as not directly applicable to descriptive analysis. Regardless of the source, a language that does not provide for subject input is not likely to yield uncomplicated sensory responses. Subjects are influenced by the information given to them, and are much less likely to question it, because of its source. While it can be argued that such approaches are merely intended to help panel leaders or the subjects, the temptation is very strong to use this approach rather than allowing subjects to use their own terminology.

To the student of the history of psychology, descriptive analysis can be considered as a type of introspection, a methodology used by the school of psychology known as structuralism in its study of the human experience (for a lengthy discussion on this topic, see Boring, 1950; Marx and Hillix, 1963; Harper, 1972). Structuralism required the use of highly trained observers in a controlled situation verbalizing their conscious experience (the method of introspection). Of particular interest to us is the use of the method of introspection as an integral part of the descriptive analysis process and specifically the language development component.

However, the obvious difference is that products are included (in descriptive analysis) so that the subject's responses are perceptual and not conceptual. In addition, the subjects are encouraged to use any words they want, provided they use words that are a common everyday language, and that they define the meaning of each word-sensation experience, if for no other reason than to ensure that they will be able to score the products using a terminology with which they are familiar. While each subject begins with his or her own set of words, they work as a group, under the direction of a panel leader, to come to agreement as to the meaning of those words; that is, the definitions or explanations for each word-sensation experience, and also when they (the sensations) occur. All of these activities require time; in the QDA® methodology, there can be as many as four or five sessions, each lasting about 90 minutes, and are essential if this sensory language is to be understood and the subjects are capable of using it (and the scale) to differentiate the products. These training sessions help to identify attributes that could be misunderstood (and will be by some subjects), and also enable the subjects to practice scoring products and discussing results, on an attribute-by-attribute basis, under direction of the panel leader. Of course, all this effort cannot make subjects equally sensitive to all attributes. In fact, when evaluating products, subjects rarely, if ever, achieve equal sensitivity or complete agreement for all attributes, nor is this ever expected (if this did occur one could rely on the *N* of 1!). The effectiveness of this effort can be determined only after a test has been completed; each subject has scored the products on a repeated trial basis, the appropriate analyses have been completed, and decisions can be reached that are consistent with what is known about the product variables and are consistent with the results of the analyses. The idea that there should be a specific number of attributes is questionable, as is the issue of whether one has the correct or right attributes. How does one know that all the attributes have been developed or that they are the right ones? In fact, such questions as these are beside the point as they are implying that there are correct answers (determined by the panel leader or possibly some higher authority). The answer to the former is empirical (and in part answered in much the same way as one determines the number of angels that can be fit on the head of a pin). The answer to the latter also is empirical; that is, given a set of product variables, do some attributes exhibit systematic changes as a function of those variables. One of the newer methods, Free-Choice profiling, requires no subject screening or training and allows subjects to use any words they want relying on statistics (e.g. Procrustes Analyses) to decide which attributes are related (statistically) to each other (Williams and Langron, 1984). However, in more recent publications in which the method was used, it was stated that about 5+ hours of training was reported as necessary to obtain useful results (Marshall and Kirby, 1988). This method would appear to be suggesting that questions as to the number of attributes or their correctness are not at all relevant, that in fact, it makes no difference what words subjects use, that the appropriate statistical analysis will yield the answer(s). This method will be discussed further in the next section.

Words used to represent sensations are nothing more than labels developed by the subjects after frequent samplings and discussions; they provide a common basis for their scoring an array of products. There is no reason to assume that these words represent anything beyond that; for example, that each represents a unique sensation (see Stone, 1999 for comments on this issue). It has been suggested by O'Mahony and co-workers (Ishii and O'Mahony, 1990, 1991; O'Mahony *et al.*, 1990) and by Civille and Lawless (1986) that the words represent concepts, and that for a descriptive panel to be effective and the results useful, concepts must be aligned; that is, that subjects must agree on all the sensations (or attributes that represent those sensations) to be included in a concept. Ishii and O'Mahony (1991) stated that "... to understand fully the mechanisms involved in formation of the ad hoc descriptive language it becomes necessary to consider the mechanisms of concept formulation." However, one must be careful to not confuse the issues associated with the search for these underlying mechanisms as having anything other than a very indirect effect, at best, on the descriptive process.

Sensory evaluation, as treated in this book, is an applied science that deals with measuring responses to selected products or product attributes. Those measures are used, directly or indirectly, to describe or predict consumer behavior. There is little impetus or value to deal with cognitive mechanisms that may, or may not, explain that behavior. Using unobservable (and usually unmeasurable) "intervening variables," "underlying structures" and "hypothetical constructs," does little to clarify sensory issues and assist in the decision-making process. The search for those mechanisms that explain a behavior after it has happened is an academic activity, where practical value and usefulness need not be measures for success. As yet, no evidence has been presented that would support the ideas of these authors about concept formation and alignment improving the reliability or the validity of a descriptive test. If anything, the converse would be true; that is, that any theory about concept formation and alignment must fit the empirical evidence. One could hypothesize that the process by which subjects discuss their judgments for each attribute and the definitions for those attributes could be considered as concept formation and alignment. This is an integral part of the QDA training process (Stone *et al.*, 1974); however, attaching a label to this activity seems quite unnecessary other than for academic purposes. It also introduces circular thinking in that the construct is used first to describe an observed behavior and then to explain that behavior, much the same way as Freudians use the construct of id, ego, and superego to first describe and then explain behavior. It is surprising that so much attention and effort is given to the terminology itself, as if there is a true, correct language which, when identified, will somehow make results magically correct and respected by everyone. As stated at the beginning of this discussion, the terminology is simply a set of labels that a panel has agreed enables them to fully communicate their description of the sensory properties of the products being evaluated. The label likely represents a complex perception integrating many qualitative and quantitative aspects of the product. For example, increasing the amount of sucrose in some products can influence perceptions for attributes in addition to perceived sweetness. To assume some innate correctness or relationship between a label and an ingredient or process oversimplifies the issue and ultimately misleads the researcher.

It should be kept in mind that the subjects will not agree completely on all the sensations that are perceived any more than will there be complete agreement on all the attributes; the sensations are themselves interactive, leading to multiple words to represent them. In addition, the individuality of each subject (in terms of sensitivity, motivation, personality) further adds to the complexity of the process. During the first few training sessions, it is not unusual for a panel to have as many as 80–100 words. During the subsequent training sessions, this list may be reduced by as much as 50% as the subjects evaluate and discuss their responses and realize that many of the words have a common sensory basis. However, the number of attributes will always be considerably more than is necessary from a strictly mathematical viewpoint; for example, scorecards for many foods will have thirty or more attributes. This should not be surprising if one considers that there will be attributes for each modality; that is, for appearance, aroma, taste, texture, and aftertaste. The fact that there are many more attributes than is needed should not be unexpected or of concern because not all subjects will be equally sensitive to all attributes. Rather, one should be more concerned about having too few attributes, such that subjects are not able to differentiate product differences. It is better to have too many attributes and rely on the analysis to establish which ones were used to differentiate the products.

In addition to a descriptive language and definitions, it is useful but not essential to have references for use in training or re-training subjects (Stone *et al.*, 1974; Stone and Sidel, 1998; Muñoz, 1986; Rainey, 1986). Here too, one finds different opinions as to the types of references and how they are to be used. For example, Muñoz presented a comprehensive list of references and how they are to be used (in texture analysis), including their respective intensity scores for scale extremes. Unfortunately, these references are based on commercially available products, all of which are variable in the normal course of production, let alone the intended changes based on changing technologies, ingredients, and/or market considerations. The author then advised the reader that these references and their intensities may change for the aforementioned reasons, in which case the original references and their intensities will have to be redetermined! So what then is the value of such references? References have a value by providing a sensory context, helping subjects relate to a particular sensation (or group of sensations) that is not easily detected or not easily described. However, references should not, by themselves, be a major source of variability, introduce additional sensory interaction/fatigue, or significantly increase training time. In most training (or retraining) situations, the most helpful references usually are a product's raw materials. Of course, there will be situations in which totally unrelated material will prove helpful to some subjects and it is the panel leader's responsibility to obtain such materials. There also will be situations in which no reference can be found within a reasonable time period. Training should not be delayed just because a reference cannot be found. While most professionals agree that references are helpful, there is no evidence that without them a panel cannot function or that results are unreliable and/or invalid. We have observed that so-called expert languages usually include numerous references, and subjects take considerably longer to learn such a language (if they ever do) than they do a language developed by themselves and using everyday language (this is evident in the 14+ weeks of training required in the Spectrum method). This should not be surprising, if one thinks about it. After all, references are themselves a source of variability; they introduce other attributes unrelated to their purpose, and increase sensory interactions and the more technical they are the more difficult it is to relate to an actual product. Also, pre-test training with simple references leads subjects to expect both qualitative and quantitative perceptions in the products they will evaluate. Where those simple references do not translate well in the complex product, and the subjects embark on a search for that perception, the result often is a "phantom" (i.e. it is not there) product attribute. Therefore, the panel leader must consider the use of references with appreciation for their value as well as for their limitations; and must decide when and what references will be used. In our experience they are of limited value; they may be used in the language development/training but not in the initial sessions as they could confuse the subjects. In re-training or when adding new subjects to a panel, they are helpful in enabling these individuals to experience what the other subjects are talking about and possibly to add their comments to the sensory language.

Some comments also are warranted about data analysis, although more information is provided later in this chapter. A descriptive test yields a large sensory database (in comparison with a discrimination or an acceptance test) including both univariate and multivariate components and, as such, it permits a wide range of statistical analyses to be done. One of the main features of the QDA methodology (Stone *et al.*, 1974) was the use of statistical analysis of the data, which represented a significant development for sensory evaluation. With the availability of statistical packages and of PCs, panel leaders have unlimited and low cost resources, providing an online capability for obtaining means, variance measures, ranks, pair-wise correlations, and for factor analysis, multiple regression, cluster analysis, discriminant analysis, and so forth (the chapter by Powers, 1988, provides an extensive review of many current procedures and practices).

As with any readily available resource, statistics often are misunderstood and/or are misused, particularly when responses are highly variable or when the panel leader uses multivariate procedures without determination of the quality of the basic data. In other instances, factor analysis and/or clustering techniques are used during training as a basis for excluding subjects who are not in agreement with the panel or to eliminate attributes that the panel leader believes are not being used to differentiate products. Powers (1988) and Lyon (1987) described such an approach during training as a means of reducing the number of attributes on the scorecard. One must be careful about using procedures that, *a priori*, decide which subjects or attributes will be used. After all, the subjects are still in training and to have them score products and use the results as a basis for reducing either, or both, may be premature. One of several objectives of training is to enable subjects to learn how to evaluate products using the words that they determined were helpful to them (at that stage of the training). To proceed from one session to another and substantially reduce the list of attributes is communicating a message that there is a correct list of words and with a little patience it will be provided. This approach could lead to a group of subjects who are more likely to agree with each other, but how does one know that those who agree are correct. Using factor analysis to directly reduce the number of attributes is troublesome, particularly during training, because it assumes a cause and effect relationship for those attributes correlated with a specific factor and such assumptions are risky. After a test one can use multivariate procedures to help not only in explaining results but also to identify specific subjects and attribute problems that can be addressed before the next test, but there is much greater risk if one does this before training is completed.

In summary, the descriptive test is a very dynamic system in which the panel leader must make numerous decisions when organizing a panel, through screening, training, and product evaluation. Without sufficient knowledge, inadequate or incorrect product decisions will be reached.

II. Test Methods

In this discussion, we focus on those methods that are described in the literature in some detail so as to enable the reader to assess their usefulness. The methods are classified according to whether the results are qualitative or quantitative, although it is recognized that one could be transformed to the other. As shown in Table 6.1, five methods are assigned specific names, one qualitative and four quantitative, reflecting a relatively wide range of approaches to descriptive analysis. A sixth method, designated as diagnostic descriptive analysis, is included because it represents a broad category of methods. A number of different procedures fit within this designation. Experts are listed here as qualitative for illustrative purposes, although it is recognized that numerical values can be assigned, making the information quantitative as in the case of wine evaluation (Amerine *et al.*, 1959).

Table 6.1 Classification of descriptive analysis methods

Qualitative	Quantitative
Flavor Profile®[a]	Texture Profile[b]
Product experts (perfumer, flavorist, brewmaster, etc.)	QDA[c]
	Spectrum analysis[d]
	Free-Choice profiling[e]
	Diagnostic descriptive analysis[f]

[a] Cairncross and Sjöstrom (1950), Caul (1957).
[b] Brandt *et al.* (1963), Szczesniak *et al.* (1963).
[c] Stone *et al.* (1974, 1980).
[d] Meilgaard *et al.* (1991).
[e] Williams and Langron (1984).
[f] Cross *et al.* (1978), Larson-Powers and Pangborn (1978), Lyons (1987).

A. Flavor Profile®

The Flavor Profile® method (Cairncross and Sjöstrom, 1950; Sjöstrom and Cairncross, 1954; Caul, 1957) is the only formal qualitative descriptive procedure and is probably the most well known of sensory test methods.

The Flavor Profile method utilizes a panel of four to six screened and selected subjects who first examine and then discuss the product in an open session. Once agreement is reached on the description of the product, the panel leader summarizes the results in report form. Subjects are selected for training based on a series of screening tests, including sensory acuity, interest, attitude, and availability. This selection process is common to all formal descriptive methods, and, in principle, one can find little disagreement with this approach. In practice, however, the sensory acuity tests are concerned only with basic taste and odor sensitivity, skills that appear to have minimal connection with product evaluation (Mackey and Jones, 1954). Nonetheless, they do provide some form of differentiation of individuals based on acuity. For Flavor Profile this database is combined with the attitudinal information, and six subjects are selected for further training, which includes instructional information about the senses as well as direct experience evaluating selected products.

For this method the key individual is the panel leader, who coordinates the testing and reports results. This individual assumes a leadership role, directing the conversation and providing a consensus conclusion based on the results. This role as panel leader can have significant consequences without some independent controls. Subjects could be led to a conclusion without being aware that this had occurred. In addition, the six subjects take turns serving as the panel leader, which could have a further influence on results. Nonetheless, as a sensory test, the method had considerable appeal because results could be obtained rapidly. The subjects meet, as a group, for about an hour to evaluate a product, reach a consensus about its sensory properties, and provide the requestor with a result. The developers of the method emphasized that there would be confidence based on the collective professional judgment of the panel and this would obviate the need for statistics.

One modification to Flavor Profile that elicited considerable interest was the dilution procedure recommended by Tilgner (1962). The purpose for the method was to be able to evaluate products in which flavor interactions were minimized by means of diluted samples and comparisons with full-strength samples were not possible. The method aroused considerable interest when first introduced, but this interest was not sustained. The major weakness appeared to be the failure of the method to demonstrate the value of the dilution results compared with those from finished products. In a later publication, Tilgner (1965) described results from a series of products using the method but not addressing the more practical issue of application. In spite of this omission, the method represented an attempt to broaden the scope of Flavor Profile. Tilgner also instituted a number of other modifications, including the use of a five-point intensity scale and statistical procedures for analysis of results. These changes were in a direction that was consistent with the more typical sensory test; however, the use of the dilution method appeared to be primarily applicable to research.

B. Texture Profile®

Chronologically, the next descriptive method of importance was the Texture Profile® method developed at the General Foods Research Center (Brandt *et al.*, 1963; Szczesniak, 1963; Szczesniak *et al.*, 1963). This method represented an advancement in descriptive analysis from a structural point of view; however, conceptually it did not take into account the behavioral issues, which in our experience limits its usefulness. By structure, we refer to the development of the descriptive terminology, the scales for recording intensities, and the word/product anchors for each scale category. However, once this structure was completed, the product evaluation procedure used a Flavor Profile approach with panelists discussing results in order to reach a conclusion.

Brandt and co-workers (1963) defined a texture profile as "the sensory analysis of the texture complex of a food in terms of its mechanical, geometrical, fat and moisture characteristics, the degree of each present and the order in which they appear from first bite through complete mastication." This definition could be applied to any descriptive analysis; in this situation, the focus is on texture, which implies independence of responses from other sensations. We will come back to this particular issue later.

In developing the method, the objective was to eliminate problems of subject variability, allow direct comparison of results with known materials, and provide a relationship with instrument measures (Szczesniak *et al.*, 1963). The authors claimed these objectives were accomplished through the use of standard rating scales for each texture term and specific reference materials to represent each scale category for each of the terms. At the outset, texture terms and definitions were compiled, sorted, and categorized. This information included both scientific/technical and popular terms, the latter from laboratory or field situations in which common usage terms were used to describe textural sensations. This led to the development of a classification of terms that were believed to encompass texture sensations. As shown in Table 6.2, the information was organized into three main categories and subsets within each of these. All of these terms were defined; for example, hardness was defined as the force necessary to attain a given deformation and viscosity is defined as the rate of flow per unit force. The technical nature of these definitions should be meaningful to the chemist, but one might question their perceptual meaning to a test subject. For each parameter, a scale of five, seven, eight, or nine categories (depending on the specific parameter) was developed and for each category (of a scale) there was a specific product that represented that sensation. For the hardness scale, a panel rating of "1" was derived from a specific brand of cream cheese, "5" was a giant-size stuffed olive, etc. Except for the chewiness scale, the authors stated that the distances from point to point were equivalent; however, no data were presented in support of this claim.

While some workers questioned definitions for some of the parameters (see the discussion by Sherman, 1969), the method required subjects to score products according to these aforementioned parameters. It was claimed that comparison of results with the specified references enabled product formulation to occur according to known physical and chemical parameters (Szczesniak *et al.*, 1963). Having a reference (high and low) for every scale may seem like an ideal means of focusing

Table 6.2 Relationship between textual parameters and popular nomenclature[a]

	Mechanical characteristics	
Primary parameters	*Secondary parameters*	*Popular terms*
Hardness		Soft, firm, hard
Cohesiveness	Brittleness	Crumbly, Crunchy, brittle
	Chewiness	Tender, chewy, tough
	Gumminess	Short, mealy, pasty, gummy
Viscosity		Thin, viscous
Elasticity		Plastic, elastic
Adhesiveness		Sticky, tacky, gooey
	Geometrical characteristics	
Class	*Examples*	
Particle size and shape	Gritty, grainy, coarse, etc.	
Particle shape and orientation	Fibrous, cellular, crystalline, etc.	
	Other characteristics	
Primary parameters	*Secondary parameters*	*Popular terms*
Moisture content		Dry, moist, wet, watery
Fat content	Oiliness	Oily
	Greasiness	Greasy

[a] Reprinted from *J. Food Sci.*, 28(4), (1963), 388. Copyright © by Institute of Food Technologists. See text for further explanation.

responses (and minimizing variability); however, it will not eliminate variability as noted in the introductory discussion of this chapter. In fact, human behavior is variable from day to day and from subject to subject, hence the need for more than a single subject for a test. Responses obtained from a panel are analyzed statistically to separate main effects (e.g. the variable being tested) from other effects or other sources of variability. Measuring this variability provides greater insight into behavior and greater understanding of the response patterns of a subject and a panel to a product. Training subjects to be invariant is behaviorally unrealistic, and is the primary cause of the failure of quality scales to find application in sensory evaluation.

The use of products as scale anchors also presents its own set of problems. These products are not invariant and change over time as a function of marketing and other considerations. Normal production variation will cause a subject's response to a product to be offset to some (greater or lesser) extent as a function of that variability. It also is reasonable to expect that a subject's liking (or dislike) for a reference will further impact response behavior. Finally, extensive use of references during a test will cause sensory fatigue. Possibly, experienced subjects overcome this latter difficulty by limiting their tasting of the references. Obviously, the solution to this problem is to avoid use of such references.

A second concern with this method is the, *a priori*, decision as to the attributes (chewiness, hardness, and so on) to be used. There are inherent risks in experimenter-assigned attributes; the subjects could ignore a perception or use one or more of the listed words to "represent" the particular perception. While a survey may have elicited these aforementioned texture attribute (see Table 6.2), these are not necessarily the only ones or these most appropriate to reflect texture perceptions for a particular product. It is not a question of right and wrong attributes, but rather an issue of risk. Training subjects to use a specific set of attributes and comparing these responses with instrument analyses yielded a high degree of agreement or repeat measure reliability. However, the question of appropriateness and validity has not yet been addressed from a sensory point of view.

A third concern associated with the method is the separation of texture from other sensory properties of a product such as color, aroma, taste, and so forth. As a rule, perceptions are interdependent, and the exclusion of some attributes from a scorecard does not eliminate their perceptions. In effect, the subject is likely to use other attributes to acknowledge these perceptions, and the visible manifestation is increased variability and decreased sensitivity. In addition, these other perceptions will influence the responses to the textural perceptions and vice versa. The reader should take note that this particular problem, a perception with no place for it on the scorecard, is not unique to this method. It is a weakness of every sensory test that requires the subject to respond to a limited set of product descriptors. However, it is a more obvious problem when subjects can only respond to a single sensory category; for example, texture but not color, taste, aroma, or aftertaste. By measuring responses to all perceptions, the experimenter can derive a more complete picture of the product's sensory properties. One can gain an appreciation for this by examining the results from a factor analysis output. The descriptors are not grouped by modality; that is, by aroma, appearance, etc., but rather there will most likely be a mingling of them. In other words, there is considerable overlap of the attributes, independent of how they were grouped on the scorecard.

It is important for the sensory professional to recognize these limitations to the method to more properly assess the results in relation to other sensory information. This criticism does not mean that the method is invalid or is not useful. The sensory professional must be able to assess the weaknesses and strengths of each method relative to the particular problem under consideration. From a purely technical point of view, there is considerable appeal to the direct link between specific instrumental measures of the rheological properties of a product and the responses of a panel to specific sensory attributes, for example, texturometer units and hardness sensory ratings (Szczesniak *et al.*, 1963). One would expect these relationships to be stronger if all the sensory properties of the products have been measured.

C. Quantitative Descriptive Analysis (The QDA Method)®

Development of the Texture Profile method stimulated interest and research on new descriptive methods and especially methods that would overcome the weaknesses previously identified – reliance on qualitative information, use of product attributes established by the experimenter, reliance on a limited number of subjects and so forth. Further interest in descriptive methods developed as a result of the growth of new products and competition in the marketplace for products with unique sensory properties, as well as by advances in measurement and improved data processing systems. The QDA method (Stone *et al.*, 1974; Stone and Sidel, 1998, 2003) represented an opportunity for sensory evaluation to satisfy these needs; however, it also was a substantive departure from existing methods in the sense that the approach was primarily behavioral in orientation, with a consensus approach to language development (no expectation that all subjects will be equally sensitive), use of replication for assessing subject and attribute sensitivity and for identifying specific product differences and defined statistical analyses. It was determined that the method would be more than a simple rephrasing of the test questions or the use of a particular scale. In effect, the method required a different approach (at that time) to the concept of descriptive analysis, beginning with the subject selection procedure and concluding with communication of results in an understandable and actionable manner. The development of the method evolved from a number of considerations, including:

responsive to all the sensory properties of a product;
reliance on a limited number of subjects for each test;
subjects qualified before participation;
able to evaluate multiple products in individual booths;
use a language development process free from leader influence;
be quantitative and use a repeated trials design;
have a useful data analysis system.

These features of the QDA methodology are discussed here to enable the reader to determine how the method can be applied to their particular needs.

1. Responsive to all the sensory properties of a product

The QDA methodology provides a complete word description for all of a product's sensory properties. By products, we mean that it can be an existing product (currently in the marketplace), an ingredient, an idea, or it can be an entirely new product for which there is no existing competition. A complete description of all of a product's sensory properties is essential if product similarities and differences are to be fully documented. One cannot expect to train subjects, for example, to ignore the appearance/color of a set of products. Although the neural pathways for each of the senses are unique and well defined, considerable interaction occurs at high centers of the brain and these sensations culminate in the behavioral responses that are not unidimensional in character. In addition, the previous experiences of the subjects also will have an influence on their responses. Thus, the response of a subject to the sweetness of a beverage will include the interactive effects of all sensory attributes such as color, aroma, and so forth, as well as past experiences. To ensure that product flavor, for example, is fully accounted for, it is necessary to also measure other attributes, as well. If there is no opportunity to express a sensation, then most likely it will be embedded in another response, resulting in increased variability for that subject.

For these reasons, it was necessary to ensure that no limitations were established with regard to perceptions for a product and subjects were encouraged to use as wide a range of language as possible. For example, subjects evaluating a fabric could include one or more aroma measures if those attributes were perceived. The verification procedure for all perceptions is covered in more detail in a subsequent discussion. Implicit in this discussion is the applicability of the method to any type of product – food, beverage, shaving cream, fragrance, fabric, furniture polish, paper towel, microcomputer, and so on.

When training is initiated, the subjects are given instructions that they can use any words to describe a product, they are encouraged to use words that they understand and can explain to their fellow panel members, and no restriction is placed on the number of words except that preference or preference-related judgments, such as good, bad, etc., are discouraged. Subjects are instructed to examine the product and write on a blank pad (or type on a screen) attributes describing what they perceive. The panel leader asks each subject, one at a time, what they wrote and then lists these on the board for all to see. This procedure is followed for two or three products and check marks are placed adjacent to attributes already listed. Subjects are more willing to verbalize attributes once they have written those attributes on the paper. The panel leader also collects these sheets to verify whether all written attributes have been listed on the blackboard. Rarely does one subject contribute a high percentage of attributes to the list; it takes the combined effort of the panel to provide a comprehensive attribute list describing the products introduced during training. This is one reason for recommending at least eight to twelve subjects to participate in language development when a new scorecard is being developed. In a typical situation as many as 80–100 words will be listed within the first two training sessions (each session lasting about 90 minutes). By the second of these two sessions, subjects are encouraged to group the words by modality and in the process, they identify the duplication of sensory experience; however, this consolidation continues throughout the four or five training sessions necessary to arrive at a completed scorecard. Throughout this training, the subjects are encouraged to be sure that they have fully accounted for all the products' sensory properties. To ensure that the subjects respond to all the sensory properties, they must evaluate as many of the test products as is possible during the training.

2. Able to evaluate multiple products

Evaluation of more than a single product in a test is intended to capitalize on the subjects' skill in making relative judgments with a high degree of precision. As is known, humans are very poor judges of absolutes but very good judges of relative differences. Thus, a test involving several products will capitalize on the subject's skill in making precise judgments about relative differences. The multi-product test also is very efficient, first by providing a much more complete context of how products differ one from the other, and second by providing information on more than a single product. In view of the effort required to qualify and to train a subject, it is good business practice to achieve optimal output from the investment. Of course, more products in a test provide more information to analyze; however, available data processing systems minimize this problem.

3. Subjects qualified before participation

Each subject must be qualified prior to participation following a standardized protocol, and this requirement must be met for each test regardless of prior test experience. At the very outset of testing (see Chapter 2), there are certain requirements for all subjects regardless of the test type; for example, a subject must be available, and to be considered for screening tests, must be a user or potential user of the product or of the product class to be evaluated. This qualifying condition is necessary because the individual will have repeated exposure to the product, and those individuals who do not like or would never use the product tend to be less sensitive and more variable to product differences. Whether this is due to the individual's dislike for the product (and therefore lack of attention to differences) or represents a true difference in sensitivity is not known; however, the crucial point is to eliminate these individuals during screening. For descriptive testing, subjects also must demonstrate their ability to perceive differences within that class of products. This is an empirical measure of a subject's skill. For new subjects, one expects a minimum of 65% correct across the trials (use a test with a $p = \frac{1}{2}$ outcome). Selecting 65% correct as a minimum requirement for training was an arbitrary decision; one can raise or lower this, based on the number of subjects who meet this criterion. Empirically we observe that subjects with poorer skills; for example, 50–55% tend to be more variable and less sensitive in subsequent product tests. Other qualifications include the ability to verbalize and to work as a group (both are important to the success of the language development process), and finally the ability to perform during actual testing. Of course, with experienced subjects for which performance records exist, the need for re-qualification is minimized and their performance in actual testing becomes the primary criterion. In the process of screening and then training, the subjects develop a thorough familiarity with the products and with the differences among them. These activities, when combined with replication, enhance the likelihood of finding differences.

A basic strength of this descriptive method is the ability to independently verify (after each test) that individual subjects perceive differences among products on attributes in a reliable manner. This is directly measured with a one-way analysis of variance from each subject for each attribute. The need to monitor the performance of each subject in each test reflects an awareness of the sensory limitations of man. There is no guarantee that an individual will always perceive differences among products on all attributes. By establishing a formal, data-based selection procedure, the system becomes less dependent on a limited number of subjects.

4. Use a limited number of subjects

All descriptive tests use twenty or fewer subjects, and the QDA® methodology recommends ten to twelve; although there have been situations in which fifteen to twenty subjects have been used. If the panel leader has technical knowledge as to the expected differences, for example, very small, then more subjects could be used or the replication could be increased. When there are fewer than ten subjects, the overall contribution of each subject to the total variability increases accordingly, such that too much dependence is placed on too few subjects. This dependence is not lessened with replication. Alternatively, increasing panel size to more than twelve; for example, to twenty, can present other kinds of problems and most of these relate to scheduling the subjects. For example, there should be no more than ten to twelve subjects in a training session so a panel of twenty will require two sessions. In addition, the panel leader must ensure that the training results from both groups are integrated before testing is initiated. A panel leader must decide on the number of subjects based on past experience (the empirical evidence relative to the subjects and the products). Experience with many trained panels leads to the recommendation that ten to twelve is an optimal number of subjects for almost all products. One final note of caution concerns reliance on the same subjects for all testing, which also is not recommended. Such a practice will create a variety of problems including elitism, atypical response behavior, test fatigue, and so forth. Instead, one should develop a pool of qualified subjects (as discussed in Chapter 2).

5. Use a consensus language development process free from leader influence

The success of a descriptive test is, of course, also dependent on the sensory language developed for the products being evaluated. The subjects use the language as a basis for differentiating the products. To be useful, the language must be easily learned and meaningful in terms of its applications in product development, quality control, in relation to consumer preference measures, and so on. We concur with Andani *et al.* (2001) that a vocabulary derived from consumers is more likely to provide a better representation of product characteristics as perceived by those buying and consuming products. Developing a language is an iterative process, and depending on the product, it could take as much as 7–10 hours (in 60- to 90-minute sessions) before agreement is reached on the attributes. In addition to developing attributes, they must be grouped by modality, and the subjects must define each attribute and, with assistance from the panel leader, develop an agreed-upon evaluation procedure. The definitions serve as a guide for the subjects during testing to minimize confusion over the meaning of each attribute (a source of variability). Linking attributes with definitions enables the subjects to proceed very rapidly and misunderstandings are minimized. As a further aid in language development, reference materials also are identified and are made available during the training. The reference material can be an ingredient, a product, or some other material that "represents" the particular sensation and the attribute (or attributes) used to describe that sensation. In most instances, ingredients are useful as references; however, not all sensations will have a reference and some references will provide more than a single sensation. The combination of definitions and references is important in helping to standardize the language development process, especially when training new subjects or retraining existing subjects who are experiencing difficulty differentiating products with a particular attribute.

There is no limit to the number of attributes that subjects can use provided there is a consensus amongst the subjects as to their meanings and their order of occurrence. Theoretically, this could result in 100 or more words being used to describe the products. In practice, however, the number of words initially is quite large but subsequently is reduced to some smaller subset. As part of the training, the subjects will score many, if not all, of the products and in the ensuing discussion they identify those attributes with a common sensory basis thus resulting in about a 50% reduction in the final number of attributes.

In this language development process, the panel leader's function is almost entirely non-participatory, to minimize influencing the subjects. The panel leader's responsibility is to decide which products will be evaluated in each session, to facilitate conversation between subjects, and to provide an operational framework for each session based on previous results and the project objective. The panel leader must also determine when group discussions are finished and the panel is ready to evaluate products – the data collection process. This language development process is, therefore, very dependent on the skill of the panel leader. The subtleties of leader influence can never be totally eliminated; however, a key to minimizing a leader's influence is to keep this person as an impartial observer and to never convey the impression of knowing what attributes should be used or what are the expected product differences. To further minimize panel leader or subject-to-subject influences, actual product evaluations are done in a conventional sensory booth according to the procedures developed during the training sessions.

If a language is already available, then it is necessary to familiarize the subjects with the attributes and the definitions, but always in concert with the products. This is a more rapid process, particularly for the experienced subject, requiring as few as two or three 90-minute sessions. For inexperienced subjects, however, the time required to learn an existing language can require as many as four sessions. There is no rule as to the number of sessions required; with experience, the panel leader will develop a sense of the amount of time required and be able to plan accordingly. Once subjects are satisfied with the attributes, they proceed to product evaluation. New perceptions or a request to change an attribute and/or a definition is the collective responsibility of the panel. If an individual subject indicates a sensation is not accounted for, then the panel leader must ask the panel to reconvene for discussion. The subjects are reminded of this additional responsibility at the outset of each test. This particular aspect of descriptive analysis permits the communication process to remain current and provides for flexibility in the use of different words to connote the same sensation but, through the definition, to maintain a specific anchor regardless of the label. In the succeeding sections, the quantification process is discussed relative to verifying that the subjects individually and as a group perceive the sensations and differentiate between products with a measured degree of reliability and face validity.

6. Be quantitative and use a repeated trials design

The need for quantitative information is essential in descriptive analysis. It is no different than any analysis, whether it is physical and/or chemical, it must be replicated. Surprisingly, this lack of replication continues without much objection by requestors (who should know better). Since considerable emphasis is placed on results derived from a limited number of subjects and a much larger number of attributes, one must be very confident about the reliability and validity of the responses. Earlier descriptive methods, such as the Flavor Profile, were criticized because of the difficulty in understanding the meaning of the words in the description and the lack of a true numerical system (and statistical procedure) for assessing product differences based on those descriptions.

For QDA, the issue of quantification was addressed at two levels, the first was the use of an appropriate measurement technique (or scale) and the second was the use of repeated judgments as a basis for establishing individual subject reliability.

A line scale was selected because it provided the subject with an infinite number of places in which to indicate the relative intensity for an attribute (within the constraints of the actual length of the line), numbers are not used thus avoiding number biases, and finally, each subject could mark at whatever location on the line provided the subject was consistent within him or herself. With use of a repeated trials design and the analysis of variance, concern about specific scale location for a response is of less importance than are the twin issues of reliability and sensitivity to product differences. From a measurement perspective, use of a line scale was consistent with the concept of functional measurement and the graphic rating-scale approach of Anderson (1970) and in part on the trial and error process described by Stone *et al.* (1974). While line scales, in various forms, have been used for product evaluation for many years (see Baten, 1946; Hall, 1958), the philosophical approach developed by Anderson and co-workers proved to be especially useful. The scale shown in Fig. 6.1 is a 6-in. line with word anchors located $\frac{1}{2}$ in. from each end. In metric terms, the line length can be 15 cm to be fully effective, with anchors located at approximately 1.5 cm from each end. The scale direction always goes from left to right with increasing intensity; for example, weak to strong, light to dark, or some similar designated set of word anchors. The subject's task is to make a vertical line across the horizontal line at the point that best reflects the relative intensity for that attribute (for that product). The specific length of the line was selected based on limited research. For example, it was observed that extending the line to the full length of 8.5 in. × 11 in. paper did not increase sensitivity and there was a tendency for variability to increase. Making the line shorter than 6 in.; for example, 5 or 4 in., also reduced sensitivity. Although these observations do not constitute an exhaustive evaluation on the appropriate scale length, the evidence to date (examination of responses from several thousand tests) clearly supports the continued use of a 6 in. or 15 cm line. On the other hand, shifting the anchors to the ends of the line would have a more dramatic effect on responses; response patterns would take on the character of a true category scale and greater departure from linearity. For computational purposes, the distance along the line to the mark is measured to yield a numerical value for computation. However, successful use of this particular line scale is dependent on the instructional set and the frame of reference provided to

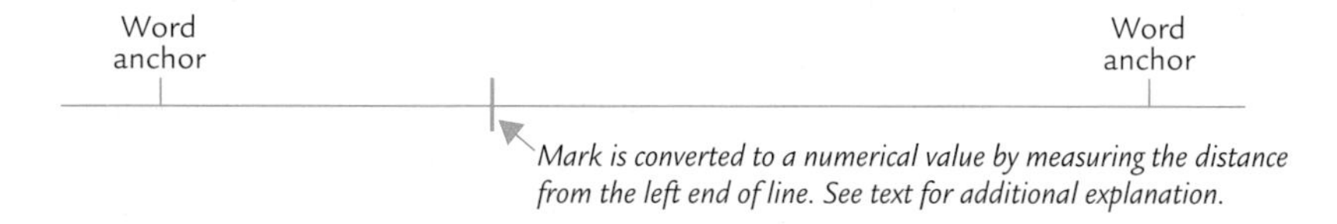

Figure 6.1 An example of a graphic rating scale (or line scale) used to obtain relative intensity measures from the subjects.

make the scale "functional." During language development, subjects are familiarized with the scale and practice its use, with particular attention given to the anchor terms relative to specific products that will be evaluated. Functional measurement requires that the subject experience what constitutes the extremes in intensities for many of the attributes in the context of the products that will be evaluated. This procedure helps to minimize end-order effects (avoidance of the extremes) and encourages full use of the scale to express product differences. Subjects are not penalized if they use less than the full scale. The primary emphasis is for the subjects to be as consistent as is possible and this is encouraged in the product scoring during training. Adding a constant does not change the relationship between products, so concern about where a subject marks a scale is of minor importance. Forcing a subject to use more of the scale or to move to a specific location is disruptive, it will alienate that individual, and as mentioned previously, this action is suggesting to the subjects that there is a correct experience and a correct response.

Empirically, this procedure was found to be very easy to use and subjects were able to complete a scorecard (containing as many as forty attributes) within a few minutes with a high degree of reliability. In early applications, use of a third anchor at the scale midpoint was common. However, removal of the center anchor was observed to reduce variability by 10–15%, which represented a substantial improvement in sensitivity and the current scale has only the two anchors.

As mentioned earlier in this discussion, the elimination of numbers from the scale and from the subjects' responses eliminated two sources of bias; avoidance of (or preference for) particular numbers that have negative (or positive) connotations. The second source of bias was the subject who changed use of numbers over time. This latter situation was noted by Ekman and Sjöberg (1965) in their review on scaling, and can be especially troublesome because one might not know if this change reflected a product difference or true bias. During training in the use of the scale, numbers are not discussed and the subjects are not told that the scale has numerical content. They may infer that the marks are converted to numerical values, but that is not the same as being told so by the panel leader.

The use of the subject's own word anchors also contributes to the utility of the scale and the linearity of the responses. The responses are used directly in statistical analysis; that is, no transformations are necessary and the monitoring of response patterns is directly achieved.

A related issue is the reliability (i.e. reliability) of the responses, which is directly addressed by having each subject provide responses to the products on more than one occasion. The importance of this particular requirement cannot be underestimated. It represents an internal check on the response system, enabling the panel leader to determine individual subject and panel consistency (from trial to trial) and to establish a numerical measure of performance. Repeated judgments extend the time required to complete a test; however, this additional time is well worth the effort. From an empirical point of view, about four trials from each subject for each product appears to be optimal. Of course, amount of replication will depend on the estimated product variability and magnitude of differences among products, the stage of product testing, as well as the expected subject sensitivity. Here again, the panel leader may decide that additional replication is or is not warranted. For example, if the test is during the early stages of product development, then fewer replications could be adequate to provide directions. Alternatively, if the development effort were at a final stage, then more replication would be appropriate. We observed that beyond four replicates, little or no obvious improvement in sensitivity was achieved. For example, in a test of six products, each subject would evaluate each product four times yielding a total of 240–288 evaluations for the panel (assuming ten to twelve subjects) for each attribute, which would be a sufficiently large database on which to reach conclusions with confidence about product differences.

On several occasions, it was possible to evaluate test results after four, six, eight, ten, and twelve replicates. The evaluations included typical statistical measures such as means and standard deviations, individual and mean ranks, and analyses of variance, and in each situation, the conclusions have not changed. In some instances, the level of statistical significance changed; however, the conclusions about product differences were not altered. Observation of results after only one replication yielded a less clear result for some attributes (about fifteen to twenty of them) but with most decisions unchanged for all other attributes.

The experienced panel leader will develop guidelines regarding the appropriate number of replications. These guidelines must take into account the nature of the problem, product variability, the anticipated degree of difficulty, subject skills, and the expected use of the results. But one point should be very clear, it is extremely risky to rely on descriptive information for which there are no repeated judgments.

7. Have a useful data analysis system

The analysis of variance (AOV) model is the most appropriate statistical procedure for analyzing scaled responses from a descriptive test. Use of the AOV model in sensory evaluation was discussed in Chapter 4, and the reader will find it helpful to review that information before proceeding. In a QDA® test, the subjects evaluate all of the products on an attribute-by-attribute basis on more than a single occasion. In design terms, this represents a treatment-by-subject, repeated measures design. The introduction of replication adds an additional level of complexity to the computation; however, from a sensory point of view, replication is especially helpful in directly characterizing the reliability of response patterns, as noted in the previous section. This does not mean that sufficient replication from a limited number of subjects enables one to automatically generalize to the population, but rather that there is confidence that the differences are due to true product differences and are not random occurrences. With this in mind, it is appropriate to focus attention on some of the more fundamental questions that need to be resolved before product similarities and differences can be considered and conclusions and recommendations made. These questions include:

1. Are individual subjects consistent from trial to trial and will additional training be required before the next test?
2. Is the level of panel performance consistent and will additional training be required before the next test?

3. Are individual attributes providing useful information and will additional training be required before the next test?
4. Are responses to product differences consistent across all subjects?

These questions are answered through several different statistical computations, such as means, standard deviations, rank order, and AOV. For example, a subject's ability to distinguish between products can be examined by means of a one-way AOV on a scale-by-scale basis. The magnitude of the difference between products and the consistency of the scores for the products from trial to trial is reflected in an F ratio and its corresponding probability value. The smaller probability values (e.g. 0.01, 0.001) reflect greater differentiation among products and a higher level of consistency and this can be considered as a measure of that individual's performance (for each attribute for that particular set of products). A subject whose probability values were very small (e.g. 0.01) would be considered as sensitive and consistent in contributing to the differences among the products and would be a good performer compared with the subject whose probability values are very large (i.e. close to unity) and who, thus, contributes little to the overall discrimination among the products. By comparing probability values for all subjects, one also develops a more complete picture of the panel's level of performance.

As shown in Table 6.3, probability values derived from such an analysis are very informative by themselves and when combined with that subject's individual product means, rank orders and contribution to interaction. For purposes of this discussion, we focus on the use of the one-way AOV probability values. Responses from subject 831 yielded values of 0.00 for attributes A and B and 0.06 and 0.31 for attributes C and D. The corresponding values for subject 833 were 0.68, 0.59, 0.01 and 0.09, respectively. Subject 831 differentiated amongst all of the products on all four attributes; however, the contribution to differences amongst products was smaller on attribute D (where the value for D was 0.31). Alternatively, subject 833 contributed much less to the differences amongst products on attributes A and B, and contributed much more for attributes C and D.

Further insight into performance is achieved by examining such measures as the means, the standard deviations and the product ranks for each subject. The latter are obtained by transforming the intensity measures to ranks and examining them versus

Table 6.3 Probability values for individual subjects derived from a one-way analysis of variance on a scale-by-scale basis

Sensory characteristic	Subject				Panel
	831	832	833	834	
A	0.00[a]	0.19	0.68	0.00	0.04
B	0.00	0.02	0.59	0.06	0.01
C	0.06	0.09	0.01	0.02	0.00
D	0.31	0.38	0.09	0.43	0.38

[a] Entries are the truncated probability values; see text for additional explanation. These values were excerpted from a larger database and are used here for illustrative purposes.

the panel ranks keeping in mind, that in those situations where the means are close it is reasonable to expect that there will be less agreement in the ranks than if the means were very different from each other. This information is used to evaluate panel performance and to identify those attributes that did not provide satisfactory product differentiation (e.g. see D versus C in Table 6.3). The latter problem may be due to the subjects not yet in good agreement as to the meaning of the attribute or using the scale in the direction prescribed; however, subject 833 was able to use the attribute to differentiate between the products. Prior to the next test, the panel leader might want to request that subject 833 describe (to the rest of the panel) the basis for product differentiation using that attribute. This discussion could lead to improved understanding as to how an attribute is used (by each subject and the panel) and better product differentiation by all the panel. For this attribute, product differentiation was not very good, the probability value was 0.38 and, depending on the remainder of the test results, this attribute should be a candidate for discussion before the next test.

The panel leader examines the pattern of responses to develop a clear understanding of what should be done before the next test. To what extent is each subject contributing to product differences (e.g. more than half, less than half)? Are the lack of differences a result of increased variability from incorrect scale use (a crossover interaction), is it a true lack of sensitivity or are the product differences so small as to be unimportant? Answers to these questions must be obtained before reaching product conclusions and before initiating the next test. Table 6.4 provides additional examples of the use of summary statistics (in this instance, the means and variance measures) to gain further insight to subject response behavior and future training emphasis. In this example, subject A exhibited minimal contribution to product differences primarily because of variability in the responses; the standard deviations were relatively high (8.3–9.4) compared to the means (13.4–16.9). Alternatively, subject B, with identical means had smaller standard deviation values (4.0–4.8) and thus made a greater contribution to product differentiation. Subject C showed a different response pattern; the mean values

Table 6.4 Hypothetical means and standard deviations for assessment of subject/panel performance[a]

	Attribute XYZ	Mean	SD	Probability[b]
Subject	**Product**			
A	1	14.8	9.4	
	2	16.9	9.1	0.41
	3	13.4	8.3	
B	1	14.8	4.8	
	2	16.9	4.7	0.05
	3	13.4	4.0	
C	1	24.8	18.5	
	2	20.5	14.0	0.25
	3	38.0	19.0	

[a] See text for detailed explanation of the tabular values.
[b] Probability values from the one-way analysis of variance.

were larger and not in the same order as reported for subjects A and B. The standard deviations also were much larger; however, product differentiation was better as measured by the probability value of 0.25 versus 0.41 for subject A. Subject B exhibited the largest contribution to product differentiation because he/she was less variable and would be a useful tutor in the next training session. Subject C, on the other hand, was considerably more variable, yet contributed to product differentiation, to a greater extent than subject A. However, it should be noted that subject C also ordered the products differently suggesting a possible crossover interaction. Here too, attention must be given to attribute definition and scale direction.

Some additional comments about subject performance are appropriate here. The first is a reminder to the reader about not using performance data to justify removing that subject's data and re-analyzing results. Eliminating subjects (and their data) is not an acceptable course of action. The second is to keep in mind that what appears to be unusually high variability from a subject could reflect product variability and/or poorly controlled preparation and handling practices. The tendency to assign variability solely to the subject is usually unwarranted. Each product type and manufacturer will have its own unique profiles and variabilities, and panel leaders must use their data files to formulate subject performance guidelines and not apply a rule arbitrarily and without fully appreciating the consequences.

In this way, the panel leader is able to isolate individual response patterns and from this information develop a sense of what needs to be done to improve panel performance as well as determine the relative quality of the database. This approach is considerably more demanding of the panel leader; however, the weight of the results justifies this degree of effort. Once there is satisfaction with the performance of the individual subjects and scales, then it is appropriate to evaluate product differences.

The data are analyzed using a two-way AOV general linear model showing both subject and product effects. Subject-by-product interactions are also estimated when the experiment includes repeated judgments. These results can be summarized in typical AOV tables (Tables 6.5 and 6.6), with main effects tested against both error and interaction mean square. Table 6.5 contains the *F* ratios using the error or the interaction terms; the panel leader selects the appropriate *F* value.

Table 6.5 Analysis of variance for a specific sensory characteristic

Source of variance	df	Sum of squares	Mean sum of squares	Versus error[a]		Versus interaction[a]	
				F-ratio	Probability	*F*-ratio	Probability
Samples[a,b]	4	10718.89	2679.72	28.49	0.00	47.81	0.00
Subjects	8	8441.71	1055.21	11.22	0.00	18.43	0.00
Interaction	32	1793.55	56.05	0.59	0.95		
Error	126	11848.07	94.03				

[a] Main effect of samples is significant; main effect of subjects is significant; interaction (sample × subject) is non-significant.

[b] See text for additional explanation.

Table 6.6 Analysis of variance for a specific sensory characteristic

Source of variance	df	Sum of squares	Mean sum of squares	Versus error[a]		Versus interaction[a]	
				F-ratio	Probability	*F*-ratio	Probability
Samples[a,b]	4	1567.43	391.85	2.95	0.02	1.16	0.34
Subjects	8	14877.14	1859.64	14.01	0.00	5.54	0.00
Interaction	32	10730.41	335.32	2.52	0.00		
Error	126	16712.64	132.72				

[a] Main effect of samples is significant; main effect of subjects is significant; interaction (sample × subject) is significant; main effect of samples (with new error term) is not significant.
[b] See text for additional explanation.

For these results, interaction was not significant and no further consideration of interaction was necessary. Note that there was a significant subject effect, reflecting differences in scale use by the subjects; however, this difference in scale use did not interfere with perception of product differences. When interaction is significant (Table 6.6), indicating differences in the way subjects interpret or measure a given attribute, the test against interaction is used. It can be seen that this resulted in a loss of significance for products. The other analysis and the response patterns must be studied to determine the cause of the problem. It has been suggested that this switch from one value to another (error or interaction mean square) represents a shift in the particular mathematical model, and that there is some risk; however, we never rely on a single statistic, and the approach described herein is extremely helpful and inappropriate business decisions have yet to be encountered.

An alternative approach would be to consistently use interaction mean square for testing significance of product differences. One problem with this approach is that there will be instances where product differences appear significant when tested against interaction, but not when tested against residual error. To have both available enables the panel leader to make the appropriate choice.

Individual interaction values can also be computed for each subject on each attribute. This provides another measure of degree of agreement among subjects, and between subjects and the panel as a whole. As a measure of this, the interaction sum of squares is partitioned in such a way as to determine how much each subject has contributed to the interaction F ratio for the panel. In this case, a high F ratio (and small probability value) for a subject is indicative of subject–panel disagreement.

Knowledge about interaction is important in understanding the nature of disagreements between individual subjects and a panel. As depicted in Fig. 6.2, two types of interaction are of particular interest. In the first type, crossover (A), the subject or some subset of a panel reverses the products compared with the panel; that is, product A was perceived as more intense than product B while the panel as a whole perceived the opposite. This may reflect a true difference in perception (i.e. bimodality), or it could reflect confusion in scale use by the subject, either of which would not be readily apparent without direct examination of response patterns. The other type of

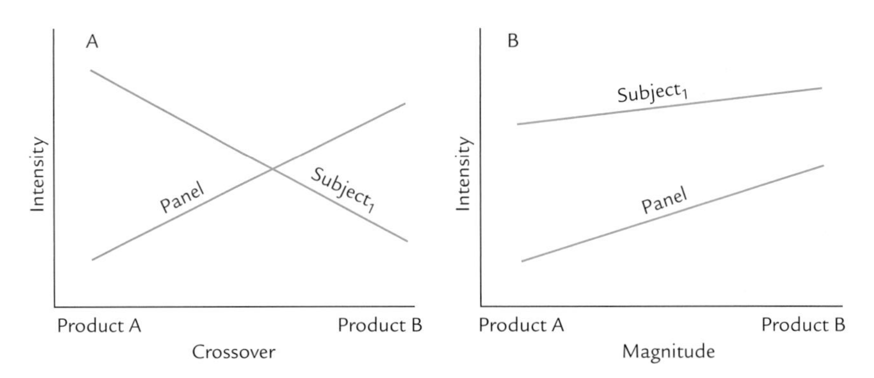

Figure 6.2 Examples of two different kinds of interaction that can occur in a sensory test: (A) represents the classic crossover type of interaction; (B) demonstrates a more subtle problem, called magnitude interaction.

interaction, referred to as magnitude, is shown in (B). In this instance, there was no confusion about which product was most intense; however, the magnitude of the difference between products was relatively small for subject 1 versus the large difference for the panel as a whole. This latter type of interaction is of less serious consequence (compared with crossover), and conversion to ranks minimizes the effect of that difference. A subject's magnitude interaction may reflect differences in subject sensitivity and/or scale use. By differentiating these types of interaction, the panel leader is better able to evaluate test results, anticipate consumer perceptions and work with those subjects that show a greater tendency toward crossover responses. We use a proprietary statistical analysis to better identify subjects contributing to crossover interaction and to quantify the severity of the crossover on a subject-by-attribute basis. Significant product differences are first determined for the attribute. Subject scores are then converted to ranks, as are the panel means, and a sum of squares computed for each subject. The computation reflects the accumulated rank distance for product means that are significantly different (based on total panel) and ranked by the subject in a different order than the panel. The example shown in Table 6.7 identifies Subject #3 as having the largest crossover score, and this is consistent with scoring Product E2 lowest for this attribute whilst the panel scores it significantly higher than the other products. Subject #2 also has a crossover score, albeit lower (32 versus 71), because Product E2 is ranked second highest for this attribute. The remaining subjects score Product E2 highest and reverse product E1 with S, or S with Pilot, comparisons which the panel result does not identify as significant, and consequently the calculated crossover scores for these subjects is 0.0. Summarizing crossover scores during training provides the panel leader with useful information about subject and attribute performance, and during final data analysis is helpful for identifying potential problem areas when assessing consumer behavior. Interaction in relation to multiple range tests and significant differences between products will be discussed in more detail later. For a more complete exposition on the statistics of interaction, the reader is referred to McNemar (1969), Winer (1971), and McCall (1975).

QDA data lends itself well to multivariate analyses to better understand subject performance and attribute relationships. The data in Fig. 6.3 are examples of the former

Table 6.7 Means, ranks, and crossover scores for sweet aroma

Product	Panel mean	Subject means							
		1	2	3	4	5	6	7	8
Prod E2	35.79[a] a	48.3	26.3	12.8	41.0	46.7	34.0	45.5	31.7
Prod E1	30.15 b	42.5	26.5	17.3	33.8	32.3	28.2	40.5	20.0
Prod S	27.90 bc	36.2	22.2	22.7	34.0	26.5	27.5	38.0	16.2
Pilot	25.85 c	36.0	16.8	15.2	33.7	22.7	27.3	37.5	17.7
Mean	29.92	40.8	23.0	17.0	35.6	32.0	29.2	40.4	21.4
N	192	24	24	24	24	24	24	24	24

	Subject ranks							
	1	2	3	4	5	6	7	8
Prod E2	1	2	4	1	1	1	1	1
Prod E1	2	1	2	3	2	2	2	2
Prod S	3	3	1	2	3	3	3	4
Pilot	4	4	3	4	4	4	4	3
Crossover score	0	32	71	0	0	0	0	0

[a] Panel means designated with the same letter not significantly different based on Duncan multiple range test.

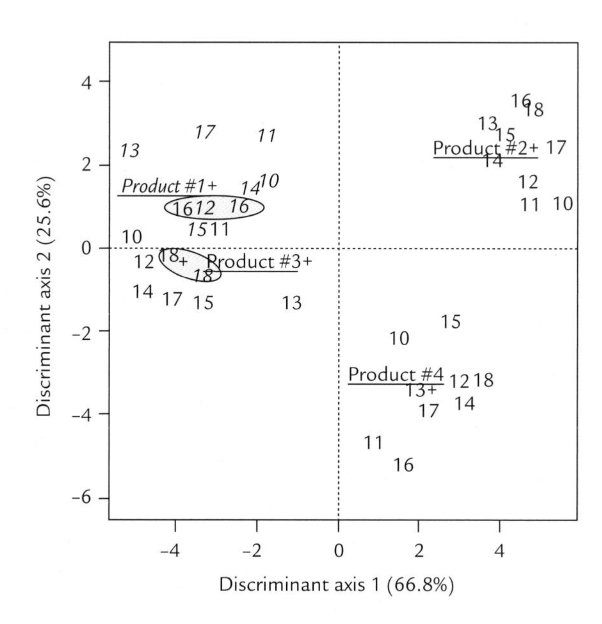

Figure 6.3 Subject discrimination of products across attributes.

and the data in Fig. 6.4 are examples of the latter. Examining Fig. 6.3, we see that the subjects discriminated the test products quite well. The panel scored Products #1 and #3 most similar to one another, where Subject 16 scored Product #3 more similar to Product #1 and Subject #18 scored Product #1 more similar to Product #3. The information provides insight about what may occur in consumer testing, and an area for

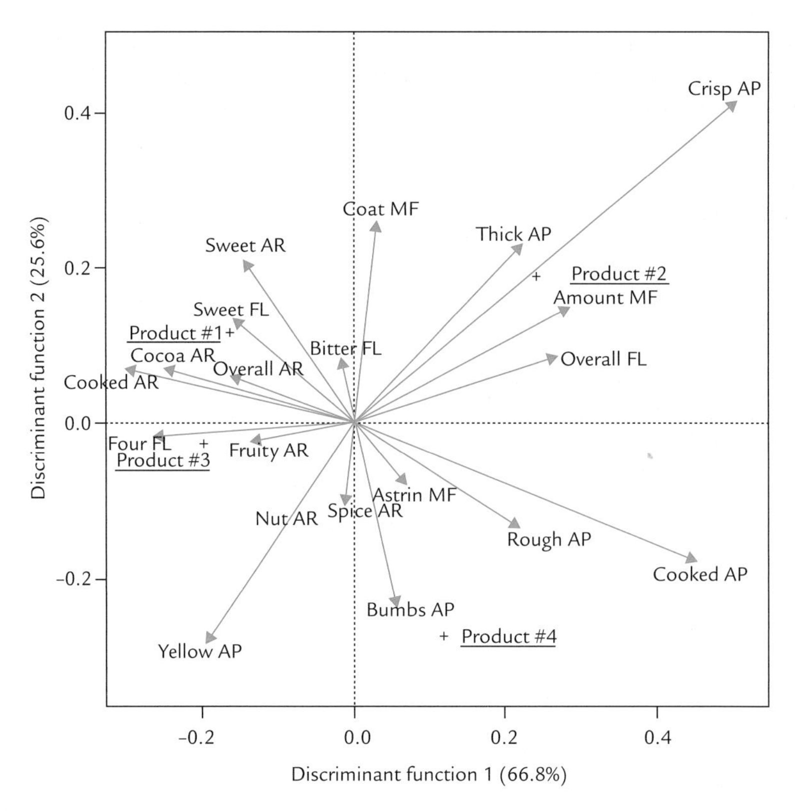

Figure 6.4 Attribute factor loadings.

follow up with the panel. Figure 6.4 allows identification of these attributes, which most differentiate the different products to the panel. For example, Product #1 can be characterized as aromatic with a sweet, cocoa, and overall aroma scores; Product #2 is characterized for its thick and crisp appearance and high scores for mouthfeel; Product #3 has a fruity aroma and flour flavor; and Product #4 can be differentiated on several appearance measures.

The AOV model also enables the panel leader to determine whether the mean scores for several products differ from one another in sufficient magnitude to justify considering them different at some stated (and low) level of risk. The analysis does not specify which products are different and one must do additional computations after the F test, sometimes referred to, as multiple-range tests. There are a variety of these tests and some needless controversy has developed concerning which one is most appropriate. The tests are not interchangeable and different tests can lead to different conclusions regarding significant differences among products. This does not mean that one test is more or less correct, but rather that they reflect different philosophies with regard to risk and minimizing decision errors. These tests include the following: Duncan, Newman–Keuls', Tukey (a), Tukey (b), Scheffé, and Dunnett. The first three tests and the Scheffé test are most commonly used in sensory tests. In effect, one computes a critical value and those mean differences that are greater are considered significantly different. The formulae are quire similar to those shown here. For additional discussion on these computations, see Winer (1971) and Bruning and Kintz (1977).

a. Duncan

The computation is as follows

$$\text{Critical differences} = k_r \sqrt{\frac{ms_e}{n(\text{per group})}}$$

where k represents values derived from table and r is the number of means being compared (number of steps apart). The Duncan procedure uses a protection level for α for the set of samples being compared, rather than an α level for the individual pairs of samples within the test. This approach minimizes the risk of a Type 2 error, but may concomitantly increase the risk of a Type 1 error.

b. Newman–Keuls'

The computation is as follows:

$$\text{Critical difference} = q_r \sqrt{\frac{ms_e}{n(\text{per group})}}$$

where q represents values derived from table and r is the number of means being compared. The Newman–Keuls' procedure emphasizes ranges rather than differences; the computations are the same as it is in the Duncan test, but the values q derived from the table are different and the result is that larger differences (between means) are required before statistical significance is achieved. In effect, the procedure provides greater protection from risk of a Type 1 error.

c. Tukey (a)

The computation is as follows:

$$\text{Critical difference} = q_r \sqrt{\frac{ms_e}{n(\text{per group})}}$$

where q represents values derived from table and r is the number of means. The Tukey (a) or HSD procedure uses a single value for all comparisons based on the total number of means involved, and larger differences are, therefore, required before statistic significance will be achieved. As Winer (1971) has noted, this test has lower statistical power than the Newman–Keuls' and Duncan tests.

d. Tukey (b)

The computation is as follows:

$$\text{Critical value} = \frac{\text{critical value } N - K + \text{critical value Tukey (a)}}{2}$$

This procedure represents a compromise between the two previous tests; the critical value changes with the number of means being compared and provides protection from Type 1 error.

e. Scheffé

The computation is as follows:

$$\text{Critical difference} = (a - 1)F\sqrt{\frac{2ms_e}{n(\text{per group})}}$$

where a is the number of groups to be compared and F is the tabular value for F with appropriate degree of freedom (df). The Scheffé test yields a single value for use in determining the significant difference between any two pairs of sample means, and as can be seen, uses the F value and further minimizes risk associated with Type 1 error to the greatest extent.

f. Other tests

Other possible tests include the Fisher modified least significant difference (LSD) and Dunnett tests. The former test is, according to Winer, suitable for comparisons planned prior to data evaluation, while the latter test is designed for use when one is comparing products to a control.

Winer (1971) prepared a tabulation of these alternative tests using a common data source for comparative purposes. The ordering was Scheffé, modified LSD, Tukey (a), Tukey (b), Newman–Keuls', and Duncan. The author felt that the Tukey (a) test had much to commend it, including broad applications and relative ease in computation. A similar type of comparison was made by Bruning and Kintz, but no recommendation was made. Rather, these authors simply identified significant and nonsignificant occurrences, using a common database.

Another test that can be applied is the Bonferroni t (Myers, 1979). This test, like Tukey (a) and Scheffé, is especially protective of Type 1 error. It takes into account the problem of the change in Type 1 error with multiple contrasts, and is especially applicable where group sizes and variances are unequal. Thus, if a test objective were to identify the product that is perceived as different for an advertising claim, then the Bonferroni t will be the method of choice. The emphasis of these tests is on minimizing Type 1 error; however, this objective needs to be considered relative to the test objectives encountered in many business situations. As discussed in the chapter on discrimination testing, most product work (e.g. ingredient substitution, cost reduction, matching a target, and so forth) is concerned with minimizing the risk of perceiving a difference between products and reducing the risk of a Type 2 error. Therefore, it will be more appropriate to use either the Duncan or the Newman–Keuls' tests for determining which means are different. However, even these latter procedures entail some risk, which is only appreciated after a thorough examination of all data, including subject response patterns.

If we consider the results shown in Table 6.8, this concern will be more fully appreciated. These data were derived from a QDA test involving twelve experienced

Table 6.8 A comparison of Duncan and Tukey (a) result for significant differences

Characteristic[a]		Mean[b]	Duncan	Tukey (a)
A	100[c]	29.7		
B	50	27.1		
C	25	26.9		
D	0	21.7		

[a] The particular characteristic is not germane to the problem (see the section on language in this chapter).
[b] Entries are mean values in a scale of 0–60. The two-way AOV revealed a significant *F* ratio, $p < 0.005$, and there was no significant interaction.
[c] Added ingredient at 100, 50, 25, and 0% of normal; that is, the current production was the 0 product.

subjects, four products, and thirty attributes; each product was evaluated once in each of four sessions (AM and PM for 2 days), with a total *N* of 48 judgments per product.

Based on the Tukey (a) test, products A, B, and C are not considered different from each other, and products B, C, and D are not considered different from each other (the Duncan brackets are used here for ease of communication). Based on the Duncan test, products A, B, and C are not considered different from each other, which is consistent with Tukey (a); however, products B and C are considered different from product D. Further insight into this "discrepancy" can be gained by examination of the way the individual subjects rated products B versus D and C versus D. For example, considering products B versus D, eleven subjects rated B as more intense than D, and the magnitude of the difference, on the average, was 5.9 scale units, whereas only one subject rated D as more intense than B and the magnitude was 0.7 scale units. It is difficult to accept a Tukey (a) no significant difference (NSD) decision in this situation, considering the responses from the individual subjects and the average magnitude of that difference.

In this particular instance, which involved ingredient substitution, a primary objective was to minimize detection of a difference. Stating that there was no significant difference between the control and 50% replacement would be very risky (since eleven of the twelve subjects stated there was a difference). Examination of the C versus D comparison revealed a somewhat less clear picture. Seven subjects rated C as more intense than D, and the magnitude of the difference, on average, was 11.6 scale units; five subjects rated D as more intense than C and the magnitude was 3.8 scale units (on average). Recommending a significant or nonsignificant difference was more difficult. The number of subjects favoring either product was almost equal, and the only source of hesitation in reaching a recommendation was the magnitude of the difference. The sensory professional would need to discuss the situation with the product specialists, as well as to evaluate any other sources of product information before reaching a meaningful business decision.

This particular situation occurs often enough that one should never be complacent about results and it is a reminder that no one statistical measure will be totally satisfactory in explaining product similarities and differences. It can be argued that this approach to the evaluation of data is time consuming and not practical in a typical busy, company testing environment. This argument is, at best, a weak one because it fails to acknowledge the purpose for a test, and the importance of making correct and supportable recommendations. Sensory professionals cannot afford to make recommendations about products that are not consistent with all the results. At this stage, a conclusion is reached about product differences and a written document is prepared, summarizing the results in both a technically and visually acceptable format. Technical documentation typically follows a specific report format (appropriate for that company) that most often includes a listing of means and variability measures. However, this method of communication is rarely satisfactory, as it is relatively easy for numbers to be misinterpreted.

This problem represented a challenge (to the authors), leading to development of the now familiar "spider webs" or sensory maps/pictures. The intention was to display results that did not rely directly on numerical values (Stone *et al.*, 1974). As shown in Figs 6.5 and 6.6, the visual display is achieved by plotting the relative

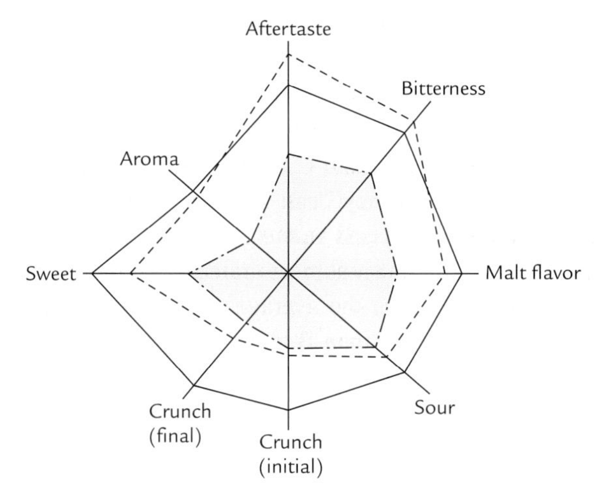

Figure 6.5 Visual display of the sensory attributes based on the results of the QDA test. For each attribute, the relative intensity increases as it moves farther away from the center point. See Fig. 6.4 and text for additional explanation.

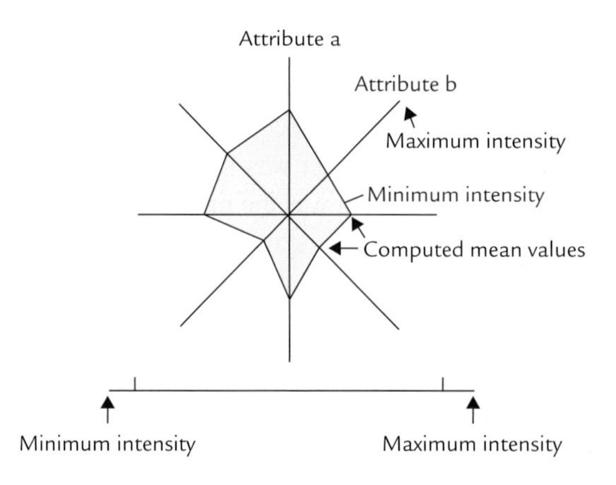

Figure 6.6 A schematic diagram with explanation of the procedure used to prepare the visual display (sometimes referred to as a spiderweb) of QDA results.

intensity values for the various attributes on a series of lines (or spokes) that radiate from a center point. These radiating lines can be envisioned as the attribute scales without the anchors. Currently, the most useful approach is to display attributes in groupings; for example, all the appearance attributes regardless of whether product differences were significant. The problem of deciding which attributes should be grouped could be resolved through factor analysis or some other procedure (see e.g. Powers, 1988; Petty and Scriven, 1991); however, subsequent testing of a related group of products could lead to quite different results, including significances for attributes that were previously non-significant. Some displays have included confidence levels. It should be clear there is no one way that is best for displaying results. The primary objective is to convey, in as simple a way possible, the specific differences in a set of products. Visual displays such as the one shown in Fig. 6.6 have proven to be extremely useful without compromising numerical significances. As a further step in the process of displaying and communicating product information, products can be added, one at a time, in a layering approach. By layering the plot, all possible combinations can be presented and discussed. Figures 6.7 and 6.8 are results from an evaluation of appearance and aroma, and mouthfeel and aftertaste attributes for cognac and brandy (the French and American designations, respectively). This display makes it easy to convey information to requestors and the plotting program now includes options for displaying a significance designation for each attribute (Stone and Sidel, 1998) and by simplying "clicking on the plot," one can add or remove any product quickly. To enhance the communication process, meeting participants are provided with the scorecard, definitions and products, enabling them to experience the results in a meaningful way. It is encouraging to note how frequently this approach is used to display sensory information other than that obtained using the QDA method.

D. Spectrum™ Descriptive Analysis

This method was developed primarily from the Flavor and Texture Profile methods and a description can be found in Meilgaard *et al.* (1999); see also, Rutledge and Hudson (1990). The selection and screening for subjects follows those described previously for Flavor Profile; that is, there are standard threshold and recognition tests along with interviews to determine the individual's interest in being a part of the panel. Discrimination testing also was proposed as an alternative or as an additional part of the subject screening process.

The training activities, as described, are quite extensive, reflecting the basic Flavor and Texture Profile procedures, with particular reliance on training the subjects with specified standards of specified intensities. The training process is very lengthy, requiring 3–4 hours per week, for a period of 14 weeks. This extensive training time is described as necessary so as to enable the panel to be universal; that is, to be able to evaluate all types of products. Whether one can, in fact, train subjects to be qualified as an "expert" in all products is an interesting idea but it remains to be demonstrated whether it can or should be done. It also is possible that this extensive training time is related to the use of reference standards and specific intensities for those standards in an effort to develop "universal scales."

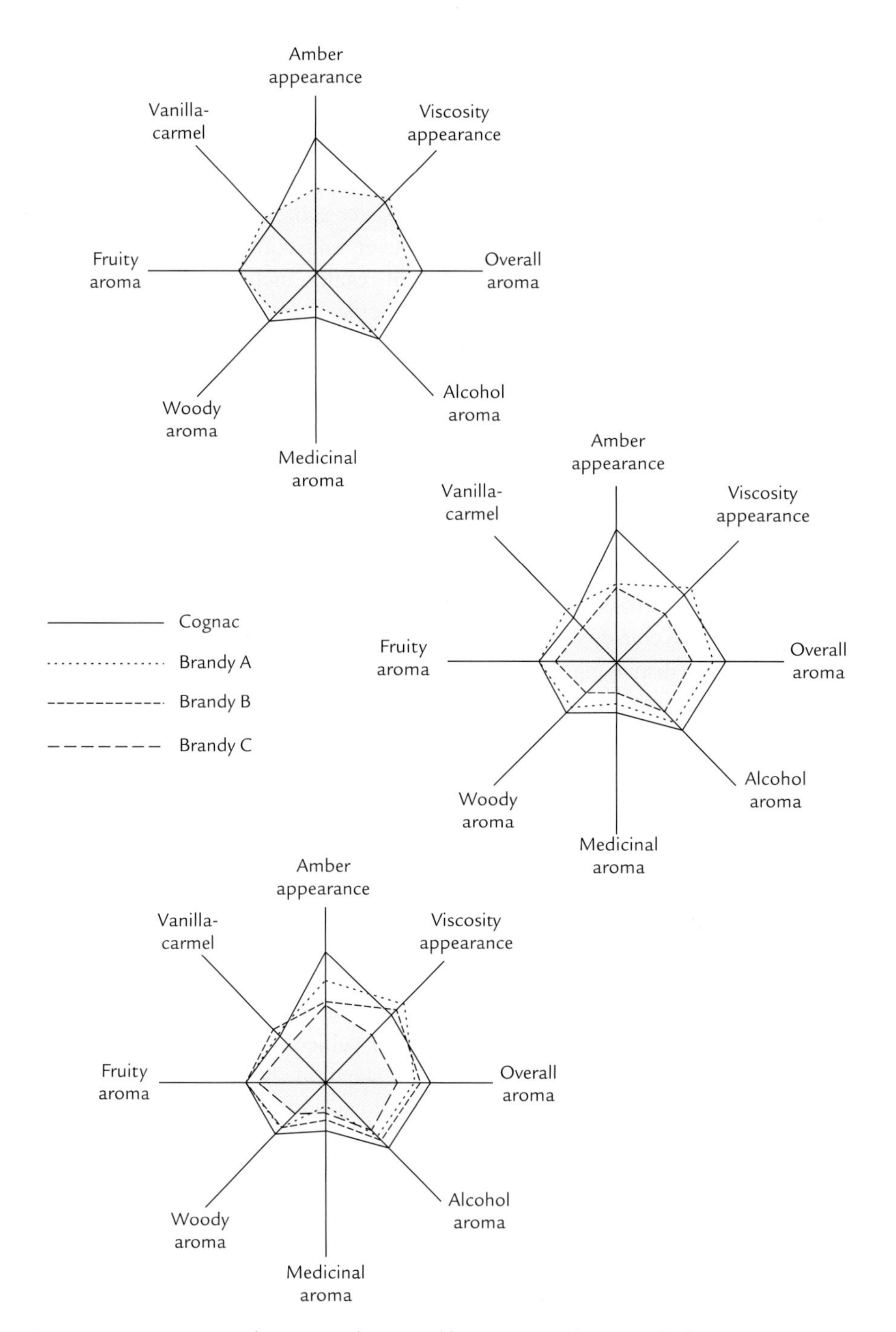

Figure 6.7 Appearance and aroma attributes used by a QDA panel to score the four cognacs and brandies. The upper figure shows two of the products, the middle figure adds a third product, and the lower allows for examination of all four products that were evaluated. See text for further explanation.

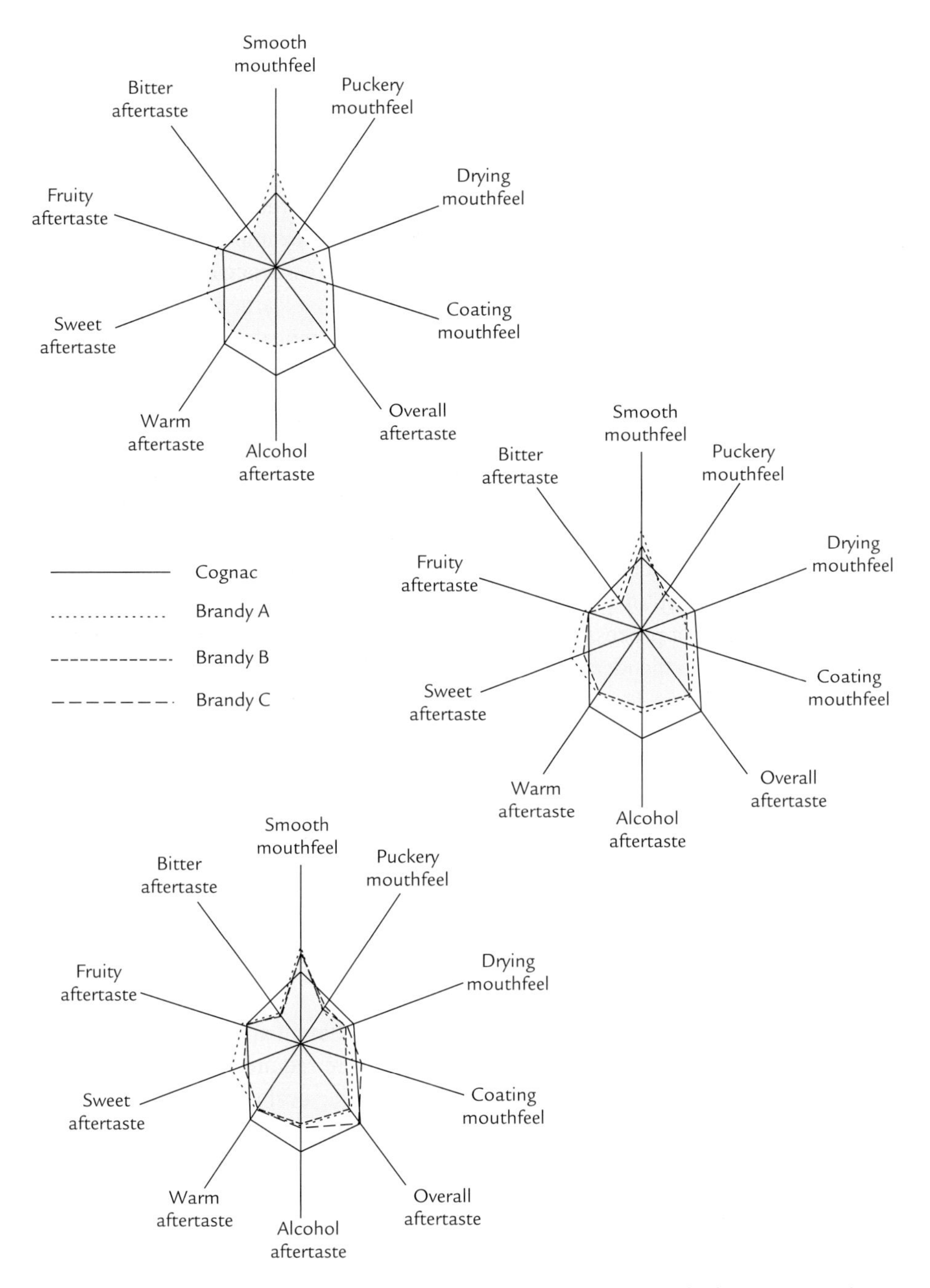

Figure 6.8 Mouthfeel and aftertaste attributes used by a QDA pane to score the four cognacs and brandies. See Fig. 6.5 and text for further explanation of the display.

Although the concept of universal descriptive scales may appeal to some, the reality of individual differences in sensory physiology and behavior runs counter to the notion of universal perception and related scales. Chasing rainbows is best left to phenomonologists, rather than the legitimate activity for the sensory scientist.

Boelens and Boelens (2002), discussing olfaction from the perfumers perspective, stated that "it is highly unlikely – in fact, practically impossible – that two human beings would describe the odor of a pure chemical compound in exactly the same way." We concur with Lawless *et al.* (2000), who observed that "It is widely believed, although rarely [if ever] demonstrated, that trained panelists in applied descriptive analysis techniques, such as the Texture Profile or the Spectrum Descriptive Analysis technique, can be calibrated and anchored to physical examples to stabilize and equate their scale useage." That subjects can be taught to associate a specific stimulus with a specific response demonstrates nothing more than a learned activity, a learned "trick." It may be an effective way for demonstrating repeatability of a behavior; however, it tells us nothing about what is perceived or the validity of the activity for evaluating products.

As noted in the introductory segment of this chapter, the variable nature of standards and the efforts of the subjects to adjust their perceptions to the assigned numerical values make it clear as to why the required training time is so long. The panel leader has an active and direct role in this training effort which it is claimed is reduced as the panel develops its confidence in its task and requires less direction.

To evaluate an array of products, this previously trained panel goes through a language development process similar to that described for QDA, but with considerable attention given to the identification and use of specific references to represent the various attributes. Here too, the panel leader has an active role in directing what the panel does and what are acceptable responses. Depending on one's perspective, the strengths or weaknesses of the method is in the number of descriptive words and associated references taught to subjects.

Recommendations for test design, data collection, and analysis are similar to those already described for the QDA method.

E. Free-Choice Profiling

Williams and Langron (1984) described a radically different approach to descriptive analysis in which no subject screening or training were required and subjects could use any words they wanted to describe the products being evaluated. In addition, each subjects' words were unique to that subject as was their scorecards. This approach was presented as an alternative to the protracted time required to train subjects to develop a language and to achieve agreement amongst the subjects using conventional descriptive methods. The authors claimed in discussing other methods, that "complete agreement between assessors is often very difficult, if not impossible, to obtain." The issue of protracted time is reasonable if all methodologies required 3 or more months as prescribed for the Flavor Profile, Texture Profile and Spectrum Descriptive Analysis methods. However, for training, the QDA method, for example, requires only 7–10 hours spread over a single week if one is working with an inexperienced group of subjects, or less if the subjects are experienced. The second issue also warrants comment. Whether it is necessary to have all subjects achieve "...complete agreement..." has yet to be demonstrated. At any point in time, it is very unlikely that all subjects will be equally sensitive to all attributes. Such an achievement would enable each test to require only one subject (our old friend, the *N* of 1). This particular issue also has been raised by O'Mahony and co-workers (1990) and Civille and Lawless (1986) in their discussions about concept development and concept alignment.

The method, as described, requires the experimenter to spend time explaining the testing procedure to the subjects, including instructions on the scoring of the attributes. Unfortunately, the example used by these authors identifies seven of the ten subjects as individuals with years of experience tasting port. Therefore, the time advantage of the method may be non-existent. It is interesting to note that in a more recent publication (Marshall and Kirby, 1988), the method is described in terms of training time, which included a pre-test of the subjects' texture vocabulary followed by ten half-hour training sessions. The individual results and the panel results are then analyzed using a generalized Procrustes analysis. This type of factor analysis analyzes data until an acceptable result is achieved; it is a highly experimental procedure, one that should not be considered without full appreciation for the consequences. As Huitson (1989) noted, the analysis always produces a result that might not be justified based on examination of the database itself. Using a random number generator, this investigator obtained a result as good as that obtained by Marshall and Kirby (1988). Taking into account that the procedure does not yield attribute means (or variance measures) for products without training time, and the aforementioned question about the use of Procrustes analysis, it is difficult to see any advantage derived from this method.

F. Other Methods and Developments

Descriptive methods continue to be described in the literature since publication of the first edition of this book, further evidence of the growing popularity of the methodology. It is clear that this popularity derives from the seeming ease with which results can be obtained and their usefulness in a variety of business applications. For the most part, these methods are more diagnostic in character and/or are variations of established methods.

Cross *et al.* (1978) described a procedure whose objective was to provide more standardization for those investigators measuring meat quality and at the same time "could identify certain textural properties of meat," but also would have more general applications. A comparison with the Flavor Profile and the QDA methods shows many common features in terms of subject screening and qualifying, the use of references, subject feedback during training, and data analysis. However, the method had the panel leader participate in product evaluation and the attributes that were used were selected in advance by the experimenter without the opportunity to change based on subject input.

Larson-Powers and Pangborn (1978) described two approaches to descriptive analysis as part of a larger investigation on the scoring of sweeteners. The first test included the use of a reference product against which the other products were evaluated.

An unidentified reference also was included as an internal measure of subject reliability, and a degree-of-difference scale was used with samples scored relative to the reference. The second test used a unidirectional line scale anchored from none to extreme. Unfortunately, the latter approach was used after four sessions with the anchored procedure, so that a direct comparison of the two methods must be viewed with caution. The authors reported more significant differences with the anchored procedure. Since there were fewer responses with the latter method, it could account for the difference. The products were presented simultaneously, and some additional variability might also be expected (hence fewer significant differences). While one may consider the presence of a reference as contributing to stability of the judgments, this assumes that the references do not change (from the start of testing to the end) or affect sensitivity, and that subjects will not be confused by the presence of this additional sensory input.

The introduction of so many additional sources of variability must be carefully considered relative to the reported advantage in subject skill and product differentiation. For some product categories, for example, salad oils, salad dressings, cigarettes, the problems of sensory fatigue and the removal of residual flavors make this particular approach impractical. Whether this is superior to direct scaling with no references was not demonstrated in the study; however, it does identify further opportunities for research. In our experience, testing without a reference has always shown a higher degree of reliability and optimal differentiation between products, but only when qualified subjects are used. The results by Lyon *et al.* (1978) and Zook and Wessman (1977) using the QDA methodology were consistent with this conclusion. Nonetheless, research of this type must be continued if the descriptive methodology is to be optimized.

The need for modifications allowing statistical treatment of Flavor Profile data has been recognized since its introduction (see Hall, 1958; Jones, 1958). Supporters of the profile method (Miller, 1978) addressed the issue of statistical treatment by suggesting a mathematical procedure for transforming profile data into numerical values. The reason for the transformation was to permit the calculation of an index (Z) derived from amplitude and total intensity. The index was reasoned to provide a single value representing overall product quality. We strongly agree with the author's caution against using this index to over-summarize a complex sensory phenomenon and we would add that the assumptions underlying this index, the method for transforming profile symbols, and the resulting computations should be treated with equal caution.

The developers of the Flavor Profile also have discussed a new version of the methodology (Hanson *et al.*, 1983) called Profile Attribute Analysis®. The method addressed the lack of scaling by incorporating seven-point numerical scales that permits statistical treatment of responses. This has long been needed as those still using the method have made numerous modifications to obtain intensity judgments. However, if the change is nothing more than the addition of a scale and a procedure for calculating a quality index, the method will continue to be of limited use as a descriptive tool. To reflect contemporary knowledge of behavior and measurement, consideration should be given to modifications in subject screening, language development, the evaluation procedure and the role of the panel leader.

We noted earlier that the Spectrum method is often positioned as a hybrid based on Flavor Profile and QDA; in a similar vein, Stampanoni (1993) introduced another hybrid of the two, which she refers to as "Quantitative Flavor Profiling." Several other authors, including Lawless and Heymann (1999), refer to generic descriptive analysis (DA) for those methods having elements of Spectrum and QDA, without formal training by the developers of these method.

Other developments have focused on greater use of statistics for identification of subjects whose scoring patterns are inconsistent with the panel and for identification of attributes that are redundant (measuring the same sensation) or provide no product differentiation. The technical and statistical details of these procedures are described by Powers (1988). While it is logical to use various statistical procedures to analyze response patterns as a means of assessing subject agreement, such procedures have their risks when they are used to eliminate subjects, particularly when done during training.

In the first instance, subjects will exhibit inconsistencies in their responses during training, not only within themselves but also between each other, and one does not need any analysis to recognize this. A purpose for the training sessions is to enable subjects to practice scoring products, to identify and to resolve, as much as possible, conflicts in scoring. This resolution comes about through discussions, led by the panel leader. For QDA training, the subjects typically score two products (one at a time) and then, with a show of hands, vote on which product is further to the right for each attribute. After one or two sets of products have been scored and the votes tabulated, disagreements are more easily observed and the panel leader can direct the subjects' attention to those attributes. For some subjects, the resolution of disagreements is easy, for others it takes longer, and some subjects may never resolve a scoring difference for some attributes. This lack of resolution for some attributes should not be used as a basis for removing a subject. That same subject may be the most sensitive on many other attributes. After all, during training, the subjects are still deciding what attributes are needed, whether some will no longer be needed, and so forth. These questions cannot be answered with confidence until the range of sensory differences for that array of products has been evaluated (during training). Using responses obtained during training to identify subjects who are outliers and dropping them from a panel is not recommended. This could result in a group of subjects who agree with one another but are less sensitive to product differences. A panel leader must be careful to not use procedures that suggest there are correct responses, which will lead to development of errors of central tendency – to be safe, subjects will tend to score in the mid-range of the scale. Finally, some disagreements will arise whenever product differences are small.

After data collection, these multivariate analyses will be helpful. However, we observed that the simple one-way AOV, the individual product ranks, and the subject rankings provides considerably more information on an attribute-by-attribute basis about each subject than does a factor analysis. Not only is a direct measure of performance obtained for each subject, but one also can determine whether a subject is causing interaction, and whether that interaction is crossover or magnitude. As previously noted, this information has a direct impact on conclusions about product differences but should not be used arbitrarily to eliminate a subject so as to obtain a better result.

Similarly, using factor analysis to eliminate certain attributes is an equally risky approach, particularly when it is part of the training process. Not only is it conveying a message to subjects that there is a "correct" list of attributes, but the groupings of attributes (correlation of each attribute to each factor) may not be based on a causal relationship. Thus, the two or three attributes highest correlated to a factor could be selected, yet these attributes, in all likelihood, would not have been used by all subjects with the same degree of sensitivity to differentiate the products. There is no question that a scorecard with fifty attributes contains considerable redundancy; however, all subjects are not equally sensitive to all attributes and the scorecard must reflect this diversity. In the QDA method, eliminating attributes is considered only after three or more tests to be sure that no product differences were obtained and most all responses are at the far left of the scale, that is, little or none of that attribute was detected. Here, too, the subjects will decide whether the attribute should be eliminated, not the panel leader. In addition, the number and diversity of the attributes reflects the multivariate nature of the evaluation process and of the products. Clearly, much more research is needed before a panel leader should rely solely on multivariate procedures without first considering the more basic issues of subject ability.

III. Applications for Descriptive Analysis

There are numerous applications for descriptive information, including monitoring competition, storage stability/shelf-life, product development, quality control, physical/chemical and sensory correlations, advertising claim substantiation, and so forth. Before describing them, it is useful if we re-emphasize the role of the panel leader in deciding how best to use this resource.

Once the decision is made that a descriptive test is appropriate, it is necessary to plan the test, bench-screen the products in the context of the test and the project objectives and decide on the size of the database that will be developed. In product development, a large array of products (e.g. ten or more) could be evaluated in a single test with less replication (three) than if there were only three or four products to be evaluated. The number of replicates would be sufficient to assign a level of confidence to the results and the conclusions and to be able to differentiate the products based on the panel leader's judgment. As a result of formulation efforts, new versions of the products would be submitted for evaluation; however, there would likely be fewer of these products. For this latter test, more replication would be incorporated in the expectation that the differences would be less obvious and that the relative importance of the decisions would be that much greater. Similarly, a storage study might involve only a few products, but in each test a high degree of precision, as well as reliability with each result, would be very important. Therefore, additional care would be taken in the test plan to ensure that there was sufficient replication so that any comparisons would be made from a larger database. In addition, individual subject performance would be critical to the decisions about specific product changes, and therefore the replication per subject also would be important.

The list of applications should be considered as a general guide; a similar list could be prepared for discrimination and affective tests. For the sensory professional, the decision as to what methodology (discrimination, descriptive, or affective) will be used is addressed once the problem is understood and the objective has been stated. Because the output from a descriptive test is so extensive, there is a tendency for it to be considered for all applications; however, this should not be done to the exclusion of the other categories of test methods. The following list should be considered in that context.

1. *Monitor competition.* It is especially important to know in what ways competitive products differ; such information can be used to anticipate changes and to identify product weaknesses. Without such information, it is relatively easy to initiate product reformulation efforts based on circumstantial evidence that a change in market share reflects a changed competitive product. The descriptive information provides a primary basis and more precise direction for any proposed changes. In addition, one can map the relationships of preferences with specific attributes (Fig. 6.9) to gain more insight to how products are "perceived" by the consumers relative to their sensory differences.
2. *Storage testing.* In a storage test in which product changes occur over time, descriptive analysis at the start of the test provides a basis on which changes can be compared. A major problem in all storage tests is the availability of control product throughout the study. A product placed in some type of controlled environment, for example, a freezer, does not prevent change, and providing fresh product for comparison with the stored product introduces other sources of variability. The QDA® method eliminates the need for the control product. This particular application and the following three are all discussed in more detail in Chapter 8.

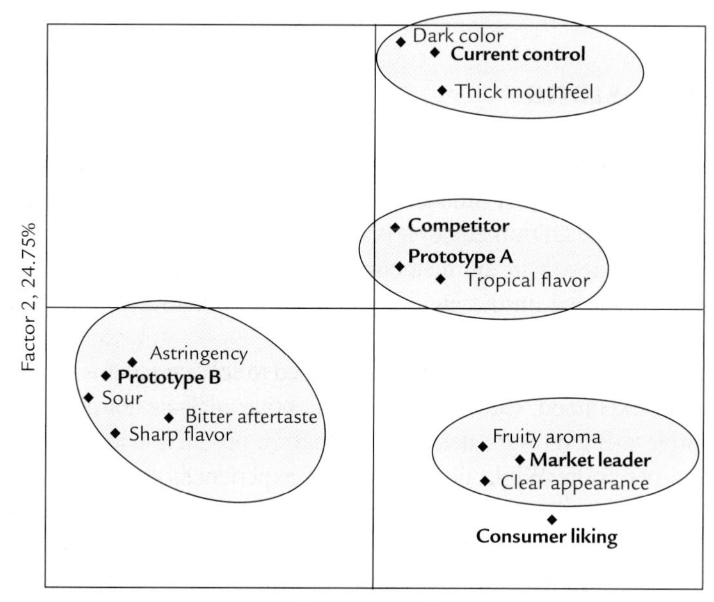

Figure 6.9 A map of sensory and preference differences. The two factors accounted for 69.91% of the differences that were measured.

3. *Product development.* Descriptive analysis is used to delineate a target product, determine whether experimental formulations match that target, and provide precise sensory information about the finished product. This latter function could be used to support advertising as well as be of value in setting quality control specifications. It also can be used in evaluating the usefulness of a new ingredient. For an example of this application, see Clark (1991). Chapter 8 of this book describes the use of a trained sensory panel to provide a descriptive analysis of the products included in optimization research. The statistical analysis relates the consumer, trained panel, and analytical (if included) data sets to determine combinations of sensory and analytical attributes that best predict optimal consumer liking. The descriptive panel is used also for the follow-up research to evaluate test products until one or more satisfy the optimized sensory target.
4. *Quality control.* Descriptive analysis could be used to identify the sensory limits for a product as well as to track long-term trends (see Stone *et al.*, 1991). It is be impractical as an online capability because of the large numbers of products that are evaluated on a daily basis in a manufacturing facility. However, it can be adapted for use in quality control applications (also discussed in Chapter 8).
5. *Physical/chemical-sensory relationships.* Descriptive analysis is especially helpful in identifying specific product differences that can be related to differences in various instrument and chemical measures. Once identified, these differences can be explored in more detail, again using the descriptive model (also discussed in Chapter 8).

It is possible to identify other applications for descriptive analysis; our primary goals here are to increase the reader's awareness of the options.

IV. Conclusions

In this discussion about descriptive analysis, the development of the methodology has been traced from the use of a product expert through the more formal and rigorous approach applied in the QDA method. It is reasonable to expect that there will continue to be changes and growth in the methodology and in its applications. In particular, emphasis must be placed on the importance of the quantitative aspect of descriptive analysis.

Quantitative descriptive methods are not intended to solve problems in an hour. Such problems, in all likelihood, require neither descriptive analysis nor any other sensory test. Descriptive methods were designed to analyze products with a high degree of reliability and precision. While the opinions of experienced staff obtained in bench screening may provide clues to a particular problem and in some instances will solve a problem, this would not constitute a basis for rejecting formal and rigorous sensory analysis of a problem. Similarly, efforts to replace the trained panelist with the consumer, as suggested by Cardello *et al.* (1982), does a disservice to both sensory evaluation and to consumer testing. Neither is intended as a substitute for the other and it is quite risky to confuse their respective tasks and their skills. These latter investigators observed that there were clear differences between the two types of panels, a not unexpected finding. Similarly, and equally not unexpected, differences can be expected when different descriptive training methods are applied (Lotong *et al.*, 2001). This issue is not trivial for the sensory professional, and requires a clear understanding of the test objective and an appreciation for those screening, training, testing and data analysis procedures most likely to achieve the test and business objective.

Descriptive analysis is a sophisticated concept in the sensory analysis of products. It has evolved from the opinions of the expert to a more rigorous and scientific approach to measuring perceptions. The QDA methodology, in particular, emphasizes the behavioral basis of the judgment process and combined with a rigorous approach to assessing response reliability, provides a level of sophistication heretofore not possible in sensory evaluation. However, it would be naive to assume that descriptive analysis is the only category of test methods or that the methods are optimal. Certainly in the case of the QDA method, changes continue to be made as more experience is gained in the use of the method as well as from new developments in measurement and related fields of investigation.

Continued and successful application of descriptive analysis requires an appreciation for the basic principles and test guidelines described herein. In our experience, this will result in a higher level of awareness of the methodology and a greater role for sensory evaluation in the decision-making process.

Affective Testing

7

I. Introduction

Acceptance testing is a valuable and necessary component of every sensory program. In the product evaluation process, acceptance testing usually, but not always, follows discrimination and descriptive tests, which have reduced the number of product alternatives to some limited subset, and precedes larger-scale testing done outside of research and development by others, such as marketing research. This evaluation task is referred to as acceptance, preference, or consumer testing, labels that can have different meanings depending on one's experience and professional responsibilities. From a sensory evaluation perspective, however, acceptance testing should have

Sensory Evaluation Practices 3rd Edn
ISBN: 0-12-672690-6

a specific meaning insofar as the purpose for the test, how it will be done, who will participate, and how the results will be used.

By acceptance testing we mean measuring liking or preference for a product. Preference is that expression of appeal of one product versus another. Preference can be measured directly by comparison of two or more products with each other, that is, which one of two, or more products, is preferred. Indirect measurement of preference is achieved by determining which product is scored significantly higher (more liked) than another product in a multiproduct test, or which product is scored higher than another by significantly more people. There is an obvious and direct relationship between measuring product liking/acceptance and preference. To be most efficient, sensory evaluation should emphasize measuring product liking/acceptance in multiproduct tests and from these data determine preference. Scaling methods allow us to directly measure the degree of liking and to compute preferences from these data. While the reverse is possible (Guilford, 1954), it is more complex, time consuming, and costly. Later in this chapter we will have more to say about the relative merits of these two measures of acceptability. The hedonic continuum is another frequently used expression for product liking and may be considered the more generic representation of the affective process. As Young (1961) noted, the hedonic continuum represents "the sign, intensity and temporal changes of affective processes...," and it is these changes for a set of products that we are interested in measuring. The hedonic continuum will be discussed in more detail in the section on specific methods.

This particular information, the measure of liking, is logical and necessary before substantial capital has been invested in equipment, production and distribution, advertising, and so forth. Obviously, we would be reluctant to invest in a product if we knew that it was not liked because of a sensory deficiency! Therefore, we organize a test methodology that will give us an estimate of product acceptance based on what Cardello and Schutz (2004) refer to as its intrinsic (e.g. ingredient and process related) sensory properties. This measure of sensory acceptance does not guarantee success in the marketplace, since extrinsic variables (Cardello and Schutz, 2003) such as packaging, price, advertising, market segmentation, and so forth will have an effect. However, it does provide us with a good indication of the product's potential as a product without any other of these accompanying features that we expect will enhance its acceptance in the marketplace. Also, the sensory acceptance test neither measures purchase intent nor infers share of market; these topics are beyond the scope and responsibility of sensory evaluation. In that sense, the sensory response is a passive measure; that is, no action is inferred from the respondent. Since most sensory acceptance tests involve limited numbers of consumers, they cannot represent all segments of interest to marketing, it would not be strategically useful to obtain measures of purchase intent and/or related types of responses. It is possible to obtain a more action-oriented measure by use of the food action rating scale (FACT) (Schutz, 1965). This scale requires the subject to estimate frequency of consumption (or use) of a product. Once more, the information will be helpful as one proceeds from the smaller- to the larger-scale testing models.

Sensory acceptance also can and should be measured as a function of product usage in a normal consumption situation, as would occur in a home-use test. If development efforts have yielded a large number of formulation alternatives, it is a responsibility of sensory evaluation to identify which product or products warrants further attention; that is, which one (or more) most closely matches the project objective. In addition to reducing the number of alternatives, the results of the test will also provide an indication of expected reaction with consumers relative to commercially successful products. This latter information can prevent or at least alert project staff that larger-scale tests may not be warranted without reformulation. The value of sensory acceptance testing is obvious, and over time a reliable and valid database should be developed for key products and their competition. With such a database acceptance, norms can be established for key products, further enhancing the usefulness of the sensory acceptance model.

It also is important to emphasize that the sensory acceptance model is neither a substitute for larger-scale consumer tests nor is it a competitive alternative. The sensory test should not be used in place of the larger-scale consumer test when the latter is needed. A frequent misconception is that use of one type of test will replace the other. Often, however, other factors influence the decision as to use of the sensory acceptance test. Of these, the most important are budgetary and timing. Sensory acceptance tests can be organized and fielded at a fraction of the cost and time of larger-scale tests. When budgets are restricted or are depleted, the temptation to substitute the sensory acceptance test (for the larger-scale test) is very strong. This is a more common occurrence as a sensory acceptance database is developed and its credibility is established. Its very success can and will lead to some misuse.

Of course, there will be situations in which the sensory test is the only test that can be done; for example, the product's sales cannot justify the expense of the larger-scale test. It is a responsibility of the sensory professional to review each request, to ensure that the specific problem warrants use of the sensory acceptance test and to provide a realistic framework for any conclusions derived from this latter, smaller-scale test. The sensory professional should make every effort to limit the extent to which there is misuse, through communications with requestors and with brand managers. The sensory test is a small-panel test; that is, usually fifty to seventy-five participate, while the marketing research test involves more than twice that number, and often in more than one geographic location. The sensory test focuses on the product, and determining the best product(s) for the consumer target, whereas marketing research focuses on populations and identifying consumers to whom the product will have the most appeal, and developing the means to influence those consumers (Carter and Riskey, 1990; McDermott, 1990). Clearly, these are two separate but related activities that complement one another, and rely on different testing procedures.

In subsequent sections we describe the various types of acceptance tests – central location, home-use, and so forth – within the context of accepted sensory evaluation principles and practices. This information should make it clear as to the differences between sensory acceptance testing and market research acceptance testing and the means by which they complement one another.

Considering the relative value of this information, it is surprising that there is controversy as to who should do this testing. In some companies, sensory evaluation is not allowed to do acceptance testing; such testing may be mistakenly positioned as consumer testing and designated as the responsibility of marketing research. If sensory evaluation intends to use employees as the subjects, management may argue that the employees are not representative of the target consumers or are biased and, therefore, sensory evaluation cannot do acceptance testing. The most frequently cited example is the result from a sensory acceptance test that was reversed when the products were evaluated by "real" consumers. Implicit in this statement is the notion that a test to measure acceptability with consumers is always valid but a test to measure acceptability with employees is not valid. Of course, results from two tests can differ for many logical reasons; products were manufactured at different times or locations (production versus pilot plant), test procedures, criteria for statistical significance were different, scales differed (a less critical issue), and so forth. In some instances, statistical significance is achieved in one test but not in the other; however, this result should not be surprising as the numbers of consumers tested differed. Obviously, these problems must be given professional attention and their resolution must be brought to the attention of management. While these concerns may seem trivial, for long-term development of one's sensory program, such differences must be resolved. Sensory professionals must demonstrate, to their own and to their management's satisfaction, that the procedures yield reliable and valid information. For selected competitive products there should be consistent response patterns, and results should be in agreement with results previously obtained. For example, if one product is consistently scored significantly more acceptable than another in central location tests, a similar result should be expected with an employee panel. We will discuss the issue of comparative testing as part of the sensory evaluation strategy for establishing and maintaining the sensory acceptance testing resource.

Alternatively, the sensory evaluation program may use local residents to overcome the criticism of using employees, but still find that results lack credibility. Often this can be traced to a lack of understanding of the uses and limitations for sensory acceptance information, which derives, in part, from confusion about marketing decision criteria. Almost all companies have developed management-approved consumer testing guidelines as a means of standardizing procedures and the decisions based on the results. These guidelines stipulate the number of consumers, the test method, the number of locations, and so forth, all of which are intended to minimize risk in the decision-making process and to enable managers to more easily make comparisons. Unfortunately, over time these guidelines undergo a metamorphosis into inflexible rules with no easy means of change to take into account advances in measurement, methodology, or in recruiting the right consumer. Often the decision criteria (developed three decades before the development of appropriate scales or recruiting criteria) are so onerous that product changes are very difficult to achieve. This leads the clever manager to select products and test protocols that improve the odds for him to get what he wants which may not translate to success. The situation becomes even more complicated by the unwillingness to remove questions that are no longer relevant or obtaining responses to attributes that are best obtained from a descriptive panel. As a result, questionnaires become cumbersome and the results are less sensitive, thus making comparisons even more difficult. While it is not our purpose here to analyze these practices in detail, it is important to make sensory professionals aware of the complexities and the challenges that can help explain, in part, the issue of credibility for the sensory acceptance model.

In this chapter, we describe acceptance testing using the same format that was used in the two previous chapters. As a part of this discussion, we also address a number of issues inherent in the relationship that exists between sensory evaluation, marketing, and market research. Some of these issues include the inappropriate application of sensory test methods, the use of large numbers of respondents, and the use of multiple-page scorecards. In each instance, the potential for conflict or problems in interpretation can be minimized through development of a sensory approach to acceptance testing based on the guidelines described herein. Experience has demonstrated that sensory acceptance testing is cost effective and a very useful screening tool before large-scale project commitments are made. If the sensory professional staff has established and implemented the guidelines by which the sensory program operates, then sensory acceptance testing very likely will receive no more criticism than any other methodology.

There can be severe consequences for a sensory program where the types of consumer tests appropriate for the science are not clearly delineated, the value of the sensory affective test is not clearly understood, or the guidelines for those tests are not followed. Consumer testing is not an allowed activity for some sensory programs, while other programs have been assigned to business groups that neither appreciate nor recognize the broad range of support sensory provides to R&D, Marketing, and Manufacturing. In some cases, this has led to the eventual dismantling altogether of some sensory programs.

II. Methods

The two methods most frequently used to directly measure preference and acceptance are the paired-comparison test and the nine-point hedonic scale, respectively. Other methods are described in the literature, but many of them either are modifications of these two methods or are types of quality scales; for example, excellent to poor and palatable to unpalatable. We will discuss some of these methods later with particular emphasis on those that represent opportunities (Cardello and Schutz, 1996; Schutz and Cardello, 2001) and those that represent risks for sensory evaluation. Before proceeding, the reader may find it useful to review the material on measurement presented in Chapter 3. The guidelines and rules regarding the types of scales and the permissible mathematics are equally applicable in acceptance testing. In addition, the admonition not to combine different sensory tasks, for example, discrimination with preference, is especially applicable. Not only will the odd-sample bias be especially strong, but also subjects for sensory acceptance testing who are not trained are relatively naive about the sensory task, and may be used more frequently than the consumers in marketing research tests. In the larger-scale marketing research test, consumers are current or potential users and are qualified if they have not participated in any testing in the previous 3 months (the time will depend on the particular test specification), meet various demographic and product usage criteria, and, in some situations, must be concept acceptors.

In addition to combining of difference with preference, having subjects evaluate specific product characteristics as part of the acceptance–preference test is frequently done, but it too is not recommended. The evaluation of characteristics, whether for intensity or for acceptance–preference, is quite risky for sensory evaluation because the test population is often too small to compensate for semantic differences that occur. Also not recommended is requesting the reasons for a respondent's decision, that is, what did he/she like or dislike about a product. As Payne (1965) observed more than two decades ago, open-ended questions are not worth the effort. Subjects are very likely to justify their decisions, and this often is a recital of advertising information or their expectation of what the product should be like. While such information may have meaning for marketing and advertising, it is inappropriate for sensory evaluation.

The problem with the combining of tasks in a single test is not that a subject will refuse to complete the scorecard or indicate he or she does not know how to respond, but rather there is every likelihood that responses will be confounded. Each response may consist of a component that represents intensity and one that represents affect, and each subsequent response is influenced by response to the preceding question (often referred to as a halo effect; see Chapter 4 for more information on this effect). This confounding typically results in higher than expected variability (and decreased sensitivity). We will have more to say about those issues later; however, our point here is to emphasize the importance of planning and limiting sensory acceptance tests to measure only acceptance (or preference).

A. Paired Comparison

The paired comparison is probably the first formal sensory test method developed to assess preference (Cover, 1936). Therefore, it should be no surprise that there is extensive literature about the method and especially on the topics of test design, statistical analysis, and mathematical models to help explain choice behavior in the paired-comparison situation (see Bradley and Terry, 1952; Bradley, 1953, 1975; Gridgeman, 1955a, 1959; Day, 1974). The test may involve one or more pairs of products, and the subjects may evaluate one or more pairs of products within a single session.

The method requires the subject to indicate which one of two coded products is preferred. A frequently used option allows the inclusion of a "no preference" as a third choice, while another option allows inclusion of a fourth choice, "dislike both equally." Examples of types of scorecards with instructions are presented in Fig. 7.1. The product setup for the paired test is demonstrated in Fig. 5.2. The test is relatively easy to organize and to implement. The only two orders of presentation are A–B and B–A, and subjects usually evaluate only one pair of products in a test with no replication. The preference test usually is a two-tailed test because *a priori* we do not have knowledge as to which product is preferred. However, there will be situations in which the interest is only in the preference for one of the products, in which case the analysis will be based on a one-tailed test. The hypothesis assumes that one of the products will be preferred.

Name ________________ Code ________ Date ________

Option A

Evaluate both products starting from the left. Check the box for the product you prefer. You must make a choice.

347 ☐ 602 ☐

Option B

Evaluate both products starting from the left. Check the box for the product you prefer. You must make a choice.

347 ☐ 602 ☐ No preference ☐

Option C

Evaluate both products starting from the left. Check the box for the product you prefer. You must make a choice.

347 ☐
602 ☐
Like both equally ☐
Dislike both equally ☐

Figure 7.1 Example of the scorecard for the paired-preference test, showing Option A, which limits the subjects to two choices; Option B, which includes a no-preference choice for the subject; and Option C, which includes two additional choices.

Analysis of the results is accomplished using the same computations described for discrimination testing, with $p = 0.05$, or use of Tables 5.11 and 5.14. In advance of a test, it is possible (and recommended) to compute the necessary number of respondents and the number preferring a particular product for a given confidence level. However, it does require the sensory professional to make assumptions about subject sensitivity and the magnitude of the difference. The computations, described in Chapter 5, are derived from Amerine *et al.* (1965) and from Radkins (1957). These authors provided a statistical basis for considering the risks and especially that risk associated with a Type 2 error in the preference test model. While we have emphasized this issue in the discrimination model, it is equally important in the paired-preference test.

If the test design permits a no-preference decision or the additional category of dislike for both (options B and C, respectively), then the analysis will not be as straightforward as the binomial paired-preference model. Gridgeman (1959) observed that the inclusion of ties (no-preference choice) in the preference test is useful in providing more information about the subject's reactions to the products. However, with small numbers of subjects, permitting ties reduces the statistical power (i.e. reduces the likelihood of finding a difference). Whether to permit the no-preference option is not always an easy decision. In the sensory test situation where the number of subjects is usually fewer than fifty, the no-preference option is less desirable. The more subjects who do not or cannot make the choice of, prefer A or prefer B, the smaller will be the database and the larger the difference in preference needed in order for it to be statistically significant. In tests involving a larger number of subjects

(100 or more), a substantial number of no-preference decisions will be important, for example, indicating that the products are equally preferred.

Use of the additional category (dislike both equally) is an option included to ensure that the products are liked; that is, A could be preferred over B, but both could be disliked if the subject's choice was limited to a single no-preference category. The statistical treatment of results from the test could be based on the reasoning of the previous option (ties permitted); that is, the analysis would be based solely on the number of preference responses for the two products as recommended by Gridgeman. The expectation would be for minimal numbers of respondents in the "dislike-both-equally" category; for example, about 5–10%. When this test plan is used, the proportion of subjects expected for the dislike-both-equally category, as well as for the no-preference category, should be computed for comparative purposes. Of course, having a large number of responses in the dislike-both-equally category should raise questions as to the appropriateness of the products for that test or, more importantly, questions as to the subjects' qualifications for that particular product.

Marketing research has made the greatest use of the paired-comparison preference method, either as a two-product test or as a much larger effort involving many products, which is referred to as multiple paired-comparison tests. The appeal of the test method is quite strong because of the unambiguous design, it eliminates transitivity, and the ease with which various marketing hypotheses can be assessed. For example, given different product positioning statements, will preference shift? From a sensory evaluation perspective, however, the paired-preference test (either as a single pair or as multiple pairs) is less informative and less efficient than direct scaling using methods such as the nine-point hedonic scale. The test is less informative because the response (prefer A, prefer B, no preference) provides no direct measure of magnitude of the preference; both products may be disliked. The test is less efficient because there is only one response for each pair of products, compared with a scoring method that yields a response per product. While the Scheffé method of multiple paired comparisons (Scheffé, 1952) yields magnitudes of preference in a multiproduct test, there is still a single judgment per pair of products.

In multiproduct food and beverage tests, there will be considerable sensory interaction because of flavor carryover from one product to the next. This can be a serious deficiency for the paired-preference model where simultaneous (side-by-side) product presentation is the most typical paradigm. Alternatively, memory may become a confounding variable if a sequential presentation is selected for the paired test.

In the multiple paired test, it is possible to minimize the sensory interactions through control of the time interval between pairs. While the time interval between pairs can be controlled, the extent to which the subject samples and re-samples each product cannot be controlled. As a result, there can be greater indecision, leading to a greater percentage of no-decisions which could work to one's advantage in certain circumstances (e.g. competitive advertising). Multiple paired comparisons also are especially cumbersome from a testing viewpoint and particularly with regards to product handling errors. For example, for a four-product test there are six pairs, ten pairs for five products, fifteen pairs for six products, and so forth. The time required for the test also is extended. Unless one is prepared to have these consumers participate over a longer time period (several hours or on several days), then the alternative is to use incomplete designs.

Statistical analyses of multiple paired comparisons, including the ability to convert the comparative responses to partially metric/order data and to undertake a variety of multidimensional analyses, are described in the literature (e.g. Greene and Carmone, 1970; Nunnally, 1978; Schiffman *et al.*, 1981). With these resources, it is not surprising that the paired test has remained the method of choice for individuals in marketing research, advertising, and so forth. Many of the methods for analysis are based on the binomial theorem and (except for the Scheffé procedure) do not permit the inclusion of no-preference ties. Baumgardner and Tatham (1988) recommend a trinomial approach (and *Z* test for significance) where no-preference is permitted. They concluded that the trinomial approach is fundamentally (more) correct, even though they demonstrated little difference in *Z* scores when applying a trinomial approach or using a binomial distribution and eliminating the no preference judgments. The statistics literature also contains numerous references to multinomial discrete distributions for those situations requiring them. This is a reminder to the individual contemplating such tests to ensure that the design and analysis are consistent with the model.

In this discussion, considerable attention has been directed to characterizing the relative value of the paired comparison model for sensory acceptance measurement. Despite weaknesses, the paired test is useful in certain situations. If an advertisement claiming a preference based on a direct comparison is contemplated, then use of the paired comparison is necessary. The paired test is also useful in situations where the chemical senses (taste and smell) are not involved; for example, evaluation of a large array of visual or tactile stimuli.

If there is an interest in obtaining a direct measure of acceptance, then the use of a scaling method is appropriate (Pilgrim and Wood, 1955). We now direct our attention to some of these methods, with particular emphasis on the use of a nine-point hedonic scale.

B. Hedonic Scale

For measuring product liking and preference, the nine-point hedonic scale is probably the most useful sensory method. As noted in Chapter 3, the method occupies a unique niche for sensory evaluation. Since its development (Jones *et al.*, 1955; Peryam and Haynes, 1957), it has been used extensively with a wide variety of products and with considerable success. An example of the scale is shown in Fig. 3.5. The scale is easily understood by naive consumers with minimal instruction, results have proven to be remarkably stable, and product differences (in liking) are reproducible with different groups of subjects. Not surprisingly, the nine-point hedonic scale is used extensively by many companies with considerable success in terms of the reliability and validity of the results. Since most of these studies are not published (but are discussed informally at conferences), questions about the scale continue to be asked or studies are presented purporting superiority of or to some alternative method. For example, in carefully designed studies comparing the method of magnitude estimation with the nine-point hedonic scale, Moskowitz and Sidel (1971) and Warren *et al.* (1982) independently concluded that magnitude estimation was not superior. In contrast, a study by McDaniel and Sawyer (1981) suggested that magnitude estimation was more sensitive because it yielded more significant differences. However, test design limitations raise doubts as to the significance of that conclusion. In recent years interest in these comparisons have not demonstrated any evidence for the superiority of the magnitude estimation method, and most professionals make use of (or should make use of) the nine-point hedonic scale.

Criticisms of the hedonic scale method are primarily the same issues that are directed to many methods: the use of parametric methods for analysis with a scale that is bipolar, the lack of definitive evidence of the equality of the intervals, and avoidance of the neutral category (Day, 1974). These criticisms were discussed previously (see Chapter 3); however, the practical value of the method continues to be demonstrated. The reader is reminded that the issue of bipolarity, for example, is a technical one not a consumer issue; that is, the consumer is blissfully unaware of this and uses the scorecard in a manner that suggests a scale of continuous measurement of liking. The explanation for this is probably manifested in the simplicity of the subject's task (marking a box or circling the appropriate expression) and the absence of numbers on the scorecard that might otherwise confuse or bias the subject. However, this ease of use must be preceded by an explanation given to the participants before the actual evaluations begin as to how to use the scale.

For sensory evaluation, the results from use of this scale are most informative. Computations will yield means, variance measures, and frequency distributions, all by order of presentation and magnitude of difference between products by subject and by panel, and the data can be converted to ranks as well, which yields product preferences. Vie *et al.* (1991) have recommended calculating *R*-indices for nine-point hedonic scale data. Additional information about product differences is obtained from the analysis of variance or the *t*-test, depending on the number of products and number of responses per product per subject. When one considers all of this information relative to the information from the paired test, the usefulness of the former method to sensory evaluation is understandable. The LAMS scale described by Schutz and Cardello (2001), or some similar labeled magnitude scale, may prove to be a significant improvement to the original nine-point hedonic scale. This needs to be confirmed through time and with broader use by sensory professionals. These researchers continue to explore this topic as a means for extending our knowledge of consumer preference behavior.

C. Other Methods

In addition to the nine-point hedonic scale, other scoring methods have been used and continue to be used to measure product liking and preference. Many of the most common of these methods were described by Amerine *et al.* (1965) and for the most part they tend to be associated with particular product categories or with a specific company. For example, meat product evaluation usually relied on an eight-point scale measuring product desirability or an eight- or ten-point product quality scale (excellent-to-poor); other products also made use of such scales (and continue to be used).

Some companies have developed scales that they believe are "special," that they consider as proprietary, but unfortunately do not have any scientific basis. Another variation uses the ten-point numerical scale anchored at one extreme with a frowning smiley face and anchored at the other extreme with a happy smiley face. The ends of the scale, 1 and 10, are also defined with word extremes such as, "doesn't appeal/very appealing" for appearance, and "particularly bad/particularly good for taste." Other examples include categories such as the best "food" ever, etc. These are nothing more than poorly disguised quality scales that are inappropriate for measuring acceptance–preference. Quality scales, whether devised to establish an excellent-to-poor or a palatability-to-desirability measure, should never be used with untrained subjects (i.e. consumers) let alone used with trained subjects; such individuals are highly influenced by each participant's attitude about what constitutes "excellent" quality or the more cognitive concept of desirability. The weaknesses associated with the use of quality scales in general have been discussed previously in Chapters 3 and 6, and the interested reader should review that material.

Another alternative is to rank products from best liked or most preferred to least liked or least preferred. Although these are among the least costly and most efficient multi-product tests to administer, they involve the same compromises described for paired-preference tests (i.e. sensory interaction or memory).

The face or "smiley" scale is another example of a scale (including several versions) that has been used to measure product acceptance and is listed in several recommended test guidelines [American Meat Science Association (AMSA), 1978; Anonymous, 1981b]. The scale consists of a series of faces with expressions in gradations of smiles to frowns that are intended to reflect gradations of preference. Two examples are shown in Fig. 3.6. The smiley scale was developed for use with children and/or individuals who could not read or understand the meaning of written words as presented in scales such as the nine-point hedonic scale. The origins of the scale are obscure, and there is little or no evidence that such individuals can, in fact, associate a particular face with their degree of liking for that product. For a child this can be a challenging intellectual task, especially for relatively young children (8 years and younger). The issue is not whether a child can or cannot read or can visually discriminate the different faces, but rather whether the child has sufficient intellectual skill to transfer sensory reaction to a product, to a specific face. The potential for misinterpretation is so great that it hardly seems worth the effort. Although Roper (1989) recommended against using rating scales with children under the age of 7 years, Kroll's (1990) data supported their use but demonstrated that the face scale was not better than other rating scales. Young children are often selected as subjects for sensory acceptance tests. They are consumers, they spend money and influence adult purchases (Clurman, 1989), and consequently their preferences are of increasing importance to consumer product companies. Kimmel *et al.* (1994) recommended that children can be used for discrimination and acceptance testing but there were numerous difficulties and/or challenges that needed to be managed if the information was to have any value. For example, the cognitive abilities and the actual test protocol had a major influence; requiring experimenters to be able to adapt a protocol to obtain the information without unduly biasing response behavior. Chen *et al.* (1996) used three-face, five-face, and seven-face scales to measure food preferences with 3-, 4-, and 5-year-old children. These researchers concluded that the face scales could be used but that cognitive abilities, as noted by Kimmel and co-workers, would limit experimenters to scales of three or five points. Recently, Popper and Kroll (2003) reported on their research on children's testing and reached similar conclusions as those reported by Kimmel and others. Essential to a successful outcome is the information provided just prior to the test, the orientation, and the type of scale used, paired preference or scaled responses.

Our experience with testing children using the nine-point hedonic scale has been positive; that is, expected preference differences have been obtained. First, no assumptions are made with regard to the ability of the children (from 8 to 12 years) to understand the absolute meaning of each phrase; just the relation to all the other phrases. The fact that children can read does not mean that they understand what they have read. The experimenter must explain the test procedure with examples of use and then the children can proceed with the actual test without having to first interpret the relationship of what they tasted with one of several faces. Experimenters are available to assist; however, children over 8 years usually want to proceed on their own. When children are too young to comprehend verbal instruction for the nine-point hedonic scale, a paired-preference procedure is recommended with parental participation.

We agree with Roper (1989) and Popper and Kroll (2003) that testing children provides many unique challenges in addition to the usual concern for product serving and questionnaire design. For example, to what degree should the parent be included in the test, should the child be tested alone or in a group, and should different questions and tasks be given to different age children in the same test, and so forth. We believe that use of known scales with children and pre-teens make sense provided the scales are demonstrated before a test, and depending on the cognitive abilities, either the parent or an experienced server is available to help face scales are not recommended for the reasons stated above.

Other scales, such as semantic differential and Likert scales, also have been used to obtain measures of product acceptance–preference (also see Chapter 3). Semantic differential and Likert scales are used extensively in studies of purchase decisions, attitudes, and other sentiments; they are especially applicable in the initial investigations of product concepts. Recently, these scales have found increased use in product optimization research for linking sensory perception to various measures such as situation appropriateness, and so forth (see Chapter 8). That these scales are used to measure product acceptance is very surprising inasmuch as they were not developed for that purpose (Stagner and Osgood, 1946). This should not be construed to mean that scales devised for one purpose cannot be applied elsewhere, as we have seen with optimization studies. However, in the context of measuring the sensory acceptance of a product outside the realm of optimization, these scales are inappropriate. They are intended for cognitive issues and are considered less sensitive than scales such as the nine-point scale, particularly when used with only fifty or sixty subjects. Finally, there is the interpretation of results. As noted in Chapter 3, responses from these scales can be summed and/or percentages computed, but not much else. However, their value can be enhanced in marketing and optimization studies by incorporating cognitive and sensory information in a meaningful preference map.

The just-about-right (JAR) scale warrants comment here (see also Chapter 3) as it has been incorporated into the acceptance methodology with increasing frequency. This is a method and an analysis called TURF analysis (Cohen, 1993), adapted from media research to identify or optimize a product line; that is, will a specific line extension enhance an existing line. Its use in product testing has been focused on identifying and directing technology to make attribute changes. Considering the relative insensitivity of the scale (see Chapter 3), it is a poor substitute for descriptive analysis testing.

A common feature of these scales (and others) is that they are usually adapted from other applications in the mistaken belief that what works in one situation will work in another. Sensory evaluation must take care to avoid blurring the differences between perceptual and conceptual measurement techniques. These scales should not be used in sensory acceptance–preference tests outside the realm of optimization. While they may be useful in those situations, they are not appropriate for small-scale sensory affective tests described in this chapter.

III. Subjects

The subjects participating in a sensory acceptance test should be qualified based on typical demographic and usage criteria or preference scores from survey data, if the former cannot always be satisfied. It may not be possible, or even necessary, to select subjects based on demographic criteria when employees are the subjects, and a large majority of sensory acceptance tests do involve employees. However, in recent years there has been an increase in the use of local residents in place of employees, a topic that will be discussed later in this section. Employees who volunteer to participate should be screened for their product usage and likes/dislikes. Screening is best done using a survey format similar to the one described in Chapter 2.

For employees, the attitudinal responses should be compared with data from other populations to determine that the subjects are comparable, at least in their preference toward specific products. The Meiselman *et al.* (1974) report on degree of liking for more than 300 products based on responses from several thousand military personnel can be used for comparative purposes. A summary of all food acceptance testing is now in preparation and should be published this year (Meiselman and Schutz, 2003). However, external survey data should be supplemented and eventually superseded with data obtained from one's own product testing. This information is used as a basis for selecting subjects for acceptance tests. One selection criterion, in addition to requiring that they are likers of the product, could be to use only those subjects whose attitudinal scores fall within ± 1 SD of the grand mean for all survey participants. This measure should be consistent with published data, such as the aforementioned survey. The decision as to the permissible range of scores that includes or excludes subjects is the responsibility of the sensory staff. The overall objective is to select a relatively homogeneous group, all of whom are within the norm of likers of the particular product (or product category), and to be able to exclude individuals who exhibit extreme or unusual response patterns, such as always scoring products as nines or ones. The latter do not differentiate among products and, therefore, contribute nothing of value.

This entire database should be available online. As tests are completed, results can be entered and each subject's file updated. This system is also used to select subjects for a test, ensuring that an individual will not be used too frequently. For employees, this test frequency should probably not exceed two or three tests per month for the same type of products. There is no question that these subjects will become experienced test participants within a few months; however, monitoring of response patterns will identify atypical results. For example, if the variance measures show a systematic decrease or current products are assigned scores higher than what has been experienced in the past. In most instances, a 1- or 2-month interval of no testing should be sufficient to correct this problem. Specific guidelines must be developed on a product-by-product basis. Of course, if one has available many hundreds of subjects, then test frequency can be further reduced.

Individuals who are qualified for discrimination and descriptive tests should not be used for acceptance testing regardless of their willingness to participate. The training process, especially for descriptive analysis, results in subjects who have an analytical approach to product evaluation that will bias the overall response required for the acceptance–preference task. Similarly, individuals who may possess technical or related information about specific products should not be used because of their potential bias. Objectivity must be maintained if the results are to be considered as reliable and valid.

The importance of subject selection and frequency of test participation are critical issues in relation to the question of the objectivity and face validity of the results from employee acceptance tests. There also is a risk that employees will recognize a product, especially if there are brand names or unique markings on those products. For companies that have a very limited product line, even these precautions may not be adequate. Employees may easily recognize those products that are different from their own, whether they are competitors or experimental. However, before a decision is reached as to the potential bias (or lack of) of employee acceptance test results, sensory evaluation should initiate a series of comparative studies to test this hypothesis.

The validity of employee acceptance tests is an important step in the overall scheme of the sensory evaluation program. At issue is the question of whether employee panel results accurately reflect those from a non-employee panel. Care must be taken to ensure that products, scorecards, test procedure, and so forth are matched. Products should be obtained from the same production lot; scorecards, serving orders, and test instructions must be identical. For the analysis, the use of a split-plot, one-within and one-between analysis of variance model is most appropriate (see Chapter 4). In this model, products are treated as the *within* variable while the two panels are treated as the *between* variable. Of special interest would be the significance measure for the product × panel interaction. If this interaction is not significant, we can conclude that the two panels scored the products similarly, and we accept the employee panel's results as a good estimate of the non-employee panel's results with respect to the *relative* difference between products. On the other hand, a significant interaction would require sensory evaluation to determine whether that interaction was the result of panel differences for product ranks or due to the magnitudes of difference between product means. Conversion of scores to ranks followed by rank-order analyses may yet demonstrate a consistent ordering pattern between the two panels.

Data obtained from several comparable studies would provide the basis for a correlation analysis. Although correlations are not sensitive to absolute values, they are a good indicator of whether the relative differences between products are comparable for the two panels. Statistical validation of employee panel results should be done periodically.

Satisfactory results from these studies allow substitution of preference behavior for demographic criteria in selecting subjects for acceptance tests. This approach is especially useful because most employees (and most local resident panels) cannot totally satisfy demographic criteria for all products. For example, in the military, much of the progress in development of rations and menu items was achieved through use of non-military personnel as subjects and then verified with military personnel (Peryam *et al.*, 1960; Meiselman *et al.*, 1974). This rationale is applicable to products such as breakfast cereals that are intended primarily for children. An employee panel whose acceptance scores accurately reflect relative differences similar to a children's panel could be used in the development process.

As previously mentioned, there has been a gradual trend toward use of local residents or contracting with a local agency that provides a sensory acceptance test service. This increased use of non-employees reflects the general lack of availability of employees as a result of industrial consolidations, and to some extent, concern about the credibility of results from employees. There are, however, several advantages of using non-employees including their availability with minimal delay, availability for a longer period of time, and obtaining a more accurate estimate of the cost for each test. This latter point is especially important for financial accountability for each test. When non-employees are used for a single test, detailed information on attitudes toward a wide array of products is not expected, and the demographic information becomes the dominant issue. Traditional information such as age groupings, sex, frequency of use, and so forth is used to determine whether an individual is qualified.

Because the sensory acceptance test uses small numbers of subjects, it will be important to select subjects who are within the norm of likers for the product and who can effectively use preference rating scales to differentiate among products (not all people can), if rating scales will be used in testing. When testing with consumers, additional selection criteria based on demographics, psychographics, usergraphics, and lifestyle are recommended (Carter and Riskey, 1990; McDermott, 1990). This information should be available from marketing (or from sensory optimization research, a topic discussed in Chapter 8).

It is becoming more common to have a pool of non-employees participate regularly in sensory acceptance tests in much the same way as employees. In this case, the qualifying procedures described for employees will be applicable and their responses must be monitored on a continuing basis. In this way, the reliability and validity of the results will be maintained and the sensory acceptance test will continue to be an integral part of every company's product sensory test program. Of course, when using non-employees, some monetary compensation will be necessary. For employee participation, an indirect reward is necessary; for example, credit toward lunch at the company cafeteria or some similar reward. As discussed in Chapter 2, employees must be rewarded for participation but not with direct cash payments (see Chapter 2 for more discussion on this topic).

IV. Types of Acceptance Testing

Acceptance panels, as noted previously, are used primarily as part of the product screening effort. They allow for reducing the number of alternatives by eliminating poorly performing products and for maintaining greater security (when employees are used) than may be possible in other types of consumer tests.

There are three primary categories of sensory acceptance tests; laboratory, central location, home-use. As shown in Table 7.1, these three test categories are listed in terms of types of subjects, and their respective advantages and disadvantages. To some extent, the distinction between testing in a laboratory versus in a central location is not as clear as that versus home-use testing. In the former situations, the subjects are brought to a central location for testing and the primary differences relate to the extent of the controls applied to the testing process and the environment of the test. Additional discussion about each of them follows.

A. Laboratory

Acceptance testing in the laboratory environment is the most frequently used of the various types of sensory acceptance tests. It is particularly appealing because the laboratory is usually very accessible to employees, the greatest possible control over all aspects of the test is ensured (lighting, environmental control, product preparation, and so forth), and rapid feedback of results is possible. The number of responses per product is listed as between twenty-five and fifty up to a maximum of seventy-five and we recommend at least forty per product. Since most of the tests make use of balanced designs and each subject evaluates each product, a panel actually could have as few as twenty-four subjects. It might be difficult to establish a statistically significant difference in a test with so few subjects, but it is still possible to identify trends and to provide direction to the requestor. As the panel size increases to a maximum of about seventy-five subjects, especially for tests involving more than two products, the statistical significance, credibility, and the importance of the results increase substantially. These economies are possible because of the test controls and the use of subjects who have prior test experience. Sidel and Stone (1976) provided a guide for selecting panel size based on the expected degree of difference in hedonic scale ratings (for the nine-point hedonic scale) and the size of the standard deviation. For example, a statistically significant difference at $\alpha = 0.05$ is possible for a 0.50-point scale

Table 7.1 Characteristics of different type of sensory acceptance tests[a]

	Laboratory	Central location	Home-use
Consumer type	Employee or local resident	Public (general or selected)[b]	Employee or public
Responses per product	25–50	100^{+}	50–100
Product number	Maximum of 5–6 per session	Maximum of 5–6	1–2
Test type	Preference, acceptance but not quality	Same as laboratory	Preference, acceptance, performance (intensity and marketing information)
Advantages	Controlled conditions Rapid data feedback "Test-wise" subjects Low cost	Large number of subjects No company employees	Product tested under actual use conditions All family's opinion obtained Marketing information (pricing, frequency of use, etc.)
Disadvantages	Familiarity with product Limited information Limited product exposure	Less control Limited information No lengthy or distasteful tasks Limited instructions Large number of subjects required	Little or no control Time consuming Expensive

[a] See text for additional explanation.

[b] General groups (subjects solicited at fairs, markets, retail outlets, etc.); selected groups (churches, clubs, schools, etc.).

difference when the standard deviation is not more than 1.50 with a panel of forty subjects. A word of caution is necessary: the relationship between panel size, magnitude of difference, variability (subjects, products, experiment), and statistical significance is presented as a guide. Different types of products will have their own unique requirements. For example, a manufactured product may show less variability than a natural product, which is more strongly influenced by the quality of the harvest, and so forth. In this case, the expectation of a statistically significant difference may not be realized without a sufficiently larger number of subjects (e.g. increasing the panel size to sixty or seventy). While smaller panels will yield significant differences as variability decreases, order effects and other factors also can influence results and reduce their usefulness.

As listed in Table 7.1, a laboratory panel should evaluate no more than about five or six products in a single session, and responses should be limited to acceptance–preference. Limiting the number of products to no more than five or six is based, in part, on practical consideration; for employees, their time away from their regular work. Of course, non-employees are available for longer periods of time and easily could evaluate more products. However, this depends on the kind of products; whether sensory fatigue will be a problem and how much preparation and handling is required. This does not mean subjects are not capable of evaluating more products. As Kamen *et al.* (1969) observed, consumers can evaluate as many as twelve products, provided a controlled time interval between products is allowed and only acceptance is measured.

For both laboratory and central location tests, the recommended number of products is limited to five or six, or fewer. More products could be evaluated; however, this approach would require subjects returning for a second or third session either later that day or on subsequent days. An alternative approach for tests of larger numbers of products is the use of incomplete designs (see, e.g. Gacula and Singh, 1984, and Chapter 4 of this book). If an incomplete design is used, we suggest the number of incomplete cells per subject be kept to a minimum of one-third or less (e.g. a four of six, but not four of seven or four of eight). Having subjects return to evaluate all products yields a more powerful database. One other issue that is often overlooked when using incomplete designs is the need to increase the number of subjects, and that often is a limiting factor in most test programs. In our experience having several sessions is more preferable than using an incomplete design. This way, all subjects are provided with a similar context of products. This does not mean that incomplete designs should be avoided or are inappropriate. For some products (e.g. a skin-care product), it may be the only way to evaluate it without making the evaluation process unworkable. Disadvantages of the laboratory test are the potential familiarity with the product when using employees, the limited information (acceptance) derived from the test, and the limited exposure of the consumer to the product. This latter point will be discussed in more detail in the next section.

B. Central Location

The central location test (CLT) is one of the most frequently used of consumer tests (the laboratory sensory test is a type of CLT) and especially by marketing research. The CLT is usually conducted in a shopping mall or a similar type of location; for example, a school cafeteria, a store, or an office building that is accessible to large numbers of people (the public). For this test, consumers will either be prerecruited, or if the site is a mall, an intercept procedure will be used. Prerecruiting is generally more costly because of the time required to contact prospective candidates and because the compensation for the effort needed to get them to the site will exceed the cost of the intercept procedure and any compensation given to the consumer recruited in a mall. In fact, for many products, consumers recruited at a mall are given only indirect compensation; for example, discount coupons. However, other factors must be taken into account when making a decision as to where a test will be done and how the consumers will be recruited. If a product has a relatively low incidence of usage then the mall intercept method will be more time consuming than a prerecruited test. For example, a product with an expected incidence of 10% of the population will require a minimum of 1000 contacts to find 100 product users, and not all of those who qualify will want to participate (which could be as much as 30%). Thus, the mall intercept method of testing could require considerably more time to complete when the incidence of participation is very low. If a planned mall test involves extensive product preparation and handling, then the benefit of the lower cost of the mall intercept will be easily lost as a result of the additional time required to complete the test and the additional amounts of product required. An obvious solution is the use of several malls; however, this also introduces its own set of problems, not the least of which is that the malls will be a potentially confounding source of variability. On the other hand, prerecruiting allows for testing to be completed within 1 or 2 days.

In addition to the general public, consumers may be solicited from religious and social clubs, schools, and other organizations. Groups such as these provide homogenous groups of subjects as needed, and this is an easy way to recruit. However, the reader is reminded that these people are representative of a narrow segment of the population, many of them know one another, and their response may be skewed.

For the CLT, there are usually about 100 responses (consumers) per product, in situations where segmentation is anticipated, even more responses might be necessary. This increase in the number of consumers (versus the laboratory test) is necessary to offset the expected increase in variability attributable to the novelty of the situation, inexperience of the consumer, and limitations in the test environment.

The number of products should be limited to about five or six, and possibly fewer in order to minimize test time, an important issue in the mall intercept protocol. In a mall test, participants are liable to leave in the middle of a test if the task is lengthy, unpleasant, or too complicated. However, test results have considerable face validity and credibility where the subjects are "real consumers" representing the target population, and large numbers of such tests have been used. Thus, increasing the number of subjects to 100 or more is both an advantage and a disadvantage.

Limited product exposure is sometime considered a disadvantage of the laboratory and CLT methods versus the home-use test, where the consumer will have more and longer exposure to a product. Inasmuch as the laboratory and CLT methods are used primarily for screening product alternatives and for more precisely defining the consumer segment in relation to the specific products, this should be a non-issue. Questions about the longer-term sensory effects (e.g. flavor wear-out) should be addressed in an extended use study rather than as a routine multi-product screening issue. We recall a company insisting that the subjects consume an entire container of liquid in order to evaluate the effect; however, they requested that several units be evaluated in a single session. Not surprisingly, most participants refused to complete the test and spent much time visiting the restrooms! While the need for consumption information is useful, the venue is inappropriate.

Another unfortunate practice that has increased in popularity as testing budgets are reduced is the "piggy-back" CLT test, where consumers recruited to a test site participate in evaluation of multiple products, often from different categories. Although the products may be independent, it is likely they have a confounding influence on the subject and the results. Sensory interaction and fatigue, response carryover from one product set to the next, and motivational change during the course of testing are but a few factors increasing the risk of contaminating results on subsequent products in the test session. We do not recommend the practice.

C. Special Types of Central Location Tests

In addition to the CLT described in the previous section, product acceptance information can be obtained in two additional ways. As shown in Table 7.2, a mobile serving cart or mobile laboratory can be used to bring products to consumers and still fit within the structure of a CLT.

Without question the laboratory environment provides the greatest control for a test. However, this control can be compromised to some extent in situations where access to sufficient numbers of people to complete a test is necessary. Sufficient product and supplies are placed on a cart, which is brought to the employees' work stations. An office area will be quieter and a more desirable area than a manufacturing location; however, there will still be some distractions. Conversations, traffic flow, visual contact with other employees, telephones, personal computers, and so forth will distract the subjects, and the sensory staff will need to take these factors into account when designing a test to be done at the subject's work station. As noted in the table, there should be as many as fifty responses per product and a maximum of five products in a test. As might be expected, the relative advantages and disadvantages represent a combination of those listed for both the laboratory and CLT.

Not all products lend themselves to this type of test protocol. Non-food items are more likely candidates; however, the use of hospital serving carts with appropriate heat controls will permit a wider range of food product applications. Nevertheless, the sensory tasks must be simple and require little time to complete. The potential for distraction (and increased variability) is quite high. One cautionary note should be mentioned. The economics of the mobile serving cart may have considerable management appeal. The serving cart is a temporary alternative, but it cannot substitute for a permanent facility with all the necessary controls.

The mobile laboratory represents one additional means by which the controls of the laboratory can be brought to the consumer. A motor home or trailer can be built to contain product preparation and holding facilities, booths, proper lighting and ventilation, and so forth. The unit can then be driven to shopping malls, fairs, or wherever

Table 7.2 Characteristics of special cases of the central location test

	Mobile serving cart	Mobile laboratory
Consumer type	Company employee[a]	Public (general or selected)
Responses per product	22–50	40–60
Product number	2–5	2–5
Test type	Preference, acceptance (not quality)	Same
Advantages	Cost Rapid data feedback "Test-wise" subjects	No employees Controlled conditions
Disadvantages	Limited control Limited information Familiarity with product	Limited information No lengthy or distasteful tasks Limited instructions

[a] See text and footnotes to Table 7.1 for additional explanation.

there are large gatherings of people, and the testing done in a way that is similar to that done in the laboratory environment.[1] This approach is most useful when the respondent population is unique, or one is interested in sampling school-aged children, for example. The recommended number of products that can be tested is not more than five; the number of subjects is increased to between forty and sixty. Because the subjects will be inexperienced, the tasks should be limited; however, the presence of the sensory staff should facilitate the testing activities.

D. Home-Use Tests

The sensory home-use test also is a valuable resource, providing information on product preparation, family attitudes, and so forth. This information is not obtained in the laboratory setting. For some non-food products, laboratory evaluation is very difficult (e.g. in testing disposable diapers), and home-use testing becomes a feasible and necessary alternative. Similarly, if one is testing running shoes or golf clubs, this is best accomplished before, during, and after use not in a laboratory environment.

Often the first exposure that sensory evaluation will have to a product in its proposed container is when it is going into home-use testing. Since products can fail due to problems with containers or product usage, it is reasonable to have a home-use capability to assess products in the early stages of product formulation or reformulation.

In the home-use test, there is no control of environmental as well as other test factors. Therefore, panel size should be about twice the size (50–100 families) of that used in the laboratory test. If the subjects are accustomed to sensory testing, panel size can be reduced; however, this reduction in panel size should be empirically based rather than arbitrary. We expect that "test-wise" subjects (i.e. experienced subjects who know how to test and who are comfortable in the test situation) will be less susceptible to error as a result of psychological variables associated with being a subject. Further improvements are possible by eliminating subjects who have been erratic or are otherwise so different from the norm that they may be considered representative of a small population of little commercial interest.

Home-use tests typically involve only two products, primarily because of the duration of time needed for each product to be evaluated. Extended use of 4–7 days would be relatively common. If there were interest in evaluation of additional products, test time would have to be extended and the rate of return of completed scorecards could drop substantially. This is due to many factors, for example, lost scorecards, vacations, and so forth. One obvious alternative is to have different groups of subjects evaluate different products, which as noted previously also has its own set of limitations.

As noted in Table 7.1, the products are tested under actual use conditions and the entire family's opinion is obtained. As with all sensory tests the primary focus of the evaluation is on sensory acceptance. Test design and instructions should be kept uncomplicated. While it is possible to field a home-use test in collaboration with marketing research, sensory acceptance should be the initial measure.

[1]An example of a mobile laboratory is seen with MSTS Ltd. in the UK (http://www.msts.co.uk).

The home-use test provides subjects with the first opportunity to form an opinion based on consuming or using the product (food or non-food). With foods, this test also may provide the subject with their first opportunity to actively prepare and serve the item as a normal part of the daily routine. However, it should be remembered that many of the perceptual components associated with product handling can and should be isolated and studied in the laboratory or CLT model. For example, it is reasonable to have consumers individually prepare a product and evaluate the sensory components associated with the preparation procedure before moving to the home-use environment. This identification of product use variables is important in understanding their effect on product acceptance.

The home environment allows a multitude of unique variables to have their "normal" influence during product preparation and use. In the early stages of development these variables may represent undesirable noise in the test, whereas in the latter stages they may represent a desirable resource for learning about conditions that could lead to product failure.

The home-use test presents sensory evaluation with several additional issues that need resolution that are not encountered in either the laboratory or the CLT designs. These decisions include containers and their labels, product preparation instructions, product placement, and scorecard.

Products in home-use tests usually are packaged in containers similar in size and shape to those in which the product will be sold, but with the standard graphics omitted. Often a plain container is used. There should be at least a three-digit code, a label containing usage instructions and contents, and a contact telephone number (in case of problems).

Preparation instructions must be complete in terms of how the product is to be used, along with directions for completion of the questionnaire. The importance of these instructions should not be underestimated, because they are the context within which the family members make their decision. Consultation with home economists and other specialists familiar with product usage is essential to minimize confusion and ambiguous results because of improperly worded instructions. Since there is no experimenter available to the subjects at the time of preparation and evaluation, the instructions must be unambiguous.

Product placement is a factor that is often determined by economics. Providing a participant with all products at the start of the test minimizes costs; however, even lower costs can be achieved by mailing products to the subjects. This latter approach is risky and sensory evaluation should avoid it for obvious reasons. This does not mean that mail panels are unreliable, but rather that they are inappropriate for sensory evaluation.

Providing both products at the same time also is not recommended because it enables the subjects to make direct comparisons, increases their likelihood of assigning responses to the wrong scorecard, and totally confounds the experimental design. Because these are serious concerns, the issue of cost should not be the determining factor. With employees, it is relatively easy for them to come to a specific location to receive their product and instructions, and to return the scorecard and the empty container after completing an evaluation and before receiving another product. If one is using local residents instead of employees, they still come to a central location to obtain product.

Larger-scale home-use tests that do not involve employees or a local panel require just as much concern about product placement. In these situations, the product placement may be done at the time an individual is qualified; for example, in a mall intercept recruiting drive. If recruiting is done by telephone, the product may be mailed; however, as noted previously, the potential for product misuse is very high. Product delivery directly to the home is very costly and when it is used, the tendency is to leave all products at the same time and to return when the test is completed. In these test situations, the greatest opportunity for control is achieved by having the interviewer place the first product and scorecard following respondent qualification, and on return retrieve both prior to placing the second. This process is followed until the final product and scorecard have been retrieved. Personal interviews, unlike the telephone or the mail, provide an opportunity to review the procedures with the respondent and determine whether the product was used properly (or at all), and if necessary to clarify the test procedure or product-use conditions, should there be any questions. This procedure is quite similar to that followed in using employees or a local panel. In our experience, having the consumer come to a location and given a briefing and review of the test procedure and scorecard is the best option. It enables the experimenter to minimize misunderstandings, answer questions, and improve the quality of the information obtained. Where possible, the subject can return the empty container and scorecards, receive the next product and any additional information about the test.

The primary concern in the sensory home-use test is measuring overall product acceptability. This may be obtained through use of one or more of the scales described in Chapter 3. To maintain continuity between laboratory, central location, and home-use tests, similar procedures, analyses, significance criteria, and the same acceptance scale should be used throughout (e.g. the nine-point hedonic scale).

In addition to overall acceptance, responses to product characteristics such as appearance, aroma, taste, and texture (e.g. mouthfeel) may be obtained. This information can be used as an indication of a general product problem but should not be used in the same way as a result from a sensory analytical test. As with any untrained panel, beyond the overall acceptance judgment there is no assurance that the responses are reliable or valid. Subjects will complete the scorecard but it is difficult to determine the meaning of the result. In the sensory acceptance test, the value, meaning, and interpretation of those responses are more often a source of error and conflict than a source of useful information. It is not unusual for researchers to collect pages of such information although they admittedly do not expect to learn much from it. The problem is, however, that once collected, there exists a tendency for the researcher to use this information in decisions, particularly if the other results do not meet their expectations.

Another problem associated with asking diagnostic acceptance questions is the different "psychological set" this establishes for the subject and the consequent changes in response behavior that this may cause. Overall acceptance requires that the subject view the product as a whole (a "gestalt"), without direction to what sensory aspects are considered important. Conversely, diagnostic assessment requires the subject to approach the product from an analytical perspective, and directs subjects to focus on specific sensory components. It is a rather simple task to change overall attitude behavior by focusing subjects on different product attributes. Asking diagnostic questions serves to focus attention on those specific attributes. Focusing on one set of selected attributes may result in a different acceptance response than may occur if attention were focused on a different set of attributes or if there were no focusing whatsoever. The line of questioning or set of attributes selected for a questionnaire has the potential for revealing more about the researcher's product knowledge and expectations, than providing unbiased and useful consumer information for product or management decisions. Including diagnostic acceptance questions does not guarantee data will be flawed, it simply increases that risk, and for ongoing sensory programs there is no way to determine for each test, when, and to what degree data have been compromised.

Because the subject's response in a purchase-and-use situation will not include the same diagnostic focusing as the research test, it is better to exclude that dimension from the test in the first place. With only product acceptability to attend to, the consumer has little doubt that we are interested in his or her overall attitude (like or dislike) for the product. Without the potential frustrations, tedium, and misguidance associated with asking consumers attribute questions, we can be more confident about the acceptance data obtained.

If there is interest in learning more than overall acceptance from the home-use test, it is reasonable to obtain limited information about product performance. For example, if a product was prepared and intended to serve four portions, did it in fact do so. Or, if the product was designed as a multipurpose product (e.g. a cleaner for glass and tile), how acceptable was it in its various use categories. A good product that was supposed to take 10 minutes to prepare may have taken 25 minutes; such information can easily be obtained, and should be. Although this information is obtained in addition to acceptance, it does not require an analytical sensory set, and as such should not create the same problems as those associated with sensory attribute questions.

Although a monadic sequential placement procedure may be used in conjunction with the hedonic scale, many investigators find it too difficult to disassociate themselves from a paired preference question and will persist in adding it as a final overall question. If so, the question may be phrased as follows: "Thinking about the product you tested last week and the one you tested this week, which one do you like best?" Usually this question is included to satisfy individuals in the company who mistakenly believe that the paired-preference test is the most sensitive or only valid way to measure product acceptance. Using a paired-preference question in the home-use test introduces a memory variable if the subject has to remember what was tested first, and how well it was liked, and so forth. Therefore, we do not view the paired-preference question as a satisfactory sensory technique where a monadic sequential usage procedure has been used.

A more serious problem with using a paired-preference question in conjunction with monadic sequential scaling of acceptance is created when the two measurement techniques produce contradictory results. Which technique (and result) is then to be believed! Actually both can be correct, but because they are different measurement techniques, they may produce different results. Since the paired question allows only a count of responses for or against a product, it is possible to get results similar to

Table 7.3 An example of the potential conflict between scaled and paired-preference data

Number of respondents	Hedonic scale rating		Magnitude of difference in hedonic scores (in scale units)
	Sample A	Sample B	
12[a]	1	9	8
8	5	4	1
4	6	5	1
8	7	6	1
8	8	7	1
Mean score	4.9[b]	6.6	
Number preferring each product	28[c]	12	

[a] In this example, forty subjects participated, of whom twelve assigned dislike extremely to product A and like extremely to product B, and so forth. For more information on the nine-point hedonic scale, see Section IIA of this chapter.
[b] Denotes a significant difference ($p = 0.002$). B is scored higher than A.
[c] Denotes a significant difference ($p = 0.008$). More respondents scored A higher than B.

those shown in Table 7.3. If we assume that a respondent who scored one product higher than another would also prefer that product in a forced choice situation, we may view the data in Table 7.3 as demonstrating a significant preference for product A. However, only twelve of the forty respondents scored product B higher than product A (mean score of 6.6 versus 4.9).

If only means, percent preferring, and statistical significance are reported (as is usually the case), one has a reporting dilemma. However, if only paired preference data are obtained, the magnitude of difference recorded for 30% of the panel is not obtained. This can be a critical omission. For scaled data, the number of subjects scoring one product higher than another is easily derived and clearly indicates all the important information: (1) mean differences and level of significance; (2) number of subjects scoring one product higher than another; and (3) the magnitude of difference for subgroups in the population. On this latter detail, a magnitude of difference of eight scale points is considerably larger than a magnitude of difference of one scale point.

Equipped with the information from the scaled data, a lower risk, business decision is possible than when only paired preference data are available. Since paired preference data can be derived from scaled data, their inclusion in the home-use test is unnecessary. The home-use test usually is reserved for the latter stage of sensory evaluation testing; it has a high degree of face validity and it provides an opportunity to measure performance and acceptance by family members under normal use conditions, but it may be more costly than other sensory tests, requires more time to complete, and there are no environmental controls.

E. Other Types of Acceptance Tests

In addition to these approaches to consumer testing, there are a few additional options available to sensory evaluation. One of these, as discussed previously, is to bring local residents into a sensory laboratory. This approach has been growing in use because it is convenient for the sensory staff in terms of scheduling of tests, the speed with which requests can be satisfied, and minimizes reliance on employees. However, this use of local residents has its own set of requirements that include recruiting, scheduling, budgeting, accessibility, and security. A system must be established to contact and schedule subjects along with a budget and means for compensating them after each test or block of tests. Accessibility to the test site must minimize the risk of subjects wandering into restricted areas, and so forth. Provided the sensory facilities are accessible, this can be one way of extending sensory resources, and especially those needed for acceptance testing. Participants are highly motivated, will be very prompt, and willing to provide considerable product information.

Another possibility is for a company to develop and maintain an off-premises test facility. This eliminates many of the problems associated with bringing local residents into company premises; however, it will be more costly than bringing people to the sensory facility. It may also be possible to contract with a supplier, provided they have the necessary sensory test resources.

In each case, sensory evaluation will need to assess its current acceptance test resources and anticipated volume of work before determining whether any of these options are feasible. There is no question that sensory acceptance–preference testing must be done; the questions to be answered relate to where it will be done, who will be the subjects, and what are the relative costs.

V. Special Problems

Acceptance testing, as in discrimination and descriptive testing, has its share of special problems and practices that have had and will continue to have an impact both in terms of the way the tests are organized and fielded and in terms of how the results are used. Section I contained a brief discussion about the relationship between the sensory acceptance and the larger-scale marketing research models. This differentiation of the sensory acceptance model is important because it is often mistaken for or used in place of the marketing research model. In this chapter, we have made clear the role of the sensory acceptance model and its responsibilities in the overall scheme of product evaluation. Nonetheless, situations will arise in which product information is questioned or tests are proposed that do not fit within the conventional scheme of sensory evaluation, yet the results will have a direct impact. These include the use of the discrimination model to screen consumers for a preference test, the use of large numbers of consumers to achieve a statistically valid sample, use of multipage scorecards, and the use of open-ended questions. It is our position that an awareness of these practices will be helpful to sensory evaluation and to marketing and marketing research. Once again, the reader is reminded that, in most instances, the issue is not so much that one approach is totally correct and the other is totally wrong as it is an issue of risk and the interpretation of results. Now that we have it, what do we do with it?

A. The Difference–Preference Test

In the discussion on discrimination testing (Chapter 2), the practice of asking each subject to express a preference after the discrimination response was discussed and its weaknesses identified. As a test procedure it is not recommended. Unfortunately, this same concept also has been applied to consumer testing with an equally risky outcome. The description of its use by Morrison (1981), citing work by Moskowitz *et al.* (1980) and earlier discussion by Day (1974), pointed to the continuing interest in this use of the discrimination model with consumers. We have already pointed out the basic flaw in this approach, namely that subjects require a considerable number of trials, usually more than ten, before a discriminator (and non-discriminator) can be identified. Day's discussion about the weakness of this discrimination–preference model is equally clear, and we are in agreement that this is an inappropriate procedure for measuring preference. Because the two tasks are quite separate – one is analytical and the other is attitudinal – it is not realistic to expect the naive consumer to handle both without considerable confusion and most likely a confounding of the preference judgment (remember that odd-sample bias will operate here).

B. The Curse of *N*

One of the features of the sensory acceptance test that is most often cited as a weakness is the relatively small number of consumers (usually fifty to seventy five) compared with the larger numbers used in the marketing research test (usually more than 100 and sometimes as many as 500 or more). This may be considered the curse of *N*; it appears to originate from the mistaken notion that validity is directly associated with the use of large numbers of consumers. Senior management often are more comfortable making business investment decisions when the information is based on large numbers of responses (usually from several regions of a country). There is no question that having the largest number of consumers in a test enhances the likelihood of finding product differences, and of determining which product is preferred. However, there are practical, product and statistical considerations that also must be taken into consideration before one simply increases the number of consumers in a test. Time and cost are practical problems that preclude obtaining responses from every current and potential consumer. This difficulty is overcome, in part, through the application of statistical sampling techniques that permit one to use a subset of the population and this allows one to generalize the results.

Many companies have developed guidelines for consumer testing as a means of standardizing testing protocols and to ensure that management decisions based on results are derived from a common information source. These guidelines were formulated from the aforementioned statistical procedures, taking into account the potential for Type 1 and Type 2 decision errors, the statistical power of the test, and so forth (see Cohen, 1977, for more discussion on this topic). Unfortunately, over time, these guidelines have undergone a metamorphosis and become rules, such that no product decisions are made by management unless a specified number of consumers have evaluated a product (and usually using a specified methodology). While it is not the purpose of this discussion or of this book to review marketing research practices, this particular issue directly impacts the usefulness of the sensory acceptance model and, therefore, warrants some attention.

The first comment to be made is that the sensory acceptance model is intended to screen products, to identify any products that are significantly disliked and any that closely match or exceed a specified target product. This process is completed with selection of a product (or products) that will continue on to larger-scale testing. The sensory acceptance model is not designed to obtain purchase intent information nor can it be used for issues such as segmentation or related demographic tabulations. In effect, results from the sensory acceptance test serve as an early warning system as to a product's acceptance without the embellishments of package, label, pricing, and so forth. In view of the ease with which the test can be fielded and the results obtained, it should be a highly valued resource. Empirically, we observe that results from the sensory acceptance test translate well in the larger-scale marketing research test; it is a good indicator of the future test. It is not a replacement but an effective screening system.

The question of practical versus statistical significance also must be addressed. For example, how much practical importance can be attached to a statistically significant difference of 0.1–0.2 scale units with the nine-point hedonic scale derived from several hundred consumers? It does not take very many responses, especially if there are some extreme scores, to shift a result to significance. Before accepting such a result, it is essential to examine the response patterns in some detail, preferably in the same way that one does with results from other sensory tests (see Chapter 3).

Another concern in all large-scale tests, most often ignored, is product variability. With tests involving large numbers of consumers (e.g. several hundred), there is no question that production variation has a confounding effect on preference judgments. In some situations, this variation can be as great as the differences between test products, leading to the cautionary statement that results from a test with the largest number of consumers is not automatically assumed to be more valid than one involving fewer consumers. Also, it is essential to examine results in detail and not just in the aggregate, as noted previously.

Clearly, then, the idea that the more test participants the better, carries with it risks that are different from those associated with tests involving fewer participants. For sensory evaluation, this issue of risk is less important because the sensory test focuses on product (multiple products preferably), not population projections, and is not used in place of marketing research tests.

C. The Scorecard as a Short Story

Having consumers respond to numerous product questions and complete a long questionnaire including open-ended questions are traditional practices for marketing research tests, and should not be a part of the sensory acceptance test. Multipage scorecards require a considerable amount of time to complete (compared with a single page and four or five questions), and the increase in sensory fatigue and boredom will lead to decreased sensitivity to questions in the latter part of the scorecard. Those scorecards also can reduce the number of products a subject can evaluate in a single session. The typical multipage scorecard includes a series of descriptive questions, preference measures, and a request to state the reasons for the products' preference (or lack thereof).

Asking the naive and inexperienced consumer to respond to specific descriptive attributes is very risky unless there is good reason (data) to believe that the consumer will understand the particular words. As was discussed in Chapter 6, descriptive attributes must be defined and understood, if the responses are to be meaningful. Often, these attributes are included as another check of the product. The problem with use of them by naive consumers occurs when the results are used as the basis for specific product changes. Remember that with a large N it does not take much of a difference in score to be significant! Obviously, the sensory analytical test service will have sufficient data of its own to provide for a more realistic and practical assessment of any proposed product changes.

Limiting the sensory acceptance test to measuring acceptance will reduce the risk for obtaining biased, unreliable, or invalid results. The scorecard must be a "null" instrument, having no influence on the subject's preference behavior. Including diagnostic and attribute questions increases the opportunity for various context effects to develop and subsequently affect the preference response. As reported by Mela (1989), the social psychology literature contains many examples of the influence of the contextual effects of questionnaire design on opinion survey responses. Contrary to that literature and what is known about sensory fatigue and various testing errors, Christensen *et al.* (1988) and Mela (1989) reported only negligible effects on preference scores when attribute questions are included. However, Mela's conclusions were based on twenty-nine subjects who participated in six different test conditions, and the stimuli were experimental samples uniquely different from what can be expected in the marketplace. Christensen's study appears to have not been published.

Perhaps the most inappropriate question for the sensory acceptance test is to ask the subject why a product was liked and/or why it was disliked. As we noted in Chapter 3 (see the discussion under nominal scales), this is not a recommended practice for sensory evaluation. The question will be answered by some and ignored by others, unless prompted by the panel leader. The information is very difficult to interpret, costly to decode, and generally is operator dependent. While it may have some value in the early stages of concept and prototype evaluation, it does not belong in an acceptance test. As Payne (1965) noted many years ago, open-ended questions are not worthwhile sources of information, considering the difficulties entailed in their collection and interpretation. They are not an adequate substitute for in-depth focus groups.

These procedures may have a role in market research, in the study of consumer attitudes, and so forth; however, they are not appropriate in the study of perception and the sensory properties of products.

D. The Many Ways to Ask the Preference Question

The reader will observe that emphasis has been placed on keeping the acceptance scorecard simple; that is, focusing on just the key question,... "all things considered, how well do you like this product?" In the sensory acceptance test, this rather simple task is often subverted by requests to include numerous additional questions focused on measures of liking for various product attributes such as appearance, aroma, flavor, etc. The requester of such information mistakenly assumes that this will identify the precise product characteristic requiring change when the product is less liked versus another. Regrettably, people's behavior does not often work in such a simplistic way, as noted elsewhere in this book. The perceptual process is complex, interactive, and influenced by the context in which it is functioning. As a result, responses to the attributes tend to be highly correlated with the initial response of overall liking. Review of literally hundreds of these tests confirms the minimalist nature of the results and the general lack of usefulness of the information. In fact, if the specific attribute were significantly less liked, this could not result in reformulation efforts as the attribute is generic and not specific. In other words, if a product scored significantly less liked for flavor, is it the quality, the amount, and/or the interaction of the two? A second issue is whether the respondent understands the meaning of the attribute being measured. One can argue that everyone should know what flavor means; however, descriptive analysis subjects spend between 6 and 8 hours learning how to describe perceptions and minimize confusion about the meaning of words, so the potential for confusion is very high for the untrained participant in a preference test. A similar argument can be made if the task is to measure the strength of the characteristic rather than affect. For the sensory acceptance model, measuring liking should be the only task and information about attributes should be obtained from a descriptive analysis test.

In the larger-scale market research test, these same attribute questions are present (along with numerous other questions). Here too, we believe the attribute questions should not be asked for diagnostic purposes; that is, product reformulation, for the very same reasons noted above. In some instances, the attributes are used in a related context of linking response to those obtained from a trained panel. In this instance, their inclusion serves another purpose.

As previously mentioned, asking for judgments (from naive consumers) to questions that have a high potential for misunderstanding is a recipe for trouble, leading to reduced sensitivity and high potential for incorrect interpretation. All too often, it is assumed that consumers come to a test with a thorough knowledge of the products, understanding of the task, and the ability to respond in ways that are expected by the researcher.

E. What Question Do I Ask First?

A frequently asked question is "...Should I ask the liking question first and the attributes second or should I reverse the sequence?" Setting aside the comments about attributes in Section D, the best answer is another question. What is the most important question you want to answer? If preference is the primary reason for the test, then it should be asked first since the responses that follow will be influenced by the initial judgment of liking. This is the halo effect, discussed in the testing errors section of Chapter 4. It is unlikely that a response will show a product liked very much will have one or more attributes that are significantly disliked!

VI. Conclusions

In this chapter, we have described a sensory evaluation model for measuring product acceptance. In the overall scheme, sensory acceptance represents the third and final phase of test resources along with discrimination and descriptive analysis tests. As a resource, it provides continuity between the controlled laboratory environment and the typical product use situation (home, restaurant, and so forth). The types of sensory acceptance tests include the laboratory, central location (a restaurant, at play, etc), and home-use. All of these test types follow accepted sensory evaluation procedures and practices, which include

1. All subjects are qualified based on their attitudes for selected products.
2. Tests generally use fifty or fewer subjects per test, with exceptions to reflect specific demographic requirements.
3. Product preparation, handling, and coding adhere to accepted laboratory practices.
4. Measure acceptance–preference; difference and descriptive measures are not recommended.
5. The sensory acceptance test does not replace large-scale consumer tests.
6. The sensory acceptance test is intended to minimize testing products that do not warrant further consideration.

The sensory acceptance test is a very cost-effective resource that has a major role to play in the development of successful products. Properly used, it will have a significant impact on the growth and long-term development of sensory evaluation.

Special Problems

8

I. Introduction

This chapter explores a number of topics, most of which are concerned with applications of sensory resources once a program is operational. While logic would dictate that these topics should be considered primarily by experienced professionals, our experience at many companies finds just the opposite. Often these topics are presented to the sensory staff when a program is new or the professional is new to the company. The problems are complex, they demand considerably more time and effort than, say, a request to measure the acceptability of two products, and most important, they have more far-reaching implications for a sensory program. They require considerably more planning than is needed to satisfy an individual test request. Examples include establishing instrument–sensory relationships, using sensory resources in the product development process, applications in quality control and quality assurance, procedures for evaluating product stability, for measuring perceived efficacy, providing data in support of advertising claims, and its use in the product optimization process.

As already noted, these are a challenge for a sensory program, not only because of the complexities of the problems and their potential economic implications for a

Sensory Evaluation Practices 3rd Edn
ISBN: 0-12-672690-6

company, but also because they impact professional activities in other parts of that company and usually are enmeshed in company (or individual) politics. Being able to develop information not readily available by other means has significant value (financial and/or otherwise). Whenever a project has such an impact, direct or indirect, the sensory professional must be sensitive to the needs of the management of that project insofar as success or failure are concerned and in what ways might that information have other implications. This sensitivity includes the practical questions of why this particular request, who made the request, the objective(s), and expected project completion dates. Less obvious, but equally important, is the need to establish criteria by which project success and failure are measured, the need to determine how test results will be used, and the need to assess the sensory knowledge of those who will use the results, especially if they might enhance, threaten, or otherwise change their positions about a project's success. This latter issue is critical to the success of any test that is done, but is particularly important in these special interest projects.

The sensory professional also must consider the impact on the sensory program itself. There can be situations in which the sensory program will lose credibility if no attention has been given to the details of a project and especially where there is inadequate documentation leading to a test that does not provide the expected information. In this book, emphasis has been placed on the organization and responsiveness of a sensory program – having available qualified subjects, complete test capabilities (discrimination, descriptive, and affective methods), complete test documentation, and the ability to respond rapidly to requests. The relative ease with which products can be tested may predispose the sensory professional to respond without thorough review of a problem in an attempt to demonstrate responsiveness to requests. As discussed in Chapter 4, detailed and documented knowledge about a project and the test objective(s) are absolutely essential before an appropriate test plan and design can be formulated. In some situations, this knowledge is sufficient to identify potential problems in the proposed project and to consider alternative courses of action. However, this does not prevent sensory professionals from becoming involved in complex problems with political undertones. Some examples of these are comparing results obtained from experts with those obtained from a trained panel, or comparing results from a central location test with those from a home-use test or with those from an employee acceptance test. In the case of experts versus a trained panel, there can be considerable confusion as to the points of difference between the two functions, and some managers might question the need for both, especially if both appear to provide the same information. The sensory professional must address these concerns; however, any response must be taken only after consideration of all the issues. The very first and most important step is to determine why the interest in such comparisons. The answer to that question will usually lead to further discussion including how the information is intended to be used before a decision could be reached as to next steps. Note that up to this point no decision has been reached as to what testing, if any, will be done.

All of this effort is intended to define what sensory does without making any judgment, for example, about what experts are doing. In most instances, experts focus on a company's products, and rarely do the experts evaluate competitive products, whereas a trained panel typically evaluates company and competitive products. In most instances, experts also make quality judgments (directly or indirectly) on a finite scale and the correlations between the two panels' attribute responses will, therefore, not be direct, which will make for a more complex comparison. Each panel provides information with different applications, and any comparison could be counterproductive. Of course, there is no guarantee that these suggestions will be accepted; however, it is clear that sensory professionals must recognize that there is a constant need to educate managers as to what sensory evaluation can and cannot provide and to be able to recognize requests that represent potential problems. Should actual testing be done, the rules by which success is measured must be established. The particular challenge of experts and expert panels will be discussed more extensively later in this chapter.

The ultimate success of a sensory program in ventures such as these will depend on the care with which each problem is studied and the exchange of information that must occur before considering even the most rudimentary of tests. In fact, comparisons such as these should not be necessary if a sensory program had been effective in educating management about its responsibilities. This is especially important because a sensory program's history may be new in your company and there is little positive experience to draw from.

In the following sections, a number of problems and program issues are discussed. They are not presented in order of importance, rather they reflect recent questions presented to the authors. The primary emphasis is to provide a dialog about each problem that may be helpful to the reader who at some time will be confronted with similar situations (if not already experienced some or all of them).

II. Instrument–Sensory Relationships (Not a Romance)

It is of value to develop instruments to minimize reliance on panel tests for routine evaluation of products. By routine evaluation, we refer to repetitive testing that is performed, for example, in a production facility for purposes of assessing raw materials and/or finished products. In addition to reducing dependence on panels, use of instruments, especially those of the imitative type, have provided insight into the sensory processes involved in product evaluation (Noble, 1975; Bartlett *et al.*, 1997; Bleibaum *et al.*, 2002). By imitative we refer to the definition by Noble "in which the property is assessed by a device which imitates the way in which humans perceive the sensory property." We would suggest a more specific definition; by imitative we mean the way in which the property is assessed by a device that correlates with the way in which humans respond to that property. For example, extensive studies on the mechanical properties of food, such as chewing, have led to the development of instruments that more accurately record the various movements of chewing as well as provide a mathematical explanation for these movements. However, their practical application remains to be demonstrated.

The literature provides ample evidence for the high level of interest as well as some insights to the problems of achieving a direct causal relationship between specific chemical and physical measures and product quality (see, e.g. Noble, 1975; Trant *et al.*, 1981), but the evidence to date suggests that either the information is not easily translated into a practical system or the cost is too high. More recently, the development of electronic noses and tongues has renewed interest in this topic (see Bartlett *et al.*, 1997; Bleibaum *et al.*, 2002). There is no question that knowledge of relationships between sensory and physical and chemical measures will have a significant economic impact in addition to improving product quality measurement and the associated improvement in product specifications. The use of an instrument or a system of instruments will be of a decided advantage in a number of situations; for example, in the evaluation of heat in pepper oils and similar difficult or unpleasant tasks, or in situations where a limited number of people are available and frequent and repetitive evaluations cannot be sustained. In practice today, however, it is the exception to find instrument systems functioning as a complete or even partial replacement for panel tests on any wide scale or to find panels being used as a complete replacement for instruments. This should not be interpreted as meaning that instrument–sensory relationships are of academic interest only, or that they are too difficult or impractical to apply within the framework of a manufacturing environment. A more likely explanation may be the lack of understanding about the various measures that are obtained, what is being measured, how it can fit within existing operations, and most important for management, the cost. Of the many types of physical and chemical measures, determining which ones correlate on a causal basis and directly linking these measures to specific product sensory characteristics is an important first step. If the goal is to incorporate the results into an ongoing evaluation of a raw material or as part of a process, then management involvement and commitment become critical.

Another issue that can be a potential problem is the idea that the instrument measure(s) will yield a numerical value that is directly equated with preference. As Noble (1975), Trant *et al.* (1981), and others cautioned, considerable risk is entailed in relating a specific instrument or a specific sensory measure with the hedonic response, that is, the preference for a product. The hedonic response may be expressed as a parabolic function, while the other measures could be linear, curvilinear, or sigmoidal, as depicted in Fig. 8.1. Product preference may be changed as a result of a combination of ingredient, process, and package changes; however, such changes are not likely to be explained by a single physical, chemical, or sensory measure. As additional changes (in a product) are made, the preference for a product may not change yet the analysis indicates a change. This does not mean that physical and chemical measures cannot be related to specific sensory measures or that some combination of physical, chemical, and sensory measures cannot be used to predict product acceptance; it is simply to emphasize that the problem is more complex and considerable risk is entailed in relying on a single measure to serve as a basis for determining that a product will be more or less liked. It also must be kept in mind that there are many other marketing-related factors that also will influence preference and often has a much greater effect than the product itself. All this will be addressed

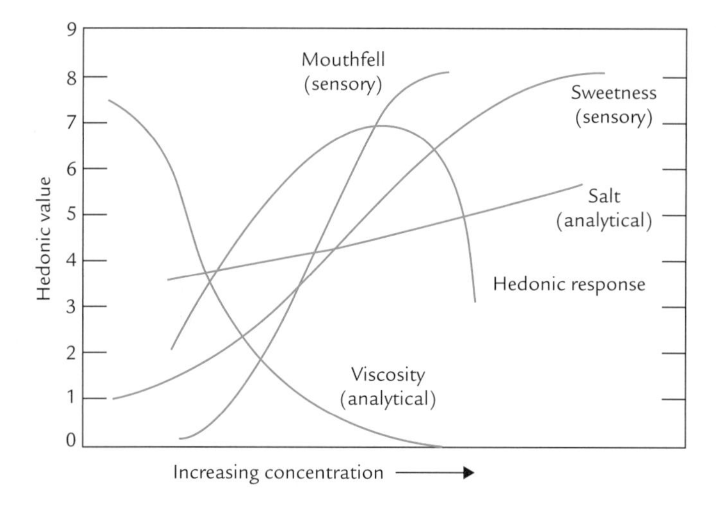

Figure 8.1 Theoretical representation of sensory and analytical measures for a product combined with the hedonic response pattern, which is depicted as an inverted "U."

in more detail in the optimization and product development sections (Sections VII and VIII) of this chapter.

For purposes of this discussion, we return to the issue of identifying the relationships among selected physical and chemical and sensory measures. At the outset, it should be clear that such relationships exist, that they are most often multivariate in nature and will be of great economic value when used, whether it is for product development purposes or for monitoring a specification. In the past two decades and after several hundred projects, we have always identified reasonably robust relationships among the various measures; that is, R^2 values greater than 0.80. At the outset of any such research, it is necessary to establish the specific objective(s) as to which instrument or instruments will be replaced (sensory or physical/chemical) and, especially, how the information will be used. For example, if the intent is to develop an instrument in place of a sensory test as a basis for raw material purchasing, then the approach will be different than using the information in a quality control process. Raw material sampling will likely be done less frequently than in-process or finished product sampling, so the type and frequency of testing would be different. Before any actual data are obtained, attention must be given to the test plan and to select the appropriate products and methods. This planning takes into account the sensitivity of the various instruments, and any other relevant background information. For example, a costly and time consuming physical or chemical measure would not be very practical, and such information should be taken into account in the planning process. Other issues that warrant attention are the criteria by which a product (raw material or finished product) is rejected, if that is a possible outcome of the test, availability of other resources in support of the test, the decision criteria, and the responsibilities for those decisions. Awareness of this information will be important in minimizing conflict about acceptable product or whatever other criteria are used and the consequences. Other information, such as estimated frequency of testing and magnitude of expected differences (derived from preliminary tests), is used to determine the scope of the effort, which in turn enables management to estimate the cost effectiveness of the entire program.

If these relationships are not yet established to everyone's satisfaction, then an investment in research will be necessary. As emphasized earlier in this discussion, sensory measures are usually multidimensional while the physical and chemical measures are typically unidimensional. A particular physical measure will be represented perceptually by several sensory characteristics; so it should not be surprising that several physical and chemical measures may be required to establish a potential causal relationship. For simple systems, it may be easier to demonstrate a univariate relationship between instrument and sensory measures (i.e. the physical element and the sensory element are more alike), but as the stimulus system becomes more complex this relationship may not hold. For example, changing the concentration of sucrose in water may be readily perceived as a change in the strength of sweetness and the relationship with a particular measure such as viscosity of the solution could be quite high; for example, greater than 0.75, this relationship would be deceptive, if the appearance or some other product characteristics also changed.

Once the decision is made to explore these relationships, it is necessary to identify the products and the methods. The sensory measure is easiest to identify – use descriptive analysis as the core of the sensory information. The physical and chemical measures are more difficult; however, we have found it best to start with current analytical methods now being used; there may be few or there may be many. We have encountered situations in which fewer than ten are used but in most companies the number of physical and chemical tests can number in the fifties, and in some instances we have dealt with several hundred measures. In as much as there is no *a priori* knowledge as to which measures are relevant, it is better to err on the side of more than too few! In fact, one side benefit of such an approach is the ability to identify methods that are providing the same kinds of information but are obtained by methods that are more or less costly. There is no question that some redundancy is not undesirable as a kind of insurance should a particular method become inoperable; however, it would be useful to know where there are cost-saving opportunities.

For products, an array of at least fifteen or more would be required, if the information is to have any relevance. Analyses of these types, involving multiple regression/correlation, require a sufficient array of product differences to yield meaningful relationships. Therefore, the products selected should represent a typical array of differences expected in this category without regard for whether the products will be well liked. In effect, it may be necessary to formulate products to stretch some of the variables; otherwise, the results could yield relatively small differences making the correlations even more tenuous. Once data are obtained, each type is subjected to typical univariate analyses to be sure that the results "make sense" based on what is known about the products. This is then followed by data reduction procedures such as principle components analysis and factor analysis to identify any underlying relationships among the measures and at the same time identify the redundancies. In most instances, we expect a reduction of about 80% from variables to factors. As shown in Table 8.1, the Factor Analysis (accomplished with a varimax rotation)

Table 8.1 The factor analysis output for the combined sensory, physical, and chemical data

	Factor 1	Factor 2	Factor 3	Factor 4	Factor 5	Factor 6	Factor 7	
Bitter Fl	0.95							
Astringent Aft	0.94							
Bitter Aft	0.94							
Overall Aft	0.93							
Astringency	0.92							
Hot Fl	0.89							
Hot Aft	0.87							
Overall Fl	0.85							
Specific gravity	0.77							
Apparent extract (AE)	0.77							
Apparent attention (AA)	−0.74							
Fruity Fl	−0.71							
Original extract (OE)	0.70							
Fructose	0.53							
Phenyl alanine		0.96						
Isoleucine		0.96						
Leucine		0.95						
Total amino acid		0.94						
Glysine		0.92						
Chloride		0.88						
Phosphate		0.80						
Glucose		0.78						
pH		0.75						
Total polyphenol	0.57	0.66						
Overall Ar		0.64	0.58					
Total organic acid		0.61				0.57		
iso-Amyl acetate			0.84					
Fruity Ar	−0.52		0.65					
Sour Ar		0.60	0.65					
Sweet Ar			0.63					
Sweet Aft				0.93				
Sweet Fl				0.88				
Fruity Aft	−0.56			0.69				
Clarity Ap					−0.84			
Color Ap	0.55				0.73			
Color	0.57				0.72			
Sour Fl						0.82		
Sour Aft						0.80		
SO_4							0.93	
Percent Variance Explained	32.20	24.92	8.73	8.48	7.34	6.94	4.28	Total 92.89

output from a combined physical, chemical, and sensory data file yielded a 92.89% resolution; that is, the percentage accounting for the differences that were measured were explained by seven factors (twenty sensory measures and nineteen physical and chemical measures of fourteen products). The individual analyses (FA) yielded 83.9 and 87.27%, respectively, each of which was interesting; however, the combined analysis provided a focus to possible connections between the different measures and those for which no connection was identified by examining the output shown. This kind of information can be mapped and examined for clues as to the relationships depicted. As shown in Fig. 8.2, the map is particularly useful when reviewed with the analytical chemist whose knowledge of the product's chemistry can explain some of the relationships. The next step would involve selecting a sensory measure such as sour flavor and identify the combination of physical and chemical measures that predict the obtained values. The result, shown in Table 8.2, identifies the combination of measures that best explains sour flavor. This process can be repeated with other measures of specific interest. Based on this information, one could focus various analyses on those measures that are most important relative to the production process and/or consumer behavior. In later sections of this chapter, we discuss use of these methods for related applications, identifying those attributes that influence consumer purchase behavior, the relationship between the important sensory measures and imagery, etc. Use of multivariate analyses is being used much more frequently with the speed and power of the PC; but with any of these tools, the opportunity for misuse is equally high (and much more common based on a quick perusal of today's literature). However, they are not an end in themselves, but rather a means for depicting relationships not readily observed through conventional analyses. All too often, the display of information is presented as the end instead of the beginning.

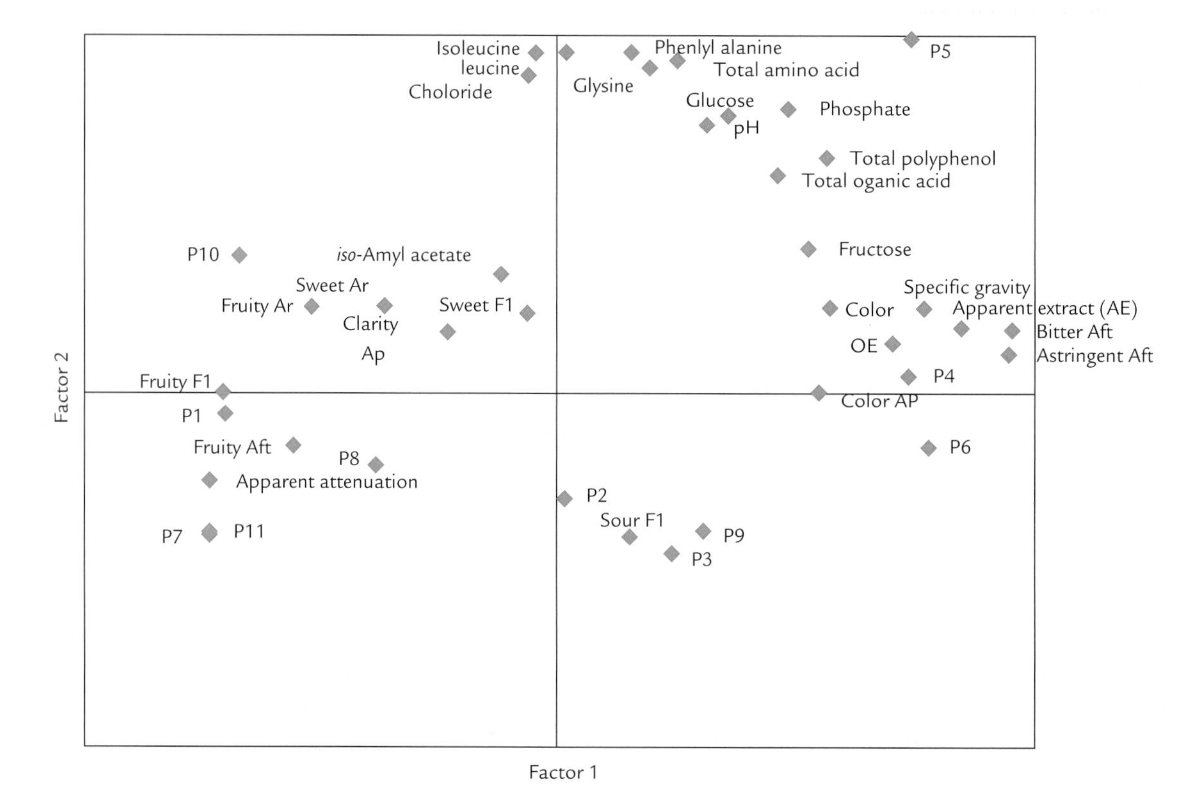

Figure 8.2 A map of the first two factors depicting the sensory and physical and chemical measures. In this map, the two factors account for 57.12% of the differences measured. See text for additional explanation.

Table 8.2 The regression analysis output identifying the physical and chemical variables that best predict the sensory sour flavor (See text for more explanation)

Model	*B*	Beta	Zero-order	Partial	% Contribution
Chloride	−0.050	−0.844	−0.438	−0.769	37
Total organic acid	0.014	0.877	0.248	0.743	36
Apparent attenuation	0.163	0.489	0.114	0.577	28
Constant	10.932				
R	0.80				
R square	0.64				
Adjusted *R* square	0.57				
Std. error of the estimate	1.65				

There is no question that meaningful instrument–sensory relationships can be identified, and should be. Both physical/chemical and sensory capabilities are sophisticated and readily available. Unfortunately, few companies have taken advantage of this potential information source. These also have considerable financial benefits as well. These programs usually originate within research and development, and often do not leave there. They should find a receptive home in many sections of a company, especially in those business units where availability of subjects and time are limited, such as quality control. Of course, the success of these programs is highly dependent on the individuals involved, the thoroughness with which the system has been studied, and there is a management commitment to the program.

III. Experts and Expert Panels

As noted at the outset of this chapter, there are numerous opportunities for a sensory program to contribute to the success of a company. There also are challenges, real and imagined, such as those presented by the comparison of sensory test results with those obtained from an expert or an expert panel. It is useful at this time to briefly describe what we mean when we state "the expert." These are individuals in a company that are known by reputation to possess detailed technical knowledge including its "taste" (used here in the broadest sense) about their companies' products. In food companies, these might be individuals who have "tasted" products daily for many years thus developing a keen sense of what a product from their company should taste like before it goes to the market. In the distilled spirits business, they may be referred to as "the nose," or some such designation; in the wine industry, it is the winemakers, in the brewing industry, the brewmasters. Their abilities were and still are highly regarded as is their impact on various technical matters (and not surprising, they are compensated accordingly). Over the years, these individuals develop specialized knowledge about their company's products that served as a primary basis for specific recommendations, for example, to purchase new ingredients, to assess the impact of new technology on finished product quality, and the marketability of a particular product (an area of some dispute!). For the most part, these individuals were successful, and although they may not have consciously recognized their actions as the forerunner of sensory evaluation, their activities constituted one of the earliest organized efforts in product evaluation. The designation of expert was acquired through practice on a regular basis, working with an acknowledged expert who was usually older and more experienced. This practice (i.e. apprenticeship) was and in most instances continues to be done on an *ad hoc* basis, that is, through participation in the evaluation process with the awareness that their judgments will not necessarily be included in any decision until such time as determined by the acknowledged expert. Furthermore, the only records of their training will be the scores assigned to products or some similar type of information.

As a result, the training varied from one individual to another, and the criteria by which an individual was certified also could change. The difficulty with this qualifying process was and still is the lack of a formal description of the qualifying criteria, that is, the scores expected for specific products, the numbers of tests and basis for qualifying or for continuing to train, and so forth. Despite these shortcomings, this system continues to be used in many companies; however, the primary roles of the expert or apprentice is most likely associated with assessments of product quality and secondarily, for the initial stages of product creation. In effect, their impact has been lessened and more directed toward specific problems.

From a sensory evaluation perspective, it can be concluded that experts functioned primarily in making judgments about product quality. Their judgments reflected not only what they perceived, but also whether the quality was within certain limits and, therefore, will be accepted by the consumer. This process is based on a mental standard, which is another weakness of the system. In spite of these deficiencies, the use of experts and expert panels continues and, therefore, the potential for comparison with sensory evaluation is very high. At the outset, sensory professionals must delineate their programs' functions – the formal procedure for screening and qualifying subjects, the analytical nature of the tests, the comparisons with competitive products, and the uses for the results. Sensory panels provide measures of the strengths of product characteristics or differences between products but do not directly assess product quality (this latter topic will be discussed in this chapter under Quality Control). Efforts to compare the two should be aggressively discouraged; such attempts rarely if ever contribute anything except an erosion of the credibility of the sensory program.

Unfortunately, situations can occur in which the comparison is inevitable, and careful planning is warranted. The request to compare the two (often stated as using both tests to increase the product information base) arises because past sensory results suggest product changes were necessary and the technical group, for whatever reasons, does not accept or believe the recommendation. Initial actions often include challenging how the results were obtained, whether the subjects were appropriate, etc. When these actions fail, the next course of action is to bring the expert or expert panel into the "picture." Once the actual decision is made, the sensory professional needs to vigorously engage the requestors in extensive dialog to delineate and document the objective, who will be tested, what products will be evaluated, and the actual evaluation protocol. Since both panels evaluate products from different perspectives, the results are not likely to be the same, and agreement must be reached as to how the information will be interpreted and applied. In most instances, the comparisons involve some type of descriptive analysis. Experts typically work from a list of terms that have been developed over many years, in association with their respective technical peers in research and product quality control. Most of these terms are technical in origin and represent existing knowledge about the chemistry, ingredients, and formulation of the particular product. In some instances, the terminology will include language obtained from an industry-wide effort.

The descriptive panel, as described in Chapter 6, uses a language that is non-technical, consumer based. We have observed situations where an expert panel focuses most of its attention on certain modalities (e.g. aroma, and scant attention to mouthfeel and/or aftertaste), with a result that appears to be quite different from that obtained from a sensory panel. Obviously, efforts to directly compare the terminologies will present its own set of challenges. In some of our unpublished research we have had the opportunity to compare results from expert, consumer, and especially, expert versus QDA panels. That research provided some very useful findings, which are discussed below.

Consumers, experts, and a QDA panel evaluated sensory attributes for an array of eighteen beverages, all except three were commercially available at the time of the test. As a result, there was a wide range of product differences, a not unexpected finding. While the primary objective was not comparing the two "panels," the database and technical interests necessitated such a comparison, using some typical multivariate analyses. Separate principle components analysis (PCA) of products across attributes demonstrated that the underlying grouping of the products and the attributes were different for the two panels. Experts organized products into two groupings, one defined by their company's products and the other by competitor products (products were not identified for the subjects). The underlying structure looked to be based on their perception of quality, or alternatively, recognition of their own products. The descriptive panel results provided more than two product groupings, which were defined by style (or flavor strength), independent of manufacturer. Product groupings for the descriptive panel were consistent with the consumer preference patterns.

It is not surprising that the results were different for the panels, especially because most expert panels (e.g. coffee, beer, wine) are used for quality control purposes, and as a result, they have limited exposure to competitive products. Frequency and type of exposure to specific products will influence the way subjects perceive products, which will also influence their evaluations.

In addition to using the aforementioned data reduction techniques, regression equations were developed using results from the expert and descriptive panels, and results from the physical and chemical analyses. We concluded that (1) multivariate analytical models predicted sensory attributes substantially better than did univariate models, (2) different models were required for the different panels, and (3) the model for the expert panel contained more variables than did the model for the descriptive panel.

These results (and others obtained in similar tests) demonstrated that the same descriptor had different meaning to the different types of panels, even when the descriptor was for a basic taste such as sour or bitter. The different meanings appear to be based on different underlying constructs (or different physical components represented by the analytical measures in the prediction equations). For many of the attributes, the underlying perceptual structure for the experts was more complex than for the non-experts, a not surprising conclusion. After all, the expert spends considerable time each day evaluating their company's products with knowledge as to the ingredients, the process, and what the product should "taste" like. Expert evaluations are accomplished from a different context than that used by the descriptive subject. The latter have no technical knowledge about the ingredients or the process, and their evaluations are based on the context of the array of products, not what a particular product is expected to taste like.

IV. Perceived Efficacy and Advertising Claims

In recent years, increased attention has been given to measuring perceived efficacy and to develop evidence in support of claims of product benefits or superiority as part of some advertising campaign. By perceived efficacy we refer to those product characteristics that provide a benefit that will be stated and/or advertised in some manner. Examples would be a hair product containing a specific chemical, or mixture of chemicals that cures dandruff, a lotion that minimizes skin dryness, and foods and beverages that promote a desired health condition based on specific nutrients. Products that are subject to defined health and safety regulations must, of course, satisfy specific regulatory requirements, such as clinical evidence substantiating the biological effectiveness of the product.

Perceived efficacy, on the other hand, addresses the issue from a behavioral viewpoint; that is, the product should be *perceived* by the consumer as providing a particular benefit. Advertising a shampoo that cleans and leaves hair with a soft feel requires evidence that such benefits are perceived by consumers (regardless of what those words mean to those consumer). A product can have both types of efficacy; however, the presence of one does not guarantee the other. Perceived efficacy does not provide one with a basis for a biological claim; however, the reverse situation would be more likely to occur. For example, developing a lotion that is effective in preventing dry skin (as demonstrated by clinical evidence) would have a greater likelihood for market success if the user also perceived it as effective in keeping their skin moist and not dry or some similar benefit. Ideally, the product's sensory characteristics are consistent with the consumer's expectations for that product. Failure to appreciate these differences in efficacy has had far-reaching and primarily negative business consequences (e.g. needless reformulation or delayed introductions). For these reasons, measurement of product efficacy is a complex issue requiring the incorporation of behavioral measures in a biological study. In some instances the two elements will be studied separately.

Measuring biological efficacy is accomplished by means of relevant physical, chemical, and biological analyses under well-defined conditions, etc. While target consumers are the subjects in the clinical trial, their reactions to the products are usually measured by specialists. The specialists are medical and health-related people including physicians, nurse-practitioners, biochemists, and technical personnel who may also provide judgments of product effectiveness. Perceived efficacy, however, is strictly a consumer's perception and this aspect may or may not be a part of a clinical trial. It is important to separate these measures to minimize any potential bias that could arise. Knowledge of the contribution of each type of efficacy to a product's success should provide a more precise focus for advertising, and should aid in developing an optimal marketing strategy that emphasizes those product characteristics most readily perceived as beneficial by the consumer.

Using sensory procedures in a clinical trial is appropriate in those situations where the respondents' perceptions of product effectiveness will be a part of the product claim. Sensory also can contribute in those clinical situations in which no claim is planned, but judgments of product effectiveness are made by the experimenter and/or the subject, in addition to the usual biological measures. The perceptions of the experimenters (or others) can provide further insight to how a particular product is perceived to be working. In this situation, the need is for the sensory professional to incorporate measurement systems that are unambiguous and easy to use, for example, a nine-point category scale of strength (see Chapter 3 for more discussion on scaling). In many situations, scales are used that may not be familiar to the sensory professional or are adaptations from more familiar scales. For example, it is very common to find three- or five-point scales being used with quality word anchors. Experimenters are often unaware of the insensitivity of these scales, in part because it is not their discipline, and in part because they are following what was done in the past and assumed that that it is "standard." As discussed in detail in Chapter 3, three- and five-point scales are not as sensitive and are not recommended. Contributions from a sensory professional will be useful provided clinicians are aware of contemporary measurement techniques and the benefits from incorporating sensory tasks into the clinical trial.

Incorporating sensory information into a clinical trial requires a thorough knowledge of the product and the details of the trial itself. For example, what product biological benefits are being measured, when and how will the product be used, at what stage (or stages) in the trial will it be possible to obtain sensory measures from the participants, etc. The issue of how efficacy will be measured is especially critical because it will be the driving force, the major influence on the test design and that will impact the specific sensory questions asked of the respondents. Knowing what kinds of benefits and potential claims (the hypothesis) will be made before testing is started has important consequences for the sensory planning.

Planning also includes the specific sensory measures that will be obtained, the ultimate use of products, frequency of usage, and frequency of response; that is, initial and subsequent responses or only a response at the conclusion. These issues are most likely to arise in the evaluation of products such as furniture polish, room air fresheners, and skin lotions. The design must anticipate the impact of product usage over time, the extent that response changes based on initial reaction compared with changes attributable to the way the product is used or the amount of the product used. For most of these tests, the problem takes on an added dimension; that is, the product is applied to a substrate (furniture, skin, or hair), and the response is from the individual who has applied the product. It is possible to have others provide judgments about the products; however, this information would be analyzed separately. Evaluating the effectiveness of a cleaner for no-wax floors might require several different types of no-wax floors as substrates, and the respondents would evaluate all of the floors. Alternatively, each person might evaluate only his or her own floor. The specific protocol will depend on the claim that has been proposed. It is very important that whatever claim or claims are anticipated, they must be known before one can prepare a test plan.

In addition to the issue of who will provide the judgments, it is necessary to consider the nature of the response, that is, the quality or aspect to be measured. This decision also will be influenced by the claim; for example, if shine superiority is the objective, then the dimension "shine" would be measured. However, the reader is reminded that the particular dimension must be defined, or the respondent may use different criteria to assess the dimension such as "shine." As discussed in Chapter 6 on descriptive analysis, considerable risk is entailed in using terms that are not defined especially for the untrained respondent.

Frequency, amount, and location of product application (and evaluation) must also be specified and should be based on prior test results. Each test must begin with an initial evaluation. That is especially important, even for products such as biological preparations that require repeated usage for effectiveness. Obviously, a product that is not well liked or that is considered of marginal effectiveness on initial exposure is not likely to become more likeable with time. Failure to obtain the initial response could lead to a misinterpretation of results; for example, the product could be assumed to be ineffective, when the problem might be attributable to the odor, the color, or some other related property.

Frequency of response should depend on frequency of application and the time estimated for optimal effectiveness to be realized. For personal care products, the frequency must be specified in advance and controlled to the extent that misuse is minimized. That is, one respondent may use the product five times, and another respondent, three times. Missing or unequal numbers of respondents are not a problem if respondents come to a test location; however, this may not be possible depending on the product and the specific claim being tested. The fact that the product is used in a non-controlled environment or that the product is applied to different surfaces does not mean that the senses function differently or that traditional measurement techniques are not applicable. These design parameters are built into a test so that their effects can be partitioned from product effects. For most of these tests, the designs are multiple factor and require use of multivariate analysis of variance model such as treatment $\times$ subject and split plot, as discussed in Chapter 4.

When food and beverage companies want to make a claim and advertise it, whether for challenging a competitor or making a claim of parity (as good as), a different set of procedures and practices are superimposed on the typical sensory and/or consumer test.

Depending on the type of claim that will be made, all aspects of the test can be expected to be scrutinized by the legal department of the company making the claim and competitors affected by the claim, by networks that will air those claims, and perhaps even consumers influenced by the claim (Zelek, 1990). Like the clinical trial, the manufacturer will have large sums of money and perhaps even their credibility at risk; therefore, advertising research involves a high degree of exposure. Careful planning and attention to detail can minimize risk. It is reasonably easy to obtain data that will be useful and defensible without appearing too self-serving, provided proven sensory practices are followed and there are clear directions of the claim or claims that are being considered. In recent years, this topic has been given more attention and discussion (see Davenport, 1994; Edlestein, 1994; Passman, 1994; Read, 1994; Smithies, 1994, ASTM, 1998; for more on the topic).

Planning a test in support of a specific product claim requires ingenuity and creativity in addition to knowledge about sensory testing. First, it is necessary to determine whether the claim will imply a comparison (either to current product or to a competitor), whether it will directly challenge a competitor, or it will simply be a parity claim (i.e. as good as). Second, it is necessary to know whether the claim will be advertised locally, nationally, to the trade, etc. This information along with the specific statements are used to determine which product(s) will be tested, what type of sensory information will be obtained (e.g. attribute, preference), who will be tested, etc. If the claim is about a sensory attribute for a single product (i.e. not comparative), a trained descriptive panel could be sufficient or one could use a consumer "agree/disagree" Likert scale. We have successfully used QDA data where the sensory attribute(s) are defined, and used consumers where more conceptual types of attributes (e.g. natural flavor) are in the claim. In the latter case, consumers may be asked whether they "agree" or "disagree" with a statement (e.g. "the product has a natural flavor").

When there is reason to believe that a comparative or challenge claim is possible, consumer testing is necessary. For national taste test claims (claims shown on the networks, broadcast, etc.), the situation is complex and much has been written and discussed as noted above. For example, the National Advertising Division of the Better Business Bureau (NAD) has developed guidelines for testing with consumers (Smithies, 1994). For a national claim, it is recommended that a minimum of 500 consumers from the four geographic regions of the country be tested. However, this is only a guideline and one might test more or less depending on the circumstances of the specific claim, the type of product, and the population tested. A second important element is the question of who will be tested, all consumers, customers of the products, the persons who shop, etc. Passman (1994) cited some examples where the consumers were not sufficiently representative enough, thus negating the basis for a claim. This latter issue is particularly important and more discussion about this can be found in the aforementioned references.

Once a decision is reached that a claim is warranted (and this usually is based on some prior technical knowledge, for example), a preliminary plan should be prepared that includes the potential claim statement or statements, who should be recruited, where and how the products will be obtained, what kind of a test is proposed, and the specific questions that will be asked. This information is discussed with the company's legal department before any additional effort is put to the plan. Once there is agreement that a claim has merit a detailed test plan can be prepared. There is one note of caution regarding any plans; documentation should be kept to a minimum. For most all claims, advertisers and the networks will expect to review all the documents to satisfy themselves that the specific claim is justified. Test details should be complete and easy to read, with all parameters defined. If the claim is challenged by competition, they too will have access to all the same information, notes, etc. The competition can refer their concerns to the NAD and this will likely result in a long and costly process, with depositions, etc. In some situations the challenge ends in court; however, every effort is made to adjudicate the dispute via a hearing that both parties agree to. Given this background, the sensory professional should make every effort to design a study that is as simple as is possible and focuses solely on substantiating the claim and nothing more. The more questions asked, the greater the likelihood that one or all of them will yield results that are inconsistent with the core question and selective reporting is never acceptable.

Product source, like consumer source, also has its own set of challenges. All products in a test must be representative in terms of source and age with no last minute alterations. Not too long ago company A believed (technical information) its vanilla flavored frozen dessert was preferred to competitor B and decided that a national claim was justified. A few weeks prior to fielding, the competitor's vanilla flavor source was changed (thought to be based on availability). A decision was made to proceed on the mistaken assumption that the original flavor would be used once the supply returned to the original source and the results would still be applicable. Unfortunately, this did not occur. In another situation, one product is obtained from retail while the other from a warehouse, which also will negate results. All too often, a well-planned test is undermined because of a failure to check the smallest detail. Once a claim is challenged, numerous people will examine every aspect of the test looking for weaknesses, no matter how minor, that will preclude the information from ever being used.

The reader is reminded that each claim or potential claim has its own set of requirements beyond those noted here. There is no recipe for success when it comes to claims substantiation, each test is unique; however, the NAD guidelines provide a useful perspective on the current situation. Perhaps the most useful part of the guidelines is access to various case studies that enable one to read about the failures and what not to do! The reader should also note that this section does not provide recommended scorecards, scales, or methods. This is intentional. As already stated, each potential product advantage/claim has its own set of challenges. The specific claim has a major impact on what kind of test plan is most relevant, what specific question will be asked, and who will provide the responses. The sensory professional can provide the relevant test plan input, recommend the most appropriate design and insure that the fielding is done consistent with good sensory practices.

Advertising a product benefit and/or an advantage presents many unique elements that are not typical for sensory evaluation or market research. However, as noted by Passman (1994), the "survey *must* be more science and less an art." This represents an opportunity for the sensory staff to provide the science and demonstrate its value to an organization.

V. Stability Testing

In recent years, determining product stability and estimating shelf life have become increasingly more important, especially for foods, beverages, and other biologically active products. This heightened interest can be attributed to the increased use of product dating, that is, the assigning of an expiration date for product sale or use by the consumer. For products not requiring an expiration date, estimating shelf life may be driven by competitive and business issues. In either situation, there are compelling reasons for knowing what product changes occur over time and their impact in the marketplace. For the dated product (sell by, use by, etc.), there is the cost of its retrieval from the marketplace and the attitude of consumers toward a product (avoidance) that is close to or at the end of its shelf life. For a non-dated product, there can be shifts in consumer purchasing habits or a competitive advertising campaign that makes consumers more aware of sensory differences or a product is out of fashion. Quite apart from these issues, technological developments (processing and ingredients) and new packaging materials also can have an effect on product stability. The financial consequences of a business decision based in part on an inappropriate shelf life can be significant and, therefore, estimating shelf life becomes very important.

Companies have always measured product stability and generally were aware of shelf life; however, competition, technology, new packaging materials, and the placement of a product date on the package has placed an entirely new perspective on the problem. The outward manifestation of these developments has been a substantial increase in stability testing but not always with an appreciation for the complexities of the problem in terms of test design and analysis, methodology, the relationship between product change and product acceptance in the marketplace, and the economic impact of increasing decreasing shelf life. As a result, sensory resources often are overwhelmed with requests for stability and a test frequency that has no bearing on expected shelf life. A simple example of this situation is the request for products to be tested monthly for 18 months when fewer than half that number of tests would have been appropriate and no significant changes are expected for at least the first 8 to 9 months. Most sensory programs will be easily overwhelmed with nothing more than six or seven of these requests. Obviously, a process has to be developed that balances the frequency with which products are tested versus the availability of resources, but without sacrificing needed information. Test frequency will be covered in greater detail later in this discussion.

At this point, it is useful to consider some basic issues of stability testing as a means for determining a product's shelf life:

1. Over time, all products undergo change and this change is usually a deleterious one; chemical and biological changes are initiated leading eventually to either product safety concerns or product sensory concerns. Our focus is sensory.
2. Measuring stability does not, by itself, establish a product's shelf life, consumption date, or some similar designation.
3. Test planning must take into account that products will change as the testing proceeds, necessitating reliance on specific kinds of test designs (split plot, etc.).

4. Because testing is usually done over time, control product tested at the start cannot be placed in suspended animation and available for all subsequent tests, and therefore no stability test will have the perfect (unchanged) control.
5. Stability testing should be initiated only after criteria have been specified for starting and ending a test.
6. There must be sufficient product from a single lot to complete the entire study.
7. The product lot used in the sensory tests should be the same as that used for chemical and physical analyses.
8. Product sourcing must be specified and representative.

When a request for shelf life determination is submitted, it is important for sensory staff to meet with the requester and discuss all the details about the project. For example, is the request based on technology, new packaging material, competition, etc. Also, what is the current shelf life and what stability information is already available? If the product is currently being reformulated, this too should be known. Establishing stability when the formulation work is still in progress can be a waste of resources unless an objective is to identify which formulation best meets a desired degree of stability. Another issue is the basis on which a test is initiated after the initial test. Should product be assigned a specified acceptance value and if product is perceived as different should the test be stopped and new control obtained? A similar issue is raised with regard to elimination of a product/variable during a test; for example, a product that scored significantly lower on an acceptance scale on two consecutive tests would be eliminated.

Besides these criteria, other important considerations include the frequency with which products are removed from storage, the kinds of tests that are most likely to measure expected changes, and the products themselves. Typically, a technologist will request frequent testing, possibly at monthly intervals (e.g. monthly for 18 months) throughout the anticipated life of the product, and with weekly withdrawals if accelerated storage is included. On the other hand, sensory evaluation prefers to minimize the number of withdrawals, to minimize the demands on testing resources (facilities, staff, and subjects). Ideally, one should be establishing baseline information at zero time and at one or possibly two additional times, and should cluster the remaining tests around the anticipated end of shelf life. It is not realistic to precisely state the number of withdrawals because it is entirely dependent on the nature of the product and background information about it, the stability of the ingredients, and the overall project objective. Some products are not released from storage until a specific time period has elapsed; this time lapse may be necessary for the ingredients to blend, to satisfy a regulation, and so forth. So, the zero time for a product may not be the date of manufacture. Therefore, it is important that this circumstance be considered (and documented) when preparing the test design and the planned withdrawal/test dates. Frequent testing places an undue demand on sensory resources; however, it may have a potential value by identifying changes early in the life of the product. Alternatively, if the product does not reach the retail level until 1 month after production and 95% of product is purchased and consumed within 6 months, then testing frequency would focus on initial, 1 month, and a cluster of tests just before, at, and after the 6-month period. Testing at 2, 3, and 4 months would not accomplish very much relative to the sensory investment. One can easily see the testing challenge for a product with a 12-month or longer expected stability/shelf life. The converse of this situation is the refrigerated product whose shelf life is counted in days. The challenge for sensory is devising a protocol in which typical testing is modified to provide the information without sacrificing its quality. For the refrigerated product, the test will likely be limited to a single day and/or a specified time period within that day. Designing the appropriate test is possible when all the information is available.

Three additional points of discussion are the availability of sufficient product for all proposed tests, product source, and the selection of the control or reference product. Amounts of product can be determined only after shelf life, frequency of withdrawal, and types of tests (number of subjects per test, etc.) are estimated. It is especially important to have these amounts specified as soon as possible so that the responsible individual can determine if enough product is available. All too often, an insufficient amount of the product is set aside before the test is planned, leaving the project staff with limited options. A related issue is to be sure that the amounts needed are in the typical retail-sized units, not one large container. The latter will not be representative product. When insufficient product is available, some compromise will be necessary. The one most frequently selected option is to reduce the sensory database, usually by decreasing the number of responses per test, using less satisfactory test methods, providing less product per serving, or to have fewer withdrawals. While a certain amount of flexibility can be incorporated in most test plans, these compromises are not equivalent. For example, changing test methods would be a poor compromise. Reducing the number of judgments or number of subjects risks not achieving expected significant differences, while a reduction in serving portion might be a better option. To minimize this particular problem, the experienced sensory professional will develop guidelines for stability testing that will include recommended amounts of product needed for specific tests and amounts needed for a typical stability test. This may not solve the problem of the forgetful technologist, but it will minimize the frequency of occurrence.

Product source also is very important because it is the basis for all decisions regarding stability. Any test plan must always include the question "how representative is this production lot." If the lot is atypical, then there is a high degree of risk that the shelf life could be under- or over-estimated. If product is available from several manufacturing plants, a business decision must be made as to which plant or plants are to be included in the test. If products from more than one plant are being considered for the test, then the analyses will be confronted with an additional degree of complexity. While it is possible to design a test that incorporates products from different plants (considered in Chapter 4 under split-plot designs and reconsidered in this discussion), there are other considerations. For example, the number of subject evaluations will double and there will be concern as to whether the results from the plants will be compared with each other.

Another issue is the inclusion and identification of a reference (or control) in the test. For example, for foods and beverages, the practice has been to place the control in a reduced temperature (chilled or frozen) environment and assume that the product either has not changed or has not changed to the same extent as the test variables. However, all products do change regardless of storage conditions, and, therefore, it is quite unrealistic to treat the product as static. In addition, to identify the product as the control or reference will change subject response behavior (the context in which the judgment is made), a topic discussed later in this section. This presents the sensory professional with design and test protocol issues. The control is changing but not at the same rate as the other products in the test. Perhaps the simplest and recommended solution to this problem is to exclude any reference product held under conditions that are not related to the problem; for example, a product held at −20°F in an atmosphere of nitrogen. If a product is normally held at ambient conditions, then the experimental conditions would most likely encompass the norm but certainly would not include a condition as extreme as −20°F in an atmosphere of nitrogen. Without the "reference," the problem of measuring product change is addressed through appropriate scales of measurement and the use of the analysis of variance and split-plot designs, rather than attempting to have subjects score the products relative to that reference (e.g. measuring degree of difference). In spite of these concerns, designated references continued to be used along with a degree-of-difference methodology, and we offer some comments about them here.

Two popular approaches for constructing a difference-from-reference scale are: (1) to represent the reference as being at the center for each attribute, and (2) represent the reference as having a different scale value for each attribute. In both conditions, the subject examines the reference (but does not evaluate it), and then scores a test product by indicating its direction and distance from the reference.

The procedure has a number of inherent problems. Frequently, a separate reference is included with each test product, thereby doubling the number of products for subjects to examine. Also, the experimenter is assuming that the reference is invariant between experiments, subjects, and products; yet, experimenters and subjects frequently report that references vary. Finally, specifying that a reference is at the scale center for each attribute is not credible with testers who perceive the reference to be different. When the perceived attribute intensity for a reference is either high or low, displaying it at the center of the scale will compress one end of the scale while expanding the other. Compression and expansion occur whenever the reference is displayed at one location, and perceived to belong elsewhere. Adjusting judgments to compensate for the discrepancy between where the reference is depicted and where it is actually perceived defeats the primary purpose for specifying reference location. In the process, subject sensitivity is compromised as they adjust their responses to reflect their changing perceptions.

Difference-from-reference methods are popular with proponents of absolute scoring and invariant subjects and products (e.g. concept of "the" gold standard). There appears to be a belief, albeit mistaken, that a method such as difference-from-reference would be more sensitive than monadic scoring; however, this has not been demonstrated for reasons already noted. It will be more useful, reliable, and valid to evaluate the reference as another coded sample along with the test products and statistically analyze for differences. The measurement concept described in Chapters 3 and 6 for descriptive analysis is applicable.

Once product and test design requirements have been satisfied, it is necessary to select methodology. No single test method will be entirely satisfactory. Discrimination would determine whether products are perceived as different, but all products could be not different but disliked. Descriptive analysis would identify product differences but not whether the products are liked. Affective testing would provide measures of liking but not the basis for the liking.

Including all three categories of methods at each withdrawal could place a strong demand on sensory test resources, so some type of compromise would seem reasonable. A recommended test approach would be to obtain descriptive analysis and acceptance measures for each product at the start of a test (zero time). This procedure would be repeated at the estimated 50, 80 or 90, 100, and 110% of current or estimated shelf life. If, however, the acceptance measures at 80% were not significantly different from the previous withdrawal, the descriptive analysis might not be done. This would be a sensory decision. As a minimum, there would be results from four of the withdrawals in which all products (still in the test) were tested with both methods.

This approach requires more decision-making responsibility by the sensory staff, but it is a realistic approach with regard to the testing program. Unnecessary tests are eliminated and the test capability has more flexibility, which is especially important. For example, if a product at the 50% (of estimated shelf life) test shows more change than expected, a decision could be made to move the next test to 60 or 70% of shelf life to determine if the rate of change is accelerating.

An alternative plan makes use of all three types of sensory test methods. Initially (time zero), descriptive and acceptance information is obtained for all products. At the first withdrawal, there is a discrimination test of the control versus the stored products. The discrimination test is recommended only if no statistically significant differences were found at the initial evaluation. If discrimination results showed no significant differences, no further testing need be done at this time. If differences are obtained, an acceptance test of the control and different products would be appropriate to determine whether there has been a decrease in acceptability. If there was a significant difference in acceptance, the study may be terminated. The decision as to terminating the study would be based on the magnitude of the decrease in acceptance and any other available information; for example, chemical analyses indicated significant changes had occurred. If there were no significant differences, the study would continue. At this time, a descriptive test to identify the perceived differences between the control and experimental products is optional. If the products represent an established brand and if a substantial data file exists, then the descriptive test at this first withdrawal might not be worthwhile.

This procedure would be used for the remaining withdrawals, but with some modifications. If on two successive withdrawals there were no significant differences between the control and test samples, acceptance and/or descriptive tests would be implemented on the next withdrawal. This minimizes the risk associated with a control that is changing at a rate similar to that of the test products.

If significant differences were obtained from the acceptance test at the start of the project, then the test should be stopped and a new sample obtained. Similarly, if product differences are obtained from the descriptive test, a decision to proceed or to begin over (obtain a new sample) must be made depending on whether or not the differences occurred within an expected range for the product studied. Criteria for determining whether differences are "expected" or "reasonable" may be established according to the principles described in the section (Section VII, this chapter) on Quality Control. Obviously, this is an important issue; that is, the criteria by which products are considered to be within specification. The issue of re-starting the test should be communicated in advance of testing with key project staff. Failure to plan for this situation will seriously undermine the value of the program and of this particular approach to stability testing.

Finally, the criteria for project termination should require that the difference or lowered acceptance be demonstrated on two consecutive withdrawals, as a verification of the product change. While there can be great interest in completing a test, in some instances the products have changed so much as to be disliked extremely and/or subjects refusing to continue the test.

A number of test designs and analyses have been described in the literature (Gacula, 1975; Gacula and Kubala, 1975; Lawless and Heymann, 1999). In most instances, these designs, and particularly those described by Gacula, emphasize a statistical approach with only limited consideration of the sensory input. For example, the same subjects are not likely to be available for every test, and, therefore, subjects are a source of variability within each test and from one test to another. While the analysis of each test within a withdrawal is quite straightforward, the analysis across time is more complicated. The product also has undergone change and is another source of variability within and across test variables. The most useful design is the split-plot analysis (general linear hypothesis), which was described in Chapter 4. In the preparation of any design, the variables need to be specified in detail. For example, if there are three packaging materials, three storage conditions (temperature and humidity), then there will be a nine-product matrix, including the control conditions. From a single production lot, sufficient amounts will be allocated for the nine-product matrix and the actual test is initiated. The reader will find it helpful to review that section of Chapter 4 when planning a stability test.

There are some aspects of stability testing not already discussed that warrant comment. For example, it has been suggested that the control product after the initial test be a sample from current production on that day when products are removed form storage and tested. This approach is suggested to address the issue of the control product changing over time (regardless of how stored). It is stated/argued that since the product is typical of production and, therefore, representative, it should be a reasonable alternative control sample. However, it would be a weak choice since it will be a source of variability not part of the original sample lot. This could exaggerate product differences and lead to false conclusions about differences (Type 1 error). An equally challenging problem is the actual choice of the "control" from production; that is, who chooses it, what criteria are used, and so forth. This should not be an issue; the control should be treated as a variable in the test not as some specially designated sample that serves to confuse subjects, leading to increased variability and decreased sensitivity.

In some instances, stability testing is planned around products of different ages obtained form the marketplace. This procedure obviates the need for testing over time, all products available at the same time. This approach will establish the condition of products in the marketplace; however, it cannot substitute for a purposefully designed stability test. Products will be from different production lots, different distribution systems, etc. If it is intended to function as the basis for designing an appropriate stability test, then it has a value. Often such a test serves to highlight the extent of differences that exist among products in the marketplace, a topic discussed in the section on Quality Control in this chapter.

Once a stability test is completed and the results analyzed, the information becomes part of the shelf-life determination. As mentioned previously, a product's shelf life is based on several criteria including safety, sensory, consumer attitudes and perceptions, and business inputs. If a product meets all safety, sensory, and consumer preference requirements, then it becomes a business issue as to what sell-by or consume-by date will be printed on the label. For example, consumers may "believe" that a particular product is fresh and have a high purchase intent as long as the sell-by date is 3 months or less. If the actual stability results indicate that a 6-month shelf life is feasible, it would not necessarily translate to changing from 3- to 6-months as consumers might not believe it and that could negatively impact purchase intent. Similarly, the packaging material may afford a much greater degree of stability than is required, representing a potential cost savings.

All too often, decisions are made regarding stability testing without an appreciation for the potential benefits from a planned approach. Historically, decisions about product shelf life were based primarily on packaging materials and safety (and the latter is certainly paramount); however, much more can be gained from measuring stability with a design approach, taking into account ingredients, technology, packaging materials, and various consumer and sensory measures. This approach will more than recover the investment made to organize and field it.

VI. Product Development

Product development is an important function in every company. By product development we refer to such activities as the formulation of a new product (new to that company or entirely new in that market), reformulation of an existing product, use of new technology, a new ingredient or some other activity that directly impacts a product to a degree that it can be promoted to the consumer (or target market) as new or some similar designation. Interest in new products is always very high because of its contributions to profits, the opportunity to achieve growth in the marketplace, as well as the halo effects associated with the brand achieving success in the marketplace impacting other products associated with that brand. Despite this high level of interest and investment, much of it is never fully recovered because of the high failure rate, and this situation has not changed very much in the past decade (Friedman, 1990; Gorman, 1990; Fuller, 1994). As a result, an enormous amount of attention has been given to correcting this situation. It has attracted all sorts of attention in the form of people with ideas, training programs, books, symposia, etc. See Aaker (1996) for a purely marketing focus; Baker *et al.* (1988), Fuller (1994) and Graf and Saguy (1991) provide a more technical product orientation, and Lyon *et al.* (1992) offer a practical primer on using sensory testing in product development. See also the two-part article by Manoski and Gantwerker (2002) and a related article by Silver (2003) for some practical observations regarding the challenges of product development and some insights about product success and failure. Publications such as Food Product Design, Prepared Foods and New Products Magazine devote a significant portion of every issue to this topic. In the case of the latter, its focus is exclusively new products, acknowledging its importance to the growth of the food and other consumer products industries. Annual conferences focus on the topic, bringing together individuals that are suppliers of services, as well as those who describe their successes, and as noted above, giving rise to an entire industry of information sources about consumers and their needs. New methods and techniques are described, such as use of ethnographics, that are intended to directly or indirectly enhance the rate of success by getting closer to the consumer to identify unmet needs, product opportunities unique to a brand, etc. Companies also have made significant investments in personnel by hiring chefs as a means of exploiting their creative efforts. Whether these investments will improve the rate of success remains to be seen. It also is not clear that existing methods are inappropriate, only that what is new receives more interest and attention, the implication being that since it is new it must be better. While it is not the intent to provide an exhaustive review and analysis for success or the lack thereof, it is useful to comment about some of these practices as they impact the role that sensory evaluation plays in the product development process.

It should be clear, at the outset, that sensory evaluation has a very important role in product development, beginning with involvement in the early planning stages and progressing to the more typical role of evaluating products during the formulation–reformulation stages and into full-scale production. Involvement during planning is essential to identify the resources required, including a description of the target consumer, and to estimate appropriate timing for implementation of steps such as initial product evaluation, expected dates of test markets, and so forth. Although a product development project may represent a line extension or a modification of existing technology and no problems are anticipated, it is nevertheless important that sensory professionals are aware of the project plan and the proposed timetables for the key decisions. Often, an existing database for the particular product category can be accessed and be of value to technology, before any actual work is initiated. For example, a proposed line extension might include formulations previously tested, and the data (from these earlier tests) could provide an additional perspective to this planned change.

Ideas for new products are derived from a variety of sources, including employees, letters from consumers, market intelligence, new technologies, as well as from more formal approaches, many of which are described in the literature (see Prince, 1970; Meyer 1984; Bone, 1987; Fuller, 1994; Henry and Walker, 1994; Aaker, 1995; Engel *et al.*, 1995). These ideas are then evaluated, usually through use of the focus group technique; however, the focus group itself may also be used for generating new product ideas. Information about a particular concept is obtained from selected consumers, usually in groups of about ten to twelve. In some situations, the discussions are done in a one-on-one basis. The choice of technique depends on the status of the project, the nature of the topic being discussed, etc. The group sessions have the advantage that they are associated with the interactions among attendees that are not possible in the one-on-one environment. In the group environment, a professional moderator is responsible for managing the process, starting from a general introduction and then directing the participants' conversation to a particular topic, eventually to discuss the specific idea, type of product, or specific features that might be incorporated into a product. Sessions last about 1–2 hours; the information is recorded and/or video taped, and a detailed report is prepared. This information is carefully reviewed to identify positive and negative attributes and is used as an aid to better characterize the particular concept. This procedure may be repeated with other groups within the same market region and in other regions, depending on the outcome of the initial focus groups and on various market and business considerations. It is also reasonable to expect that information developed from initial groups will be used with subsequent groups. This serves as a kind of cross-validation of the information developed.

The focus group technique is extremely popular with marketing and market research professionals and in recent years, it also has become popular in the technical community. While the technique is primarily qualitative, it is popular because it is a relatively easy window into the minds of consumers who are representative of the intended customer. Focus groups are easy to organize and are relatively low cost. As a result they are often used in extreme; that is, a particular project could initiate ten or more on a single topic and would cost about the same as a product test involving 150–200 consumers. In addition, the sessions are recorded and in today's electronic environment, they are transmitted to other locations worldwide. Individual experimenters can participate regardless of their location. Developments in use of focus groups can be found in various marketing research publications (see, e.g. Quirk's Marketing Research Review, **16**(11), 2002) as well as Fern (1982), Fuller (1994), and Goldman and McDonald (1987).

In recent years, techniques such as ethnographics have been added to the qualitative tools available to the creative process, to identify product gaps/opportunities, etc. The technique allows a trained researcher to "move in with a family" and/or allow cameras into a home to fully capture how a family functions and specifically, when, where and how it uses a specific product. The process is especially attractive, in part, because it fulfills the marketing team's desires to get close to the consumer. With in-home cameras, one can directly observe the consumer (the entire family) use/prepare and consume a particular product. Not surprisingly, the process has achieved some successes but with any qualitative tool, it is subject to different interpretation based on the choice of experimenter or observer. Most practitioners acknowledge that interpretation is critical, but equally critical is the need for independent validation. Taken together with traditional focus groups and other qualitative techniques, the process of developing and refining ideas into product concepts are essential first steps. Alternatively there are those who develop a product, do no formal qualitative research and are successful, proving that proceeding "by the book" does not guarantee success. However, following the aforementioned procedures should, at the least, identify those ideas and/or concepts that are not well received sufficiently early in the process to minimize the expense of moving ahead with a concept that will not be successful.

Quantification of information obtained from focus groups should be encouraged. We have converted information from the focus group into a series of close-ended questions that are scored by a larger group of consumers. This procedure provides an independent assessment of the qualitative information.

A different perspective is achieved when a food company employs a chef to create products that reflect that individual's creative efforts. Historically companies employed technical groups (the D of R&D) to create new products. With re-structuring and mergers, much of the development effort was outsourced. Today, companies have changed, enhancing the development effort with chefs. However, the basic challenges remain, to wit, satisfying consumer expectations with positive sensory experiences. It remains to be seen whether the use of alternative approaches to product development, such as the chef as technology's creative arm, will be sustained. After all, the successful product must provide a positive sensory experience that is consistent with expectations and associations engendered first by seeing and/or smelling the product. This experience is confirmed (or not) by taste, mouthfeel, and aftertaste. The "tasting" experience reinforces the sensory and imagery expectation created by the product's visual and olfactory characteristics.

At this stage of a project, various types of research are initiated to assess concept/product feasibility. This research, which is sometimes collectively referred to as front-end research, should provide five types of information: a concept that scores well with target consumers, a measure of concept viability (validation), a list of consumer-defined attributes (most likely benefits and uses), target population demographics, and identification of an initial control or competitive product. While some of this information is qualitative, especially the consumer-defined attributes, it is very important for sensory project staff to be aware of the information or at least to know who to contact for the information. Knowledge as to what type of consumer should participate, and what products should be included also need to be defined as they will have a major impact on results. In those instances where the target consumer is not the actual target; that is, that consumer rejects the concept and/or the product, serves as an alert as to subsequent testing with that population of consumers. What is important here is to emphasize communications among all parties, especially in the early qualitative stages.

The focus group, as already noted, is an essential tool for the product development process; however, it can be overused and/or the results can be subject to misinterpretation. This happens most often when an inexperienced (or experienced but biased) individual is observing the group and assigning too much importance to some of the comments from one (or two) participants. Unfortunately, this selective listening, a trait common to individuals who hear only what they want to hear rather than the entire discussion, can have disastrous consequences for a project. Development efforts can move in the wrong direction, etc. Some individuals will field ten or more groups and collate the information but present it as quantitative without ever establishing that it is reproducible. While it is not a sensory responsibility to question this approach, it is important for the sensory professional to be aware of information sources and be able to place them within the context of the project. In most instances, however, once agreement is reached concerning concept viability, formulation efforts are initiated and sensory evaluation should have a more active role in developing quantitative information.

As we observed in an earlier publication (Sidel *et al.*, 1975),

> *The objectives of marketing and sensory testing during product development are to determine the relationship between a product concept, a control product (when available), and the experimental product for the purpose of aiding product development efforts to converge on these points.*

This is the desired goal; however, there are many pitfalls in this process and the most logical of plans frequently is changed for reasons that can be wise, and sometimes not so wise. Sensory evaluation must provide needed services, maintaining an independent but cooperative position as concepts appear to change, priorities and timetables shift, and key personnel are transferred.

As soon as is practical, testing should be initiated to establish a sensory database for the product or product category. If control product is available (identified from the concept and focus groups), then the question of what to test is relatively easy – control product and other similar products. In developing an initial database, some care must be exercised in product selection, especially with regard to formulations that may not yet be ready for evaluation. This testing may be intended to further refine the consumer language, or to understand the ways in which the products differ, and/or to provide a more precise sensory description of the concept. As noted elsewhere, product source is very important and should be documented, including preparation location and date. This information becomes increasingly more important when the concept and/or the target population shifts, about which we will have more to say.

From a strategic point of view, the most useful sensory methodology will be descriptive analysis (e.g. QDA) for several reasons. First, it provides a quantitative map of the products, delineating all the characteristics and their differences. Second, the method enables one to test multiple products, and third enables one to compare results from one test to another. As many as twenty or more products can be evaluated and the evaluations can be done in a laboratory environment or in typical use situations. Mention was made previously about product selection, and in particular selecting formulations that may not be ready for testing. Once a concept has been described, formulation efforts should result in a large number of prototypes. Some of these prototypes may be very different from others, reflecting different interpretations of the concept (or of the target product) or the creative efforts of technologists in association with chefs. One of the challenges that the sensory staff face at this stage is the difficulty of convincing developers to prepare sufficient numbers of products for evaluation without regard for whether the products are considered "acceptable." There is a reluctance of developers to provide more than two or three samples for testing. This often derives from a mistaken belief that the test results might be used to judge progress, or a desire to by-pass any sensory analysis and go directly to an acceptance test (thus saving time and money). In almost every instance this results in failure and time is lost. The value of the information obtained from a multiproduct test is far greater than a test of two or three products. Multiproduct tests have the potential for developing causal relationships that have even greater value by identifying those formulation changes that impact attributes in negative ways (e.g. increasing the strength of characteristics such as artificial, mealiness, etc. that are known to reduce preferences) or are not perceived as significantly changing the strength of specific product characteristics. This latter situation is particularly important as technologists and chefs may assume, usually incorrectly, that any formulation change (ingredient type and/or amount) should result in a one-to-one perceived change. Without empirical evidence derived from a design study such assumptions are only that.

The sensory professional must make a concerted effort to reassure the development specialist of the usefulness of having a range of products and not be overly concerned about whether they are good, bad, or indifferent. At the same time, the sensory professional may find it necessary to modify test plans to incorporate a more diverse array of products than originally intended. As discussed in Chapter 4 on errors in testing, inclusion of one or two products that are very different from others will very likely cause contrast and convergence effects. Inclusion of such products may be necessary and this would require a change in the test design; for example, blocking the serving order such that these products would be served last. In effect, the sensory professional must be flexible in terms of adapting a methodology when presented with atypical products. The decision as to which products will be included in a test should be based on bench screening and extensive discussion with the project specialists and any other project team members willing to participate. It is wrong to test only those products that represent best effort. Unfortunately, this latter practice makes it very difficult, if not impossible, to understand the effects of ingredient and process variables, and particularly those variables that affect desired attributes in a negative way. What should be kept in mind is the need to include a sufficient number of products to yield an array of differences (and similarities) that will be helpful in subsequent formulation and processing efforts. In addition, the project staff should be reminded that results of these initial tests are a part of the database and not intended as the basis for changing the concept or assessing progress of development efforts. Too often, decisions are reached about the progress of development based on tests designed primarily for other purposes (the database), and in this particular instance, such decisions could have significant consequences for the project staff. Some individuals may decide that product development emphasis should be changed or will recommend termination of the project. Once a few tests have been completed, there will be sufficient information to allow for an assessment of progress relative to the program objectives.

A brief comment is warranted about the problem of the changing product concept. Product concepts change for any number of reasons. For example, new market information may reveal that the original concept was not sufficiently well defined, additional testing with consumers may dictate a change in positioning, or competition may have changed their product. Technology may change or a realignment of marketing personnel and of responsibility may cause changes in project direction. These changes are often made with no change in budget or timetable and that clearly impacts a variety of activities, including planned sensory tests. This is an opportunity for sensory, given the responsiveness that is possible; for example, to field a series of descriptive tests in 1 or 2 weeks or small-scale acceptance tests in 1 or 2 days. The existing product sensory information will be especially helpful in this situation. If the product range (in the initial tests) is sufficiently broad, then many concept changes probably will continue to fall within the product category. However, not all changes can be anticipated and sensory evaluation cannot test all product possibilities. The product development process is never completely predictable, and sensory evaluation should accept this lack of predictability as an aspect of the work, especially during the initial planning and work stages.

Up to this point, some of the more obvious actions taken during the early stages of a new product venture have been emphasized. As these activities are formalized, the program should develop into a more orderly process. As shown in Table 8.3, events in the development process have a logical sequence (assuming there are no unanticipated diversions). However, the development process is neither logical nor is it orderly, and the ability to respond quickly, to take a flexible approach, will enhance the sensory group's credibility with product managers and management, in general. For purposes of this discussion, we have focused on three functions, market research, product development, and sensory testing. However, it is likely that product development will involve the efforts of many other groups, for example, purchasing, advertising, production, and quality control, but that their involvement will not always be continuous. The sequence of events, as presented in Table 8.3, is based on the assumption that there is an identified control product representing the concept. Two other scenarios are possible, if no control product is available or if the concept is so novel as to have no direct counterpart in the marketplace. The effect of these scenarios on the development sequence will be considered later in this discussion.

The first three steps in Table 8.3 may be considered as the source for the initial database; extensive communication about a concept will be required and bench screening of various prototypes before and possibly after sensory testing will be necessary. Once the concept has been refined (steps 4a, b), it is likely that the development staff will have refined their skills and will have several prototypes available for comparison with the control product (step 5). The most promising products are screened using the discrimination model (step 6a) or using descriptive analysis, if the differences are obvious. The descriptive model is probably most useful at this stage because an operational panel will be able to evaluate six to eight products and results available within 3 days. If the discrimination model is used, then any of the prototypes that match the control will be verified using another batch of product (step 6b). Obviously, confidence will be increased if developers can formulate the product a second time that is perceived as not different from the control.

This leads to the next step, controlled or preliminary affective testing (step 6c), which could involve an employee panel and/or selected consumers brought to a central

Table 8.3 A list of the sequence of events in the product development process when control product is available[a]

1. Market research	a. Identify product category
	b. Develop and test concept
	c. Identify control product
2. Product development	Formulate prototypes based on 1a, b, c
3. Sensory evaluation	
Descriptive analysis	Develop data base with control, competitive and prototype (or protocept) products
4. Market research	a. Refine concept with focus groups
	b. Develop market and use strategy
5. Product development	Formulate protocytes based on 3 to match control
6. Sensory evaluation	
Discrimination	a. Determine which prototypes match the control product
	b. For product that matches, verify with additional formulation
Affective	c. Test developed and control products in laboratory and at central location sites
	d. Test developed and control products in home use
Descriptive analysis	e. Define current developed product and other formulation for use in manufacturing and quality control specifications, and identify any sensory properties responsible for unsatisfactory acceptance ratings
7. Product development	a. Shift from pilot plant to test production
	b. Initiate cost reduction
8. Sensory evaluation	
Discrimination	a. Evaluate production product and impact of cost reduction
Descriptive analysis	b. Evaluate any products that fail discrimination test
9. Market research	a. Large-scale consumer tests in selected markets
	b. Evaluate advertising, package, and pricing
10. Product development	Initiate line extensions
11. Sensory evaluation	
Descriptive analysis	a. Evaluate line extensions
	b. Evaluate competitive products
Affective	c. Test line extensions and competitive products

[a] This table was developed from a previously reported article by Sidel *et al.* (1975).

location. The primary goal for this activity is to establish a baseline for product acceptance without benefit of any imagery. If the prototype product meets acceptance expectations, then home-use testing may be initiated (step 6d). By "meets acceptance expectations," we mean that the product achieves a selected liking-preference score (as a minimum) considered as necessary before the product will be considered for greater investment, a larger scale test or some other type of qualifying challenge. One of the responsibilities of sensory is to determine in advance of these tests if minimum scores are considered necessary, or if some other criteria will be used by management to assess a product's potential. Once results from the home-use test are confirmed, sensory must evaluate the product in a descriptive test (step 6e) to quantify the product profile. This information should be used by quality control and manufacturing, but it may also be used by others as product development efforts change, etc.

Assuming the product passes all requirements, the project moves to step 7, and the development effort switches from reliance on pilot plant samples to use of regular production facilities. At this stage purchasing, production and marketing will focus on ingredient cost and availability, estimated production volume, etc. It is at this stage that ingredient changes are likely to occur, leading to reformulation and retesting. Once again the discrimination model is most appropriate (step 8a); however, inherent variability in raw materials may necessitate going directly to descriptive analysis.

At this stage, the program will receive considerably more attention from management. There is an even greater financial commitment to provide product for large scale marketing research tests, for production to determine the ease with which the product can be manufactured, packaging issues (type and label contents), distribution, advertising, etc. All of this comes with an increased cost and risk. If sensory data are used in support of label or other advertising claims, then a thorough and detailed review of these data is necessary. It is also possible that the competition may introduce products, may change their advertising, or may undertake some similar action designed to offset the uniqueness of the new product. This competitive action may force a reassessment of the product and additional formulation work may be initiated. Descriptive analysis (e.g. QDA) would be appropriate for these products.

The results from these descriptive tests will be very important if project management is concerned about the competition and is contemplating reformulation. It is relatively easy to chase competition and to lose sight of the original goal. The descriptive analysis results serve as a reminder and a focal point for any formulation work. However, this reminder will be disregarded unless the sensory professional makes the effort to communicate the information in a way that is easily understood. At the conclusion of step 9, the project enters a new stage and may be transferred to specialists that move projects into full-scale production. For sensory evaluation, most of the work will have been completed and pertinent information communicated to legal, quality control, and product management.

Typically, project staff attention now shifts to the formulation of line extensions (steps 10 and 11). Here, too, the database (descriptive analysis and acceptance) serves as a frame of reference in the screening of submissions before more extensive testing is initiated. Sensory and development specialists will be coordinating their work and functioning at optimal efficiency. It is possible that some (or all) of the line extensions will bypass many of the aforementioned testing steps; a strong correlation between internal and external results serves as the basis for reducing the total number of required tests, especially some of the larger scale consumer tests. Once the product and line extensions have been introduced and are in full production, sensory evaluation should summarize all test results in a single document. Documentation is important in that it serves as a record of the range of products and product variables that were evaluated and the relation of the results to other tests (home-use, central location, and test market) and provides other pertinent information.

As noted previously, there can be other scenarios; no control product matches the concept sufficiently well enough to represent a basis for proceeding, or no formulation matches the concept well enough. In the former situation, where no control product matches the concept, the initial steps are identical with those in the first example – developing a database, refining the concept, and product formulation (steps 1–4).

In some instances, the concept can be stated in several ways and one can measure which formulation best matches which concept. With the control expected to be similar but not identical with the concept, formulation work and bench screening may actually be more difficult. For example, it may be difficult to determine how similar the products should be to the concept (we will have more to say about this in Section VIII, on optimization), and which variables should be emphasized.

It should be obvious that this scenario and the subsequent scenario are the most challenging from the development and sensory testing perspectives. The products to be included in the initial tests are not so easily delineated. If the products are not expected to match the concept, the discrimination model is inappropriate at this stage of the project (step 6a).

Acceptance testing (step 6c) will be helpful and will provide direction to the formulation efforts (especially when combined with the QDA data) and an estimate of the degree of liking for the products. The latter condition is important since the product will not match the concept. If none of the products score well in the test, for example, achieving a 7.0 ($\pm$1.0) on the nine-point hedonic scale, then some additional descriptive analysis may be necessary.

In some instances, one can have subjects develop their own ideal product using their existing descriptive scorecard. Subjects score the characteristics based on their "ideal" product. The resulting data may help identify those experimental products closest to the "ideal" and this could aid the developers in focusing their work. However, some additional comments are appropriate here. We observe that a subject's "ideal" often represents a target to aim for but subjects do not "expect" or believe it can be reached. In addition, asking subjects for their ideal as a direct question does not necessarily mean that it also is important (enough so as to have a direct effect on preference behavior). The discussion on optimization (Section VIII of this chapter) provides a description of an alternative and potentially more successful approach to identify what is necessary for a product to be ideal.

If results of the acceptance test (step 6c) meet the score specification, then the sequence of events should follow those described previously, with the descriptive data from step 6e used as the new target. Steps 7 through 11 will follow in sequence, much as occurred when control product was available from the start of the cycle.

When a product counterpart to a concept is not available in the marketplace, then it will be necessary for a protocept to be developed. A protocept is a product that represents the concept prepared with ingredients that would be available in a kitchen (if it were a food), using best ingredients. This should be prepared by a chef familiar with the project and able to provide options for further consideration. This protocept would not likely be manufactured; however, its role is very important in representing the characteristics of the concept. The protocept would be tested by market research to ensure that this best possible example of the concept is viable and it is as well liked as the concept. If it is not, then it will be necessary to repeat the process; however, preparing alternatives, increases the likelihood that a successful match will be identified within a single test versus a series of tests that are time consuming and expensive. Only if the protocept is viable should product development proceed to formulate various prototypes (step 2) and sensory evaluation proceed (step 3). It will probably be necessary to include the protocept in the descriptive analysis, to provide for a record of this type of ideal product. Protocepts that are formulated "by hand" can be difficult to duplicate, and small differences should not be cause for major concern. The descriptive data provide a basis for assessing the impact of these differences.

Continued refinement of the concept takes place (step 4) at the same time that product development proceeds with formulation of prototypes (step 5). For sensory evaluation, as before, the descriptive methodology is the most useful technique (steps 3 and 6e). As the project proceeds, some problems can occur, primarily those associated with the protocept. If it is used for too long, the subjects may consider it a control product and diverting them from their primary goal. Since it could never be matched, a substantial amount of time and effort could be wasted on this quest. Once again, descriptive analysis will help to identify the prototype that most closely resembles the protocept, which then can be eliminated. The prototype will be evaluated in a series of affective tests (steps 6c and d). If a favorable response pattern is demonstrated, the project proceeds through the remaining steps (7–11) in much the same manner as the previous scenarios.

Throughout this development process, sensory and market research must maintain a dialog, comparing test results, being very sure about the source of the products (protocept, prototype, production) relative to the results, and deciding how to best use available resources. Additional acceptance testing probably will be required to ensure that the product (in several versions) continues to meet the acceptability requirements. It also is possible that some modifications will be made to the concept to accommodate control product.

Finally, some comments are warranted about some newer developments such as optimization techniques and their usefulness in product development. These techniques have many benefits and can, in fact, enable a project team to reduce the development process time and provide a direct link between product, attitude, and imagery. It provides a technical basis for formulating a product to a specified target of consumers, but in the process it provides an extensive database about product formulations, what sensory characteristics are most important, etc. Because of the multivariate nature of the testing, the program requires more planning time; however, the actual testing is more efficient.

In the beginning of this discussion about product development, mention was made of the need for information about key decision points to be communicated amongst a team. Topics such as the criteria by which progress is judged, how, for example, sensory information is communicated, the extent of involvement of all team members in all meetings, etc. all need to be discussed and agreed to at the start. The importance of establishing a project team with direct communication links is especially important in any product development effort. All too often, such access to information is restricted unnecessarily and this leads to problems after tests are finished and reported. Projects become misdirected and failure risk is much higher than anticipated. In many projects, the role that sensory plays is not as prominent as it should be primarily because of a lack of understanding of sensory's contribution.

This brief discussion about sensory's role in product development has focused on principles and practices, in the broadest sense, recognizing that the process of developing a product is difficult, very costly, and quite unpredictable. It is difficult because business plans and strategies will change, and sensory resources must be capable of responding rapidly to these changes. Of course, having a product database will enhance sensory's ability to be responsive and to receive recognition as a contributor to the product development process. While much has been written about the product development process and much more will continue to be written, it remains to be seen how effective sensory can be in this process. Clearly, it will depend on the skill of the individual sensory professional and having the resources available when needed. Examining all of the information written about product development, it is clear that the role sensory has is never a prominent one, which could explain the poor success rate for new products.

VII. Quality Control

Quality is the basis on which most companies manufacture and promote their products. Substantial investments are made in advertising to promote product quality to the consumer. Companies also have made investments in equipment and staff to address quality from the raw materials through to retail. It is interesting to note that this investment in quality remains a challenge, as noted by Daniels (personal communication, 2000), as many as 25% of products in retail exceed company specifications, excluding physical damage. In effect, there is considerable variation among products available to the consumer at retail. The importance of this variation, as measured by preferences and purchase intent differences, remains to be demonstrated. Nonetheless, the fact that such variation can be identified raises questions about the impact of any investment in quality processes and how much variation can occur before it is noticed by the consumer. In recent years, the quality issue has been somewhat overwhelmed by food safety and food security issues, nonetheless, it remains a critical element in consumer purchase behavior and is an integral part of most all imagery conveyed to the consumer.

The word quality is used in so many different ways that it is often difficult to understand what is meant by the word, especially when used by those in R&D versus marketing or production (see Stone *et al.*, 1991). All companies maintain a quality control (QC) resource at production facilities, with support from their R&D operations. Considerable literature on quality, its definition, and how to maintain it also is available; however, only limited information has been available specifically on sensory evaluation and its role in quality control. Several publications on quality control for the food industry provide a synopsis of applications for sensory evaluation (Gridgeman, 1984; Lyon *et al.*, 1992; Hubbard, 1996). However, no attempt is made to directly address the more basic issues of what is sensory quality, how it is determined and how sensory resources are incorporated into the product quality decision-making process. Nonetheless, these references are useful and especially the former, which is part of a three-volume set on quality control. Of necessity, this discussion focuses on a specific approach to the use of sensory resources that the authors have found to be particularly helpful. It is more global, reflecting a market focus, taking into account the business implications of quality and the establishment of product quality standards. Of particular note is the explanation provided by Hawthorn (in Herschdoerfer, 1984):

> *The aim of quality control is to achieve as consistent a standard of quality in the product being produced as is compatible with the market for which the product is designed, and the price at which it will sell.*

In a symposium on "Sensory Quality in Foods and Beverages" (Sidel *et al.*, 1983), we noted that the word "quality" had different meanings and had evolved from an expert dictated concept to a more production oriented system, and gradually becoming a more consumer-influenced concept. A discussion on this issue can be found in Stone *et al.* (1991). Traditionally, "quality" implied "degree of excellence" (see, e.g. Kramer and Twigg, 1970; Wolfe, 1979; Sidel *et al.*, 1983). Used in this way, the term implied a universal, objective, absolute, and context-free criteria for establishing and judging the quality of a product. Examples of quality standards are represented by such procedures as the oil quality scale, butter and ice cream scorecards, government standards for meat, and so forth. Alternatively, consumer acceptance (and purchase behavior), which is a driving force in the marketplace, implies none of these standards. It is segmented, subjective, variable, and context dependent. The notion that an expert's opinion of what constitutes an excellent or high-quality product will invariably reflect consumer acceptance should no longer be an issue. Sufficient documentation to the contrary is directly available (McBride and Hall, 1979) or can be easily deduced by reading articles about product quality (Smith *et al.*, 1983; Stone *et al.*, 1991).

To date, most QC sensory programs have not been as successful as anticipated. This lack of success can be attributed to any number of reasons; however, it is clear that it is not related to sensory's ability to provide resources or to measure differences among an array of products from the same or different plants. Rather it appears to be much more related to organizational issues, reluctance to move away from reliance on experts and/or existing practices, and inadequate consideration given to how sensory information will be integrated with other product quality measures. Considering the amount of attention given to product quality in the technical and trade press, it is an opportunity that should not be ignored.

We believe that a successful integration of sensory resources with existing quality control activities begins first with an agreement as to what is sensory quality, and second, there is management, production, and quality control support for integration of sensory quality measures into the quality monitoring function. There is no question that sensory can provide data on raw materials and product variation within and across shifts, and provide this in a timely and actionable manner; however, the more basic issues are whether the information is relevant, that it is understood and that it will be used as a part of the quality monitoring function. To be successful, there has to be agreement as to what kinds of information will be used to define a product's quality; that is, the relevancy of the information and how it will be integrated with the other quality information. Without this information, no sensory quality control program can expect any success. As mentioned, the first step in this process is to agree as to what is product quality, how it will be obtained, whether it will include manufacturing quality, or is it entirely based on consumer quality criteria. As Hawthorn noted, quality control is based on an integration of information that must include the consumer; that is, meeting the expectations of the consumer balanced by what can be manufactured at a price that will sell and yield a profit. These elements are at the core of what should be a contemporary sensory quality control program. As already emphasized, most current QC programs are focused on production monitoring based on long established criteria. The general attitude is best expressed in the following way: since all production is sold, the system is working (i.e. consumer complaints are low), any proposed additional evaluations should fit within the existing system but at no added cost. However, the reality is quite different, as previously noted. We have observed significant preference and purchase intent differences for a single brand obtained from within and across markets. Many existing sensory quality monitoring systems are hopelessly out of date, using antiquated (insensitive) scales and experienced but not qualified subjects, so such results should not be surprising. If product quality is to be consistent with consumer expectations then a radical restructuring of the process is warranted.

Establishing a consumer-based sensory quality program is best achieved by starting from the marketplace; that is, use consumers to provide the "quality" information and integrating this information with production and raw material quality criteria. As previously noted, companies developed quality standards based on what was being manufactured and built monitoring systems around it, with input from technology and other product specialists. It has been driven by manufacturing, a realistic focus as long as the market was expanding greater than population growth, competition could be minimized and one was confident that acceptance by the consumer was consistent with the market strategy (image, price, etc.). Over time, however, this situation has changed, almost dramatically considering the competitive nature of the marketplace. It would not be surprising, for example, to learn that some companies use grading systems unchanged for over three decades without any verification that their systems are consistent with consumer behavior. Products are incorrectly downgraded or the grade of a raw material is higher than what is needed. We have observed systems where downgrading as much as 15% of a product (sold at a discount for other applications) when it was as well liked as a higher priced grade. The marketplace had changed but the "grading system" had not. The lost profits were significant. Demonstrating the changes and their financial effects was achieved by combining a sensory analysis of selected products with various consumer measures to identify which sensory characteristics were most important to "consumer quality." This procedure identified the discrepancy in grading and the basis on which the quality system could be changed and still meet consumer expectations. This was a clear example of using sensory resources effectively.

Sensory involvement in quality control must be approached carefully with the active support of management, manufacturing, and marketing, the former two being most supportive. There also must be agreement as to the product standard (or the lack thereof). The standard could be current production or it could be a written statement. However achieved, this standard is a starting point not the end point, and should be substantiated with consumer and sensory testing of an array of standard and non-standard products. The purposes for such an exercise will determine how much variation there is, which product characteristics are most important to these variations, and how much variation is possible before it causes a consumer reaction. The issue of consumer reaction must be specified, in advance; for example, it could be a significant reduction in purchase intent.

Although philosophical and procedural differences will exist between production and sensory when establishing a quality standard, the purpose for monitoring quality is universal. That is, systems and procedures should be established to minimize production or distribution of a product that deviates from the chosen standard. While "deviation from the standard" can lead to withholding a product from normal distribution channels, manufacturers recognize that some deviation is realistic (the idea of a gold standard, implying invariance, should be buried). The issue is one of degree. That is, how much deviation from the standard is tolerable before sensory acceptance and/or consumer confidence is significantly lowered. Distinguishing between sensory acceptance and consumer confidence is necessary; the consumer may recognize two samples of product as discriminably different, yet find them equally acceptable. However, a constantly changing product could affect consumer confidence. Consumer confidence is a business issue, while perceptions are a sensory issue. From a sensory perspective, it is easier to assess the effect of product variations on sensory acceptance than on consumer confidence; therefore, we have offered our warning and we can proceed to the measurement of deviations from a standard and their relationship to sensory acceptability.

The procedure used to establish a standard for production is important because it will have a direct influence on determining the degree of deviation that will be allowed and the measure of that deviation. If expert opinion were used to establish the standard, most likely the expert would establish the extent of deviation and the amount of change before quality would be lowered significantly. The expert, as noted earlier in this chapter, must rely on some type of grading systems to measure deviation from a standard (see Baten, 1946; Mosher *et al.*, 1950; Downs *et al.*, 1954; Amerine *et al.*, 1959). The weaknesses of grading systems have been covered elsewhere in this book (Chapter 3), and in the literature by Pangborn and Dunkley (1964), O'Mahony (1979), and Sidel *et al.* (1981, 1983).

When a combined consumer and sensory approach is used to establish a standard, that sensory model can be used to determine the effect on acceptance of any number of product variations. Once a model is known, this effect can be accomplished as a paper-and-pencil exploration, or it may involve testing actual samples representing a wide range of possible manufactured variables or deviations. This enables development of a scoring system that identifies which characteristics have exceeded a standard (±range) and leaves to management the decision as to what action will be taken.

Obviously, there can be considerable pressure when a product is on hold; for example, production, traffic, warehousing, and so forth will be disrupted. On the other hand, permitting product that exceeds the established specification to leave a plant and enter the retail system is more damaging and the effect will be more long lasting, although these latter effects are not directly observed, at least not in the immediate future. Over time, however, their effects can be very significant. Companies attempt to minimize this problem through a separate program, often referred to as Quality Assurance. This program monitors longer-term shifts through testing product obtained from retail outlets. But any results obtained from retail are influenced by the distribution system and related handling issues. However, the key to minimizing the long-term changes is to reduce the variations at the source. Before describing a means for developing and integrating a real-time sensory quality system, it is useful to reflect on how the information should be used and the main pitfalls to avoid. As noted above, measuring the strengths of important sensory quality characteristics is relatively easy, as is determining whether the strengths exceed the acceptable range also is relatively easy; however, it is far more challenging as to the actions recommended. In most instances, quality measures were (and continue to be) made using a scale that included acceptance/rejection and most test participants learned to avoid the latter and subsequent discussion with plant managers seeking an explanation. As we will discuss later in this section, sensory measures cannot include accept/reject judgments directly or indirectly, leaving those decisions to plant management. This minimizes conflict, and enables the process to function solely as a measuring system. Manufacturing emphasizes output and will pressure any function that impedes that flow, except of course, product safety. By shifting the decision to management, the sensory information represents what is perceived without determining that it is or is not approving release of a production lot. It is a management responsibility to address the issue of risk using a combination of sensory, physical, chemical, and business information to release a specific lot.

To develop a sensory quality monitoring system, it must be reliable and valid and at the same time rapid, uniform, consistent, and simplified (Stewart, 1971). This will require compromises from sensory, quality control, and manufacturing to achieve the flexibility necessary to operate in a production environment.

Before describing a sensory system for monitoring product quality, some additional comments are warranted about developing the "standard." A sensory model based on regression analyses is necessary to identify the important sensory quality attributes and from that information establish the limits within which products can vary but still be considered standard. Once this information has been developed, management, production, and technology need to be aware of and acknowledge that production variation results not in a single standard but rather in a family of products that "constitutes the standard." To fully accept and appreciate this concept, a set of descriptive profiles is developed from products representing the tolerance limits and from products within and outside those limits. An example of a profile is shown in Fig. 8.3. Product accept/reject decisions are based on deviations from the standard. The process of identifying the important sensory quality attributes and establishing their ranges and converting this into an operational scorecard is a

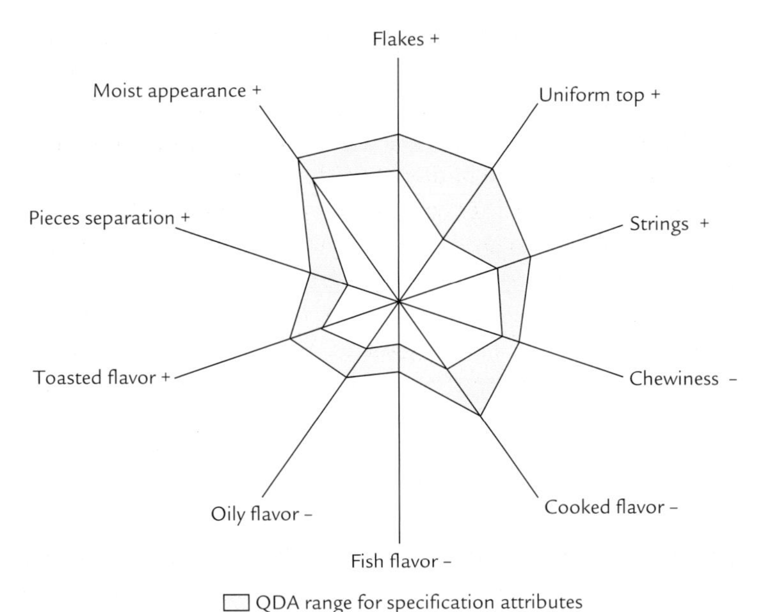

Figure 8.3 An example of a plot of the important sensory quality characteristics alone with the range within which a product can vary, but still meet the specification.

Table 8.4 A summary from a regression analysis identifying the most important analytical and sensory attributes and their relative contributions to acceptance. Based on the variance and the slopes of the individual lines, the best estimates for the ranges are determined leading to the scoring system shown in Fig. 8.4a–c and the text for further explanation

Analytical	***B***	**Beta**	***r***	**Beta × *r***	**% Relative contribution**
Color	−0.009	−0.388	−0.739	0.287	21.40
Reduced sugars	−5.508	−0.236	−0.282	0.067	5.00
Sensory					
Spicy aroma	−0.043	−0.280	−0.559	0.156	11.63
Sweet-flavor	0.075	0.265	0.241	0.064	4.77
Onion flavor	−0.085	−0.398	−0.885	0.352	26.25
Dairy flavor	0.108	0.322	0.129	0.415	30.95

multi-stage process. The initial task is to identify an array of products representing within and outside the range that would be acceptable based on current criteria. Products beyond what would be considered acceptable also are included. The second task is to obtain a sensory analysis, consumer quality measures, and physical, and chemical analyses for all the products. Through a series of regression analyses, the most important sensory, physical and chemical attributes are identified. Results from such analyses are summarized in Table 8.4. Once the attributes are identified, they are plotted versus the obtained acceptance scores and the limits established from the consumer judgments that indicate a significant change in preferences and /or purchase intent. Figures 8.4a–c (identified as the product quality index) show

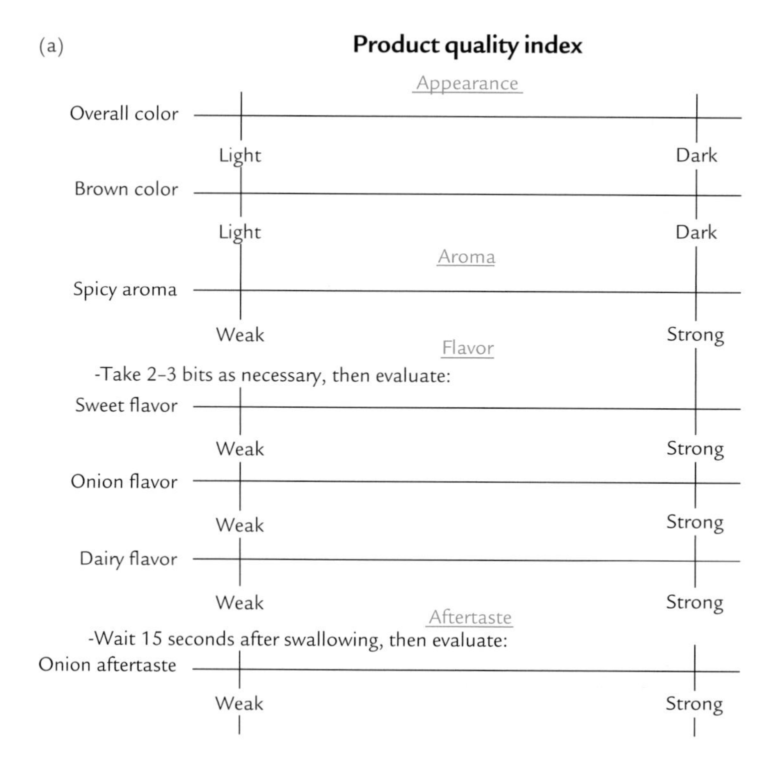

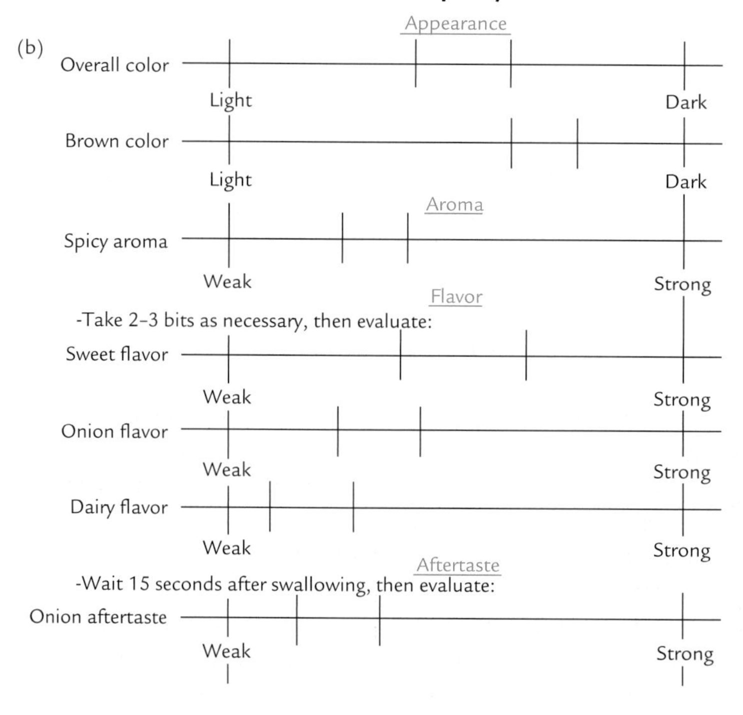

Figure 8.4 (*Continued*)

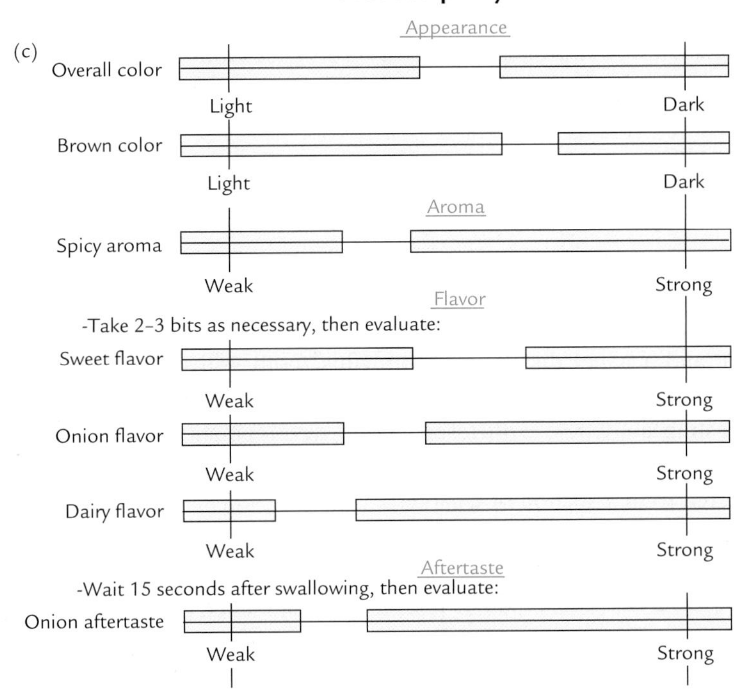

Figure 8.4 (a) The product quality index scorecard developed from the regression analysis and plots versus acceptance. See text for further explanation. (b) The index with the ranges identified. (c) The template applied to the index. A rapid scan of the template identifies which attribute scores are outside the range. See text for more explanation of its use.

the scorecard (a), the scorecard with the limits (b), and the template (c). During training, the subjects use the scorecard "a" to familiarize themselves with the attributes and practice scoring with products representing within and outside the range. The system is dynamic and representative of what is manufactured and the limits can be changed based on manufacturing issues and consumer considerations. Not surprisingly, there will be adjustments; for example, if the limits are too narrow for an attribute of less importance, the limits can be extended or the converse can be applied. What is critical is to make such decisions based on both manufacturing and marketplace information, not based solely on what can be manufactured or create limits that are too costly to achieve or result in too high a rate of rejection. In effect, one seeks to develop a dynamic system that reflects both internal and external considerations.

In addition to the delineation of the standard products, there also will be reliance on specific methods and subjects. This will require the adaptation of standard analytical sensory test methods (mostly discrimination and descriptive) to fit within the manufacturing environment. There is no universal test method for this application.

Monitoring product quality requires specific sensory test resources and the availability of qualified subjects and an individual responsible for organizing and administering the tests. The resources described here have been used successfully in manufacturing (Nakayama and Wessman, 1979) and include more recent developments (see Gridgeman, 1984; Stone *et al.*, 1991). For most evaluations, discrimination and descriptive tests will be used; however, their use will be modified to reflect the nature of the problem, the limited availability of subjects and the limited time in which to reach decisions.

1. An area for testing should be designated at each plant. It is unlikely that there will be an area as extensive as that available at research and development, but lighting and related environmental controls, booths, and accessibility are required. Typically, there would be three or four booths, a small preparation area, and a panel discussion room (this room will most likely be used as a general purpose room by others). This accommodation would allow for a range of testing activities, with research and development providing the necessary support for more extensive testing. For further detail on facilities, the reader is referred to that section of Chapter 2.
2. All subjects must be screened for testing. Guidelines for screening are provided in Chapter 5. The importance of having qualified subjects has been emphasized throughout this book and it is no less important here. It is interesting to observe the positive impact that screening (and training) have on plant personnel. Some production personnel have, for years, evaluated products as part of their daily work routine but have never been given instructions as to how to use their senses and whether the information they provided had any impact. It also may reveal that some individuals are not as sensitive as believed or, in some instances they are quite insensitive to specific characteristics. The screening procedures need to be well defined such that all subjects follow the same protocol. Usually, the R&D sensory staff develop this protocol (with suitable modifications as experience is gained).
3. Reference materials (products and/or ingredients) for discrimination and descriptive tests may be identified and their preparation and use documented (if appropriate). In our experience, only a limited number of references will be or should be necessary. For subject training, they can be helpful whether for the descriptive analysis or if the multiple-standard discrimination test will be used. Over time, discrimination and/or descriptive evaluations will be used to replenish the references. If the evaluations include ingredients, product during processing, in addition to finished product, then references may be needed for each of these test activities. Use of references should always be approached with care as they can communicate a sensory message that is not relevant to the task (see Chapter 6 for more on this topic).
4. Once subjects are screened, they proceed with descriptive training to recognize product attributes that are within and are outside of a specification. Training for multiple-standard discrimination tests involves first familiarizing subjects with the reference range and the evaluation procedure. Next, subjects evaluate sets of products and their performance is monitored. Qualifying subjects follow the same general plan as described previously for discrimination testing.

For descriptive analysis, subjects are trained according to the guidelines described in Chapter 6. Since the products will have been evaluated as part of the specification, the subjects are trained with the existing language, definitions, and any reference materials. However, it is not necessary for these subjects to be trained for an evaluation of all of a product's attributes. In fact, the results from the descriptive analysis of the products used to establish the quality standard will have identified the most important attributes and it is these attributes that are the focus of training. A typical scorecard used at plant will be limited to a single page and not more than eight or ten attributes, otherwise it will be too cumbersome to use and given an impression of complexity that is inappropriate.

5. The frequency of the evaluations and when done will be specified, as part of the initial development of the program, as will the testing protocol and related issues. Such documentation is important so as to ensure that the same procedures are used all of the time.
6. The criteria for product acceptance–rejection must be documented and agreed to by plant management. From a strategic viewpoint, it is necessary to remove from the subjects direct responsibility for placing product on-hold or for rejecting a specific lot. Subjects should focus solely on providing responses (to specific attributes) and the test administrator tabulates results and advises QC and/or plant manager as to the results. Traditionally, QC programs used a procedure that trained the individual subject to a specific score below which (or the converse) product was acceptable and above which, it was not. In addition, the subject also had to explain each judgment that resulted in product rejection. Clearly, this approach discouraged dissent, and individual subjects quickly learned to "adjust" their responses to conform, which was not in the best interest of consistent product quality. However, it did provide false evidence of the consistency of the products. It is, therefore, very important for the success of a sensory QC program to ensure that subjects are not directly responsible for the product decisions. In addition to not being directly responsible, the use of a second tier of testing will further enhance the program's success. For example, the QC manager, in concert with the appropriate plant managers, can evaluate all products that are borderline and/or outside the range and make the final decision (using all available information of which sensory will be one part).

As previously mentioned, the in-plant QC program will rely primarily on two methods, discrimination and descriptive analysis. For the former, the multiple-standard discrimination method is recommended. Product that is in and out of specification must be available during and after subject screening and training. For each test, such standards also are included. This procedure requires each subject to determine whether products are within the specified range. These tests are simple; that is, they are go/no-go tests and no other information is required. As few as three subjects will evaluate a product. If two of the three subjects state that the product is outside the specification, the product either is not accepted or is put on "hold" for further evaluation (see above note about second tier testing). Reference products should be available for the subjects at these tests. The use of very few subjects and a methodology that relies on the go/no-go decision at this stage is especially appropriate. Most manufacturing sites have limited numbers of people available for product evaluation, and still fewer to participate on a daily basis, willing to evaluate multiple sets of products.

On a daily basis, finished product also will be evaluated using a modified version of the standard descriptive test. The modifications, described previously, will include fewer respondents (two or three) and fewer descriptive attributes (six to ten). Results from the testing that established the product quality standard will have identified the attributes that are most important as well as the range of scores around each computed mean. The subjects are trained using the original protocol but only for these important attributes. Each subject scores a product once and the test administrator places the template (see Fig. 8.4a–c) on each scorecard and quickly identifies the attributes outside the range. If two of the subjects score an important attribute outside the range it is identified in the reporting to the QC manager. Here, too, some responses beyond the acceptable range are expected, and it could require two (of three) subjects marking outside the range for the three or four most important attributes to result in a hold. Note that there is no statistical treatment of the responses (there are too few and no replication) and the intent is to provide a rapid response that is not dependent on a specific numerical value. If a particular lot is put on hold and plant management cannot reach a decision, then samples could be re-evaluated by a second group of subjects or R&D could be requested to make a more complete analysis. The requirements for hold and reject will be product specific, there are no universal rules other than to be using the most important sensory quality attributes, qualified subjects, and the active support of plant management. Regardless of the path that is followed, the idea is to keep the evaluations in balance with the product and the production process.

It has been suggested that magnitude-of-difference scoring might be an appropriate methodology. In this test, the subject provides a measure of the difference from a standard. We see no particular advantage to this method; the magnitude-of-difference measure will have its own problems (what type of analysis, for one, and the second is having a standard that is reasonably constant), and it is still a go/no-go decision. For this particular application, the emphasis must be on a dichotomous outcome that is easy to understand. Experience has shown that the go/no-go minimizes the potential for conflict and/or the misuse of scores to promote a particular position.

7. As with any sensory analytical test, subject performance is also monitored. This assessment should include use of reference products and those used during training. Subjects should be aware of the performance monitoring and have the opportunity to review their records. Every effort must be made to keep subjects motivated and to help them maintain their sensory skills. Subjects who exhibit inconsistencies in their performance will have to be dropped (sometimes temporarily and then recertified). The extent of these inconsistencies will depend on the product, and especially on the magnitude of difference representing the specification.

8. A formal record-keeping and reporting procedure also is essential. Because little published literature on sensory evaluation procedures in production exists, it is important that a company have complete documentation of its systems.

The foregoing considerations should be viewed as guidelines for developing a QC sensory testing system.

There are three stages in the manufacturing process at which product quality could be monitored. The first stage covers the continuing go/no-go decisions that are made as raw materials are received, the second stage occurs during their storage, and the third stage occurs during one or more stages of manufacture. Sensory monitoring during these periods serves to minimize release of out-of-specification product. Tests at these stages should be intuitively obvious, yet surprisingly little of this testing is done. If such testing is done, relatively few records are kept, and many of the procedures have been so drastically modified as to be almost unrecognizable compared with written company protocols. While it is possible to accept tests performed in a less adequate facility, the test procedures must adhere to accepted sensory practices. Considering the importance of product quality at this stage of its life, it is surprising that so few companies are aware of the weaknesses of their current procedures and the relative ease with which these procedures can be improved. It is hoped that the guidelines and descriptions in this discussion will provide the necessary stimulus to improve the monitoring of product quality. The remainder of this section concerns the stages of manufacture where sensory tests can be readily made.

Ingredients are received in bulk from suppliers or from company-operated facilities. On receipt, they are checked to ensure that they meet the specification. The evaluation may be extensive, as in the case of analytical testing, or may be as uncomplicated as requiring a sniff or taste by an inspector. It should be understood that not all ingredients require formal sensory examination. In a formal monitoring program, the company will have developed a list of ingredients that require sensory examination, and will have developed a list of ingredients that require sensory examination, and will have established a frequency for that examination. For example, evaluation may be required for every new lot in the case of some ingredients, and every tenth lot, once a month, and so forth, for other ingredients.

Once frequency of examination has been established, the sensory test method should be specified. Here we suggest the use of an individual who has been screened, qualified, and trained to discriminate product that meets the specification. The individual may record judgments such as accept, reject, or hold. A hold requires additional and similarly qualified individuals to evaluate the material using the same test procedure. Each company must decide for itself which ingredients it will accept; however, with three trained and qualified subjects, any reject or more than 50% hold responses should be given serious consideration by management. Management may acknowledge the recommendations to reject or hold an ingredient but still approve its use based on other business reasons.

Some ingredients enter the processing system immediately on receipt and are evaluated at that time. Other ingredients may be stored for several months or longer, and a periodic assessment of these should be performed to avoid potential problems.

The procedures will be similar to those used on the ingredients' receipt. Any ingredient stored prior to use in production should be evaluated at the time of its planned introduction.

Product manufacture can range from batch to continuous operations and can involve numerous points where ingredients are added and processes occur. Mixing, blending, fermenting, and packaging are examples of some of the types of steps. At critical points, product quality must be monitored. Consideration must be given to those points where the potential for variability is high and will result in a noticeable defect in the finished product. Success at this stage of monitoring product quality requires a reasonable and cooperative effort on the part of sensory evaluation, production, and quality control. Each process is unique and an approach that is suitable for one product probably will not be appropriate for another. It will be necessary to evaluate products removed at different stages of the process and to determine whether the information is meaningful and has a relationship to finished product quality.

The discrimination model is the most useful sensory approach for evaluation of products during processing. The subjects (one to three) would make their evaluations relative to the multiple-standard method, as described previously, as the criteria for acceptance, hold, or rejection of product. Descriptive analysis may be helpful, at least during the investigative stages, to identify at which step in the process the most change has occurred. However, the most useful methodology will be discrimination because of its rapid input to the decision-making process.

For finished product evaluation, the immediate decision-making will be based on the discrimination model with multiple references representing acceptable product or using the modified descriptive procedure. Subjects will be trained to identify products that exceed the range of acceptable differences. Criteria for accepting, rejecting, or holding product will be similar to those applied to ingredients and to products during processing. Descriptive analysis should be used for selected products on a regular basis. The purpose would be twofold: to identify any trends away from the reference and to provide a day-to-day independent check on evaluation. The descriptive method would make use of the existing database, would have a limited number of dimensions, and so forth. The descriptive data are plotted against the reference standard(s) to determine whether the finished product is within acceptable limits.

It is assumed that the primary sensory evaluation group will conduct in-depth QDA analyses of the products to monitor long-term drift. The statistical methods for monitoring long-term descriptive drift are similar to the split-plot analyses discussed under product stability and experimental design (see Chapter 4).

As noted previously, much of the success of a sensory QC program depends on having management's commitment to the process, identifying the important sensory quality attributes, and availability of products representing within and outside of the standard product for training and testing purposes. Our approach relies on a combination of consumer acceptance and descriptive analysis to establish the sensory limits for a product (the family of gold standards). Another approach relies on management and a project team to select an example(s) of their company's product as a standard, and that product is then submitted to sensory analysis. The resulting description and its limits then become the documented standard against which other descriptive profiles are compared. The approved finished product should be stored and replenished as needed for training or refreshing sensory memories. These products should be included in selected tests.

Establishing and replenishing references for ingredients and product during processing is considerably more difficult. The research required to establish these references may be prohibitive, and the effort of the project team or expert judgment may be required. Once references are established and a reasonable replenishment cycle is agreed, their use in the sensory monitoring of product quality can proceed along the lines described above. It is possible that reference products and ingredients can be obtained and stored only at considerable expense. In this situation, more reliance will be placed on sensory resources at R&D to provide complete descriptive analysis of products and in the process, identify references for use in training and monitoring the sensory skills of plant personnel. In today's business environment of heightened food safety and food security, in-process evaluations will be more difficult to achieve and could quickly be supplanted by electronic noses and tongues (Bartlett *et al.*, 1997; Bleibaum *et al.*, 2002).

The approach to quality control described here emphasizes the impact of the marketplace on helping to select standards, use of discrimination and descriptive testing at the plants and a management approved plan of the decision-making process. Reliance on a single test method is not recommended, whether there is a single plant or there are ten plants. Each system in each plant will have its own unique features, but all will have sufficient commonality to provide for comparisons where needed. Statistical designs and analyses combined with contemporary quantitative sensory methodology will make QC systems valid and successful. Finally, this approach has proven to be very informative as to the various measurements currently being used. We have identified significant investments in QC procedures that were redundant with other measures, as well as having no bearing on finished product quality. While some of them may be valuable from a manufacturing control perspective, many were thought to be important to the consumer only to find that they had no impact.

From this discussion, the reader should develop an appreciation for the complexity of the use of sensory evaluation in quality control. However, the need for sensory evaluation is so great that quality control cannot be ignored. By identifying the basic elements of a QC program, the sensory professional can proceed with greater confidence than heretofore realized.

VIII. Optimization

Developing new products or improving existing products is a costly and time-consuming process. Companies are continually seeking new approaches for achieving greater success in the marketplace. In recent years, the concept of optimization has been identified as a technique that potentially can satisfy this objective. By optimization we mean a procedure for developing the best possible product in its class. This procedure implies that an opinion of best possible is provided, and in sensory evaluation this means responses for the most liked/preferred product (Sidel and Stone, 1983; McBride, 1990; Sidel *et al.*, 1994). Optimization information has considerable appeal because of its immediate and practical applications for the marketing specialist seeking a competitive advantage. For the product specialist, the information provides a focus for formulation efforts; for quality control, it provides a basis for identifying those specific product variables that require monitoring before, during, and after processing, and so forth. With unlimited development possibilities, it is understandable that optimization has considerable appeal. However, as with any new approaches, optimization warrants careful study before it can be fully embraced as a worthwhile sensory evaluation resource. In this discussion, our attention is focused on different approaches to sensory optimization, with particular consideration given to the development of guidelines for the planning and design of these tests and some very practical aspects of the testing itself. Other types of optimization programs are possible, for example, ingredient costs, processing, nutritive value, and so forth. In most instances, the particular models to be discussed are applicable. In this discussion, we focus on the sensory model but with consideration of some newer options including consumer attitudes and imagery to further enhance the usefulness of the information.

The use of optimization models received its greatest impetus from the work of Box and associates (for more detail on the method, see Box, 1954; Box *et al.*, 1978), who developed an approach to multivariate designs described as response surface methodology (RSM). This statistical design concept was especially valuable in engineering and manufacturing, in general, where it was possible to identify and control input and output parameters and to mathematically identify the combination of input variables necessary to achieve an optimal result. For example, it could be the maximal yield from a chemical or food process, achieved with the minimum input of energy within specified cost constraints. The concept of response surface has been well received, leading to a relatively wide range of industrial and research applications including its use in quality control (for more discussion on this application, see Taguchi, 1987). The use of response surface in sensory evaluation has become considerably more commonplace since its earliest applications (see Henika, 1982; Mullet, 1988; Resurreccion, 1988; Schutz, 1988).

In addition to and independent of response surface designs, developments in the behavioral sciences were providing additional statistical models that were especially appropriate for sensory optimization. Multiple regression/correlation (MR/C) techniques are sophisticated and useful statistical procedures that enable the investigator to understand the ways by which variables are related to each other, as well as to develop mathematical expressions for predicting future events based on those variables without knowing, in advance, which variables are most important. These techniques are analytical in the sense that they are able to sort information, to categorize details that can be categorized, and to identify aspects that may require further inquiry. For sensory evaluation and the behavioral sciences in general, the multiple regression/correlation techniques are especially useful because they have, as noted by Cohen and Cohen (1983) "... capacity to mirror, with high fidelity, the complexity of the relationships that characterize the behavioral sciences." In sensory optimization, we wish to identify those product variables that are important to acceptance; however, we usually do not have *a priori* knowledge about which variables should be manipulated, and therefore we look to these statistical techniques to assist us in sorting the possibilities. From this sorting, a mathematical model will evolve that can be tested and refined, leading to a predictive tool which has widespread product application. The interested reader will find useful information on the topic in Gunst and Mason (1980), Draper and Smith (1981), Cohen and Cohen (1983), and Manly (1986). Both RSM and MR/C use similar types of computations in deriving the various models (both are different types of multivariate designs).

There are some differences between the two approaches and we believe that these differences are important insofar as sensory evaluation is concerned. As already noted, an objective of optimization is to identify those variables important to sensory acceptance (or any other dependent variable; e.g. cost of ingredients) and the degree of importance for each. If important variables are not represented in a test, then the various computations will not identify them. In response surface designs, the important input variables must be specified in advance and, systematically varied, and their output measured. For sensory evaluation, it is usually not possible, *a priori*, to specify the important sensory variables and therefore the selection of products for the project becomes very important. It will be discussed later in this section. The inexperienced investigator should be aware that a result is always obtained from a multivariate analysis regardless of whether product selection or test variable preparation was correct. This also applies to data that are highly variable and exhibit little or no face validity. The analyses will iterate until a statistical significant result is obtained and in the process it may eliminate some data. There is no argument about the use of tests for outliers or with the investigator removing data for a product because it is distorting the model; however, this should be done with full knowledge of the consequences (see Manly, 1986, for some comments on these issues). In that regard, it is worth noting the recent application of a technique referred to as partial least squares (PLS) regression as a third approach, at least in so far as concerns the data analysis (Martens and Martens, 1986). The methodology was developed for econometric applications but has been applied to other fields where "the emphasis is on predicting responses and not necessarily on trying to understand the underlying relationship between variables" (Tobias, 1999). PLS procedures are particularly appropriate when knowledge about the independent variables and their relationship with dependent variables is unclear, and when there is an expected high degree of multicollinearity among the independent variables. In most instances, one wants to minimize the problems associated with multicollinearity. Also, relying on a default system without fully appreciating the consequences can lead to solutions that are interesting but may not answer the question being considered. In as much as the results from a multivariate analysis is usually the basis for further work; for example, product change, not an end by itself, one should apply it with care (an argument for all multivariate analyses). Another modeling approach that has generated interest is the use of neural networks (Bomio, 1998; Ferrier and Block, 2001). The methodology derives from an effort to incorporate large data sets for which there are no obvious relationships except that they are derived for a particular product. For those situations in which little or no sensory analyses have been done, and/or there is little understanding of the relationships between ingredients and sensory responses, this approach will have relevance. All these techniques represent advances that warrant consideration by the sensory professional; however, each must be viewed in the context of its usefulness in providing specific direction for requestors and not simply because it is new.

As already noted, for MR/C the important variables must be represented in the set of products, while RSM requires manipulation of the important variables (known in advance). If the variables only need to be represented, then we can include other products of interest, especially competitive products. This approach has the additional advantage of ensuring that the important sensory variables are included in the set of products. We assume that if our products have little or none of the important sensory variables, then certainly they will be contained in other competitive products available in the marketplace. Implicit in this discussion is the expectation that many if not all of the products will be different from each other (different because of sensory qualities and not just by formulation or by chemical analysis). If this were not the case, then one might have far fewer products (and a much smaller database), which significantly reduces the effectiveness of the resulting model; predictions would be based on a relatively limited database. Pre-testing of products will minimize the problem, but this could mean elimination of some products and the loss of the ordered matrix (especially important in RSM designs). As with many other sensory test plans and procedures, attaining the ideal design can be confounded by practical considerations. To address the issue of having so many products as would be encountered in a full factorial design, the use of partial factorials and related types of designs are appropriate. Such designs provide the means by which the variables of interest can be evaluated. To assist the investigator, several computer programs are available for these applications.

In an optimization study, a logical sequence of events is usually followed. As shown in Fig. 8.5, the process begins with the planning stage and this includes selecting the product category; obtaining products; deciding which optimization methodology will be used, defining the consumer population, and preparation of the actual test plan. It is important to obtain products that fully reflect the marketplace and whatever is available through formulation. Based on the specific optimization method chosen, the products will be screened and selected for testing. The methods used for the analyses are interpolative not extrapolative, so it is essential for the products to represent the sensory space for that product category. If one is using an RSM approach, additional formulation may be necessary to ensure a suitable matrix of products. Once testing is initiated, the project proceeds in a more systematic way. Detailed descriptions of the statistical procedures can be found in the texts cited earlier. These are omitted here because there are many alternatives (as described in the literature) and the specific steps are left to the individual investigator.

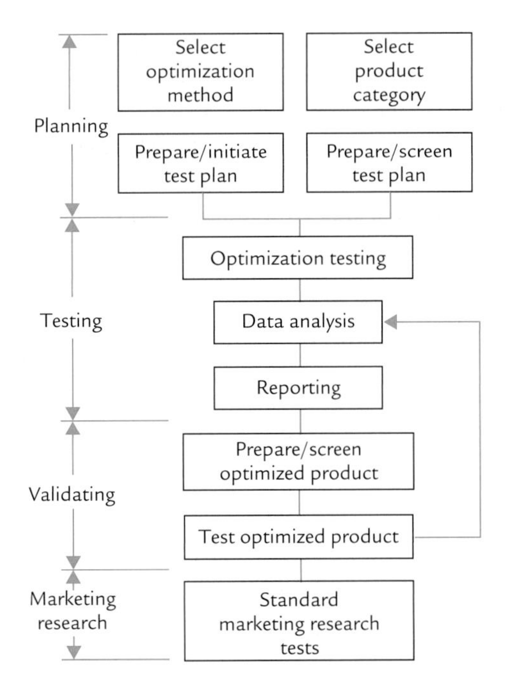

Figure 8.5 Block diagram of the major components of an optimization scheme. See text for additional explanation. Reprinted from Sidel *et al.* (1983). *Food Technol.* Vol. 37, No. 11. Copyright © by Institute of Food Technologists.

Up to this point, the emphasis in this discussion has been on the concept of optimization and some of the differences between RSM and MR/C designs. It is useful if we also consider the data derived from the testing. The sensory information is the descriptive data derived from a QDA analysis while the consumer's degree of liking for the products is obtained from the target population. Other data should include chemical and physical analyses, and possibly other kinds of consumer information; for example, purchase intent, imagery. All this information forms the database for the subsequent analyses. The first step in this process is to examine the results in a univariate format to establish that the results are consistent with expectations regarding product sensory differences and consumer preferences. While one might assume this to be an obvious first step, it is often overlooked, in part, because of use of default systems or the only interest is to obtain a significant regression equation. Unfortunately, some default systems also remove responses that are mathematically outliers, further "adjusting" results with no appreciation for the behavioral consequences. The sensory and all other product analytical data are subjected to appropriate data reduction techniques (Kline, 1994). These results are plotted and examined to verify that they reflect the product differences; once again, applying the "intra-ocular" shock test of asking if the results make sense. Attributes and analytical measures are then selected to represent the various factors and one proceeds with the relevant regression analyses. A typical output will be similar to that shown in Table 8.2, except the *Y* value would be preference or some other dependent measure obtained from consumers. Where there are preference segments, discussed later in this section, the results are related to the preference segments to identify which characteristics define the segments. For example, if there were two preference segments, one would want to examine the relationship between preferences and specific sensory attributes, as shown in Fig. 8.6. Obviously, the presence of the segments leads to development of two regression equations, etc. A linear multiple regression equation would take the following form:

$$Y = k + \text{Descriptor A } (W_a) + \text{descriptor B } (W_b) - \text{descriptor C } (W_c) \\ + \text{chemical measure 1 } (W_1) + \text{physical measure 2 } (W_2)$$

Where Y is the acceptance/preference value (dependent variable), the constant k is the equation intercept, descriptors A, B, C are the most important variables derived from the analysis, $W_{a,b,c,1,2}$ are the weightings for those variables, and sign (+, −) indicates scale direction for that variable.

The technologist then formulates products based on their knowledge of ingredient and process effects on the specific attributes and the products are tested relative to the target. Once there is confidence that significant progress ahs been achieved, a validation test would be initiated with target consumers. Acceptance testing would be an appropriate test of the model. As a measure of test-to-test reliability, two or three products from the initial study would be included.

Optimization studies would be incomplete if they identified only the important variables and their contributions to product acceptability. From these data, it also is possible to predict the combination of variables that will yield optimum acceptance. The prediction will consist of mathematical and written statements based on assumptions developed from the test data and will provide for more than a single optimal

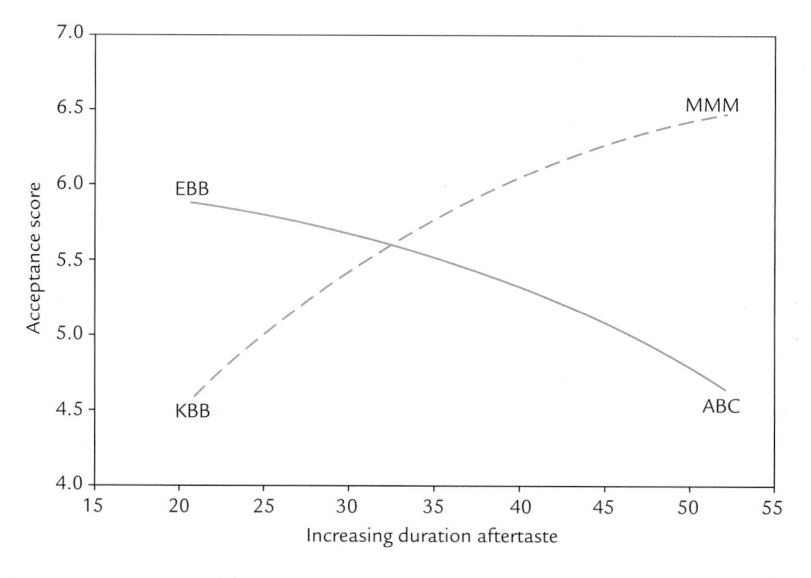

Figure 8.6 A plot showing a sensory attribute that differentiates two preference segments. See text for more discussion.

product; that is, optimal acceptance may be possible based on different combinations of the important independent variables.

For sensory optimization, proper product selection and the type of sensory information that is obtained is essential. The importance of these requirements cannot be underestimated. Product selection is difficult because the criteria by which products are selected will include sensory properties, technology, formulation differences, and marketplace considerations. It is important that the full range of anticipated sensory differences is represented in the test products; this could mean the inclusion of products that might not be economically viable but that have a particular sensory characteristic not readily perceived by other test products. Specific formulations might be included because of interest in particular process variables or ingredients. The inclusion of competitive products further ensures that a full range of sensory properties will be represented. In some instances, companies will undertake an optimization project but exclude all competitive products without realizing that it can identify the means for optimizing one's product only to discover that it is significantly inferior to other products in the market. Satisfying the sensory requirements involves bench screening and possibly some testing; however, our experience suggests that the screening is usually sufficient to yield an acceptable array of products, usually twenty to thirty. Bench screening will require several sessions with sufficient time to recover from the sensory challenge of sampling many products. This is necessary to ensure that the project staff gains a full appreciation for the range of product differences and similarities in the market relative to the project objective. In some categories, it is not unusual to start with as many as 100 or more products. This number should not be surprising if one considers the large number of formulations that are possible just with ingredient changes. As noted previously, the intention is to select an array of products that encompasses the sensory world of the product category independent of whether the products are liked.

The sensory data are developed using descriptive analysis and the consumer provides the dependent judgments, preference, purchase intent, etc. Separating the two kinds of information is critical to minimizing the halo effects and the very high potential for multicollinearity when consumers are also providing the descriptive information. It is remarkable that this reliance on the consumer for all the judgments continues with the efficiencies and availability of descriptive analysis capabilities. Similarly, the trained panel's liking responses are biased and should not be obtained.

Descriptive analysis is the most appropriate sensory tool for optimization because there is no *a priori* knowledge concerning the important sensory characteristics. Therefore, all of the sensory properties of the products should be described, and then various factor analytic techniques and regression analyses can be applied to establish the relationships between the various sensory attributes. These results can then be used in combination with the consumer responses to identify the important variables. The literature on sensory optimization provides numerous examples of design approaches (Moskowitz, 1972; Horsfield and Taylor, 1976; Henika, 1982; Schutz *et al.*, 1982; Schutz, 1983; Mullet, 1988; Sidel, *et al.*, 1994; and numerous others). Most of these investigators incorporated sensory evaluation into their tests; however, few used a quantitative descriptive analysis for the product sensory database.

However, the experiences of Schutz and co-workers and of Horsfield and Taylor were sufficiently promising. With the application of quantitative descriptive procedures such as QDA and a clear delineation between the analytical and the affective responses, sensory optimization has become more reasonable and a potentially valuable resource (facilitated by the access and power of PCs to analyze results).

By coupling the different sensory capabilities within the MR/C design, there is a much greater likelihood for identifying those product sensory variables that influence acceptance in the marketplace and that combination of variables that will lead to optimal acceptance (see Stone and Sidel, 1981; Sidel and Stone, 1983; Stone *et al.*, 1991; Sidel *et al.*, 1994). In our experience, sensory optimizations are more successful when beginning with a MR/C design approach and then to use the RSM after identifying the important variables. This approach capitalizes on the power of both designs. We would be remiss if we did not comment on the complexity of optimization from a testing as well as a conceptual viewpoint. The elements of testing have already been described, as were the challenges of design and product selection. Conceptually, optimization may appear to be an attempt to control the development process or possibly the creative efforts of specialists. It is foolish to conclude that a mathematical model will mean the end of product creativity. There is no substitute for the intellectual efforts of the specialist capable of interpreting and incorporating sensory responses into finished products that possess that combination of unique properties not possible by other means. Creativity will also be an integral part of the process, not only for the product specialist but also for the sensory professional. The purpose for the optimization model is to provide a more precise delineation of the approach that has the highest probability for success with the target population(s).

Optimization procedures continue to be of significant value and interest in sensory evaluation and since our last publication have become a staple in the consumer product industry. Studies have revealed new information unobtainable with smaller and less diverse product sets. One finding is that consumer preferences are often heterogeneous, and the heterogeneity is related more to sensory difference among products than to demographic differences among populations. We have observed this type of result on a worldwide basis, in very diverse countries, regions, and cultures. In unbranded evaluations we frequently detect different "preference groups" or "preference clusters" imbedded within the aggregate test population. Once data are obtained from the consumers, one can apply clustering procedures to the responses to establish whether such segments exist. Fig. 8.7 is an example of an output in which three clusters or segments are identified. Because the testing was done on a blind basis, the basis for the clustering is not explained by brand usage or typical demographic criteria and more often explained by other emotional and related criteria. This information, by itself, is interesting because it can help to explain why products do well in one test and less so in another, simply because of the type of person in the test. However, the real value rests in identifying product opportunities in the marketplace driven by specific sensory characteristics and related imagery. For example, some groups are differentiated by their preference for low intensity (flavor and aroma) products; others prefer attributes in one modality to the exclusion of those in another, while others prefer products that have unique attributes or intensities (see Fig. 8.6).

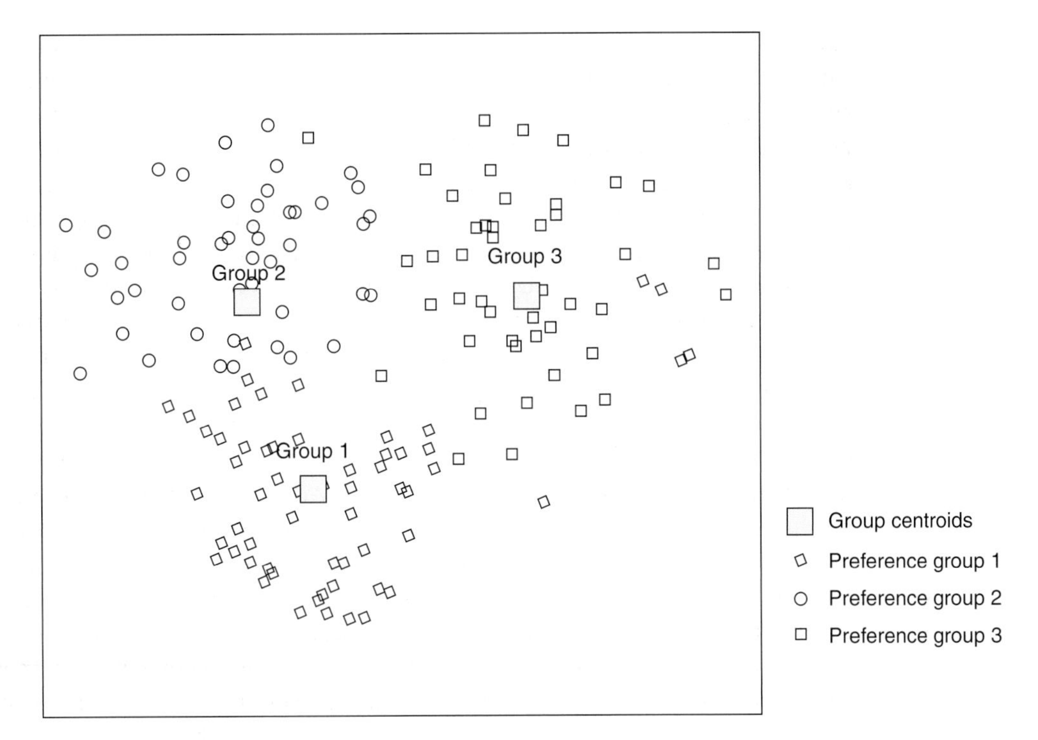

Figure8.7 Plot of the output from a cluster analysis identifying three segments.

We have observed many patterns and the task is to identify attributes important to each preference group. Once this is accomplished, a meaningful development and business strategy is possible. This may require unique products optimized for the different groups or a "bridge" product that represents a compromise between disparate preference groups. Deriving a bridge product from known preference differences is preferred to using averages from aggregate data. The latter discount important differences and results in products with little or no unique appeal. Some attributes increase acceptance with one preference group whilst decreasing acceptance with another group. When group size is equal, such attributes have no influence on aggregate acceptance, and leads to an erroneous conclusion that the attribute is unimportant or that the development changes were too small and not recognized by consumers. A worse case scenario is a test that includes significantly more consumers from one preference group than occurred in a previous test. In this case, aggregate results will represent preferences of the dominant group, which may not agree with previous results or changes in the test product. Knowledge about preference groups and the attribute intensities they prefer removes much of the mystery of why some consumer tests seem to go awry and results do not support previous research or the current hypothesis.

A basic optimization procedure limits consumer response to product liking, and models those responses to descriptive and/or analytical measures for the purpose of determining which attribute combination will result in a best liked, or optimized, product. The context provided by the products set is sufficient for deriving a successful optimization model, and this is all that may be needed. However, purchase behavior is influenced by additional factors, many of which can be, and need to be, assessed in the optimization process. The optimized product can be defined in relation to an "ideal," to specific uses defined by a situation and user group, packaging, pricing, and brand imagery. Products with diverse uses (e.g. an ingredient and spread) and used by different groups (e.g. children and adults) require an approach that addresses those issues. Usage and Attitude (U&A) data assist understanding consumer attitudes and behavior, and where this is unavailable or outdated, the optimization project must include many of the same elements. Assessing and integrating these elements provides better understanding of the wants, needs, and purchase interest of the consumer. It also improves potential for developing the right product for the right population, and identifying product-related benefits important to that population. The following paragraphs describe some of the enhanced measures we have used in our own optimization research. At this juncture, we reinforce the importance of the team approach in optimization research, as additional elements from development and marketing are included in this research.

The initial phase for this research requires gathering available information. One needs to begin with usage and attitude information about the target consumer. This information may be available from U&A data, or it may need to be developed for the research. To supplement U&A data, we recruit target consumers, mail (or otherwise provide) to them a proprietary situation usage survey (IBU® an acronym for Item-by-Use) that they complete in advance of the qualitative or quantitative testing. Consumers selected for the qualitative sessions are assigned "homework" involving one or more creative tasks (e.g. prepare a collage) to focus them on the product category, and ease them into sharing their views and opinions at two consecutive days of qualitative sessions. Information from the survey and group sessions is analyzed and is the basis for subsequent questionnaires for the quantitative phase of consumer testing.

Consumers recruited to the test location are asked to complete a questionnaire about their "ideal" product, its attributes and uses, and a series of questions derived from the IBU® consumer survey and discussion groups described above. Products are then evaluated, one at a time, in a standard CLT format. Consumers complete a hedonic question for a product followed by another proprietary questionnaire (SBU®, an acronym for Sample-by-Use). The SBU® contains questions related to the perceived intensity for sensory attributes (also measured in the preliminary "ideal" questionnaire), situation appropriateness (initially measured by the IBU®), and a conjoint linked proprietary questionnaire (SenseMark®) assessing the degree to which the products sensory cues are judged to deliver on marketing related issues such as brand, perceived value, perceived benefit, and so forth. Proprietary exit questionnaires include demographic information, lifestyle and attitude questions, anticipated category and brand purchase behavior for the immediate future, and a post-test "ideal" assessment. Information from the product evaluation and exit questionnaires provides a user profile and, where possible, a discriminate function linked to preference group membership. This information provides preference group specific screening criteria, as well as identifying whether, or how, preference groups differ in their attitudes, lifestyle, and purchase interests. It would be naive to assume that preference group members have homogeneous attitudes, values, and behavior. "Knowing the consumer" is raised to a new level of understanding with these enhancements to optimization research.

Consumer focus on the category in optimization research offers an opportunity to measure response to a variety of other issues. Packaging container sizes, shape, structure, graphics, and so forth is readily accommodated in the research, as are alternate concepts and communication options. Quantitative survey information and qualitative follow-up groups are used to further explore topics of interest for groups exhibiting homogenous attitudes and preferences. Our results have convincingly demonstrated the importance for sensory professionals to work closely with professionals in other product-related business units (e.g. marketing) in a systematic and integrated approach to product optimization. Rarely will isolation or working in an information vacuum produce the success needed to conduct this research and to compete in the marketplace of today and the future.

IX. Conclusions

In this chapter, considerable attention has been given to some applications for sensory resources, particularly for those applications in which sensory information is not the only information source, yet it often is crucial to the decision-making process. While these activities will bring attention to sensory evaluation, they require a much greater understanding. Sensory professionals cannot expect to be focusing their attention solely on a test (or series of tests), rather as much attention must be given to the basis for a problem, what are the objectives, who will make decisions and how will they be made, and so forth. In effect, sensory professionals must make the transition from servicing requests to a direct involvement in the organization and planning process. For sensory evaluation to mature and achieve respectability in the business environment, it must actively participate in the kinds of programs described herein.

In describing specific problems, we identified ways in which sensory evaluation can contribute and we purposely emphasized the planning and organizational aspects of the particular problems instead of presenting a step-by-step solution. Since each company and each product category has unique characteristics, we could not provide a detailed description for the evaluation of specific products. The reader is expected to apply the information presented in this chapter to his/her specific needs. It is important to bear in mind that the principles of sensory evaluation do not change, only their applications change. Success depends on the patience, skills, and the knowledge of the sensory professional.

Epilogue

9

I. Introduction

The emphasis in this book has been directed toward developing, organizing, and operating a sensory program within a business environment. However, the reader is reminded that the information is relevant anywhere sensory analysis of products is contemplated, or one is engaged in research on the senses. Based on the successes of sensory evaluation in food and non-food applications, it is clear that the information has value; contributing to a product's information base and contributes to that company's profits. However, the success of a sensory program does not just happen, it requires a commitment from that company's management, a commitment to support a program that offers a full range of services, has the flexibility to respond rapidly to changes in the marketplace, evaluate new methodologies, and be able to respond to shifts in product categories because of changing business plans and strategies.

Successful sensory programs require time to develop, regardless of company size. While we originally noted that as much as 3–5 years would be needed the business environment has changed and the time span reduced significantly. Most companies operate on a much faster timetable, and 1–3 years is more realistic. In this time span, a sensory professional must develop resources and demonstrate successes. This should not be construed that there will be no success before 3 years, rather it means that a reasonable amount of time is necessary to establish test capabilities within that company's culture, and initiate testing. Of course, this very much depends on the capability of the sensory staff to develop resources and apply them in a responsive manner. Program success also depends on management's understanding of what sensory can do for them.

A successful program requires at least one individual – the sensory professional – to assume responsibility for its technical and business development. Without this

Sensory Evaluation Practices 3rd Edn
ISBN: 0-12-672690-6

individual to develop and champion sensory evaluation, success is fleeting at best (Eggert, 1989; Stone and Sidel, 1995). Perhaps the most important requirement, beyond the technical issues, is the ability to think and act strategically, to be aware of business and brand strategies, to be aware of activities (marketing and technical) that impact a product's sensory characteristics.

Unfortunately, individuals working toward these goals have few role models, people or organizations, to turn to for guidance. It is challenging for a sensory professional to think beyond a test or a test method, to consider how information will be used and whether that information will enable others to act decisively. One purpose for this book has been to provide sensory professionals with guidance, to provide a perspective not available in other publications. We identified the organizational building blocks for a successful sensory program and alternative ways of combining these blocks to yield a viable resource. These blocks or components are described in detail in Chapter 2, and the interested reader may wish to review that material again. Our emphasis is based on the realization that sensory evaluation is one of the least understood and most misused functions in the research and development process.

Scientists and technologists diligently adhere (in most instances) to the rigorous rules of science in studying specific problems, yet they totally ignore these same rules when it comes to evaluation of the end point of their endeavors – a product. There has been a general lack of respect for the science (of sensory evaluation) and for test results especially when those results are inconsistent with expectations (real or imagined). This might be explained by the lack of unique instruments for sensory analysis (at least not used on a routine basis as noted in Chapter 8), and no reason to restrain anyone from ignoring results, especially when the "science" uses the eyes, ears, nose, and tongue. It is typical (and reasonable) for scientists, technologists, brand managers, etc. to examine products and discuss test results. However, when those individuals decide that the results were not what was expected and change recommendations based on their own "evaluation," is ample evidence of the challenge facing the sensory staff. This example and other abuses of sensory evaluation have been described in the literature (Pangborn, 1980). In the two decades since this article was published, some progress has been made and more companies accept sensory results regardless of the outcome, but the fundamental problem remains, that is, dismissing results as not being "very scientific." Obviously, the sensory professional must be aware of and ready to counter such claims and the risks associated with such unscientific actions. Considerably more effort will be needed to counteract the continued misuse of sensory evaluation, including the reintroduction of experts under the guise of specially trained panels, the use of expert languages (lexicons), and the movement away from properly designed studies with appropriately qualified subjects (see Stone, 1999). Sensory professionals must be able to use accepted sensory practices, and also be able to communicate effectively, if they expect to be heard and be a part of the product decision-making process.

Sensory evaluation represents a different type of challenge for managers and for scientists and technologists. This challenge is more obvious when test results are used for determining project accountability or as a measure of a requestor's performance. For example, when a developer works to cost-reduce a product without affecting sensory perception (i.e. to make a change that will not be perceived), sensory evaluation can be considered as an internal check on project progress. Each time a test results in a failure to meet an objective, some resentment of sensory evaluation will develop. History cautions us about the fate of the bearer of bad news. Although sensory evaluation is merely describing results, stating that the products were perceived as different (i.e. reading the instrument), the individuals responsible for the project could misconstrue this action as a personal rejection of their work. If the cost savings associated with the test are substantial, there will be great interest in the project, and there will be pressure to succeed. Sensory professionals must be sensitive to and think strategically about the potential impact of a test result. Care must be taken to ensure that the results are not used as a basis for measuring a developer's competence. The problem can be difficult if not impossible to eliminate entirely; however, the sensory professional should maintain regular communications with requestors and their management to be sure that the objective (the purpose for the test) is clear and unambiguous, and be sure that sensory information is not misunderstood or misused. In some instances, we have observed requesters seeking alternative testing resources in the hope that it will yield a favorable result. Requestors can be very creative in describing their particular problem so as to justify an alternative test method or test capability. While there is no way to completely prevent such a course of action, it does reinforce the importance of communications for sensory evaluation. Product and marketing research managers must have complete confidence in what a sensory professional can do for them so as to minimize risk in product marketing decisions, and most importantly, to not reject results because they do not satisfy their personal goals.

In this book, we have described numerous problems (or opportunities, depending on one's view) that are frequently encountered by sensory professionals. These problems are not confined to any specific product category; they are generic to all products. We propose alternative courses of action, presented in the context of guidelines that will enable the sensory professional to develop an appropriate course of action and lead to a successful solution. This process is highly dependent on the active (and willing) participation of a sensory professional with the equally active support of management. Sensory evaluation at the professional level remains for the strong-hearted individual.

II. Education and the Sensory Professional

Over the past two decades, there has been a significant increase in awareness of the science and the applications of sensory evaluation. Books, journals, and scientific and technical societies have organized symposia and technical programs on the science and this has had a salutary effect on the practical applications of the science of sensory evaluation. Increasing public awareness of the field as a result of a growing interest in wine and food appreciation has enhanced awareness and attracted more people to the field. All this activity has stimulated the academic community to catch up with the needs of industry, government, and academia itself, creating a further demand for qualified professionals. There are now many food science departments offering courses in sensory evaluation, and in 2002 the University of California Davis Extension initiated an online course "Applied Sensory and Science and Consumer Testing Certificate Program for Distance Learners" (www.extension.ucdavis.edu/agriculture/sensory/applic.html). Eventually, university programs will help to alleviate the shortage of trained professionals. Various technical societies and industry associations have continued their work to develop testing guidelines. In addition, workshops on sensory evaluation are offered regularly by individuals, consulting organizations, and academic institutions. The American Society of Testing and Materials Committee E-18 (Sensory Evaluation of Materials and Products), the Sensory Evaluation Division of the Institute of Food Technologists, and the Sensory Panel of the Food Group of the Society of Chemical Industry and the European Chemoreception Research Organization are the most active of the many associations concerned with sensory evaluation. Web sites in Spanish and in English also have been developed, providing an opportunity for individuals to share their interests and to seek advice (a somewhat risky step without a reasonable understanding of basic principles, but then again it comes at no cost). Nonetheless, these developments speak well for the future of sensory evaluation. ASTM Committee E-18 has been particularly active, with many pamphlets and books published (and several more in preparation). Such pamphlets and other materials have been very helpful for new professionals; but they too, come with some caveats. Some recent documents read like a cookbook with detailed recipes. This has surface appeal (all the detailed steps have a look of precision) but take no account of behavior, nor do they reflect alternative approaches, giving the impression of a static field when, in fact, it is dynamic. In some instances, the documentation was not subject to peer review but was based on the collective decisions of like-minded individuals. Nonetheless, such activities and documents are necessary if sensory evaluation is to go beyond simple tests and achieve the respect it deserves.

These activities are generally welcome, but they are not a substitute for formal academic training, and rigorous evaluation by professionals as to the relevance at their company. Individuals seeking assistance often assume that a particular method must be applied as stated in one of these documents, with no regard for the relevance of this procedure to the specific product or problem. It does not take much time or effort for guidelines to undergo a metamorphosis into restrictive rules, with disastrous consequences for a science that is not static. In many instances, the authors' intentions (when preparing these pamphlets and books) were to describe the various methods using examples of how methods might be applied (in general), but with no realization that an example would become a rule.

The past hesitancy on the part of the universities to develop an adequate curriculum has lessened and this, too, speaks to the growing importance of sensory evaluation. Because many of the supporting disciplines already exist – experimental psychology (behavior, measurement), physiology, and statistics; the addition of courses on sensory evaluation provide the student with a curriculum not easily available in the past. As more qualified professionals enter industry there is more likelihood that companies will delegate responsibility for sensory resources to individuals with the appropriate skills.

Most academic institutions have grown beyond considering sensory evaluation as a part of an allied discipline, such as flavor chemistry. Still others considered it as not much more than 3 hours of lectures in a course on quality control, of lesser interest than more laboratory-oriented scientific activities (e.g. cell biology, neurophysiology, natural products chemistry) that attract greater interest and longer-term financial support. The link with flavor (and aroma) chemistry is understandable inasmuch as the chemistry is accompanied by descriptions of the end-products in terms of their aromas and tastes. The early literature on the chemical senses devoted considerable attention to this topic (see, e.g. Moncrieff, 1951) and this trend continues (see, e.g. Harper, 1982a,b). Recent publications have provided a more comprehensive description of the use of sensory evaluation in this field and its more unique components (Fisher and Scott, 1997). Knowledge of the aroma and taste qualities of various chemicals is essential to the chemist formulating flavors and fragrances for specific application (see, e.g. Dorland and Rogers, 1977). Often this technical (expert) language was, and to some degree, still is, equated with sensory analysis leading to more confusion as to sensory's role. In recent years, more of the academic institutions and more of these companies have come to appreciate that sensory evaluation is a separate but related activity and have developed the resources and added professionals to accommodate the changes that have occurred.

Obviously, the sensory professional without formal academic training can be at a disadvantage in today's competitive business environment. First, in terms of organizing and managing testing activities, and second, in recognizing research that is directly applicable to one's own program. It is in this latter area that more discussion is warranted. There is no question that research on the physiology of the senses and studies of binding sites, etc. are essential to understanding the perceptual process at the cellular level. However, it would be inappropriate to allocate resources based on ongoing research, or to make substantive changes in an evaluation procedure without convincing evidence. Research that focuses on the mechanisms of perception are very important but the professional working in industry must deal with complex stimuli and limited timelines. For example, measuring how much of an ingredient change is possible before it is perceived relies primarily on the discrimination model. The results are very important from a business perspective. What the chemical and biological steps were or what criteria (sensory and mental processes) a subject used to reach the decision are matters that go well beyond the sensory test itself. As was mentioned in Chapter 5, the research by O'Mahony (1986), Ennis and co-workers (see, e.g. Ennis and Mullen, 1986; Ennis and Bi, 1998; Bi *et al.*, 1997; Rousseau *et al.*, 1998; Bi and Ennis, 2001; Rosseau and Ennis, 2001) has failed to demonstrate any useful links with the practical issues of difference testing and the associated decision-making process.

In the 1970s, substantial attention was given to the use of magnitude estimation, a form of ratio scaling. The technique was proposed as the correct and most sophisticated scaling technique; it would replace other scales (nominal, ordinal, and interval) in sensory evaluation and be more accurate (see Chapter 3 for more detail on scaling).

Journals publishing articles on sensory evaluation contained numerous examples of the applications for this scaling procedure. In some instances, scaling was even listed as a sensory test method in much the same way as one considered other test methods; for example, duo–trio and triangle test methods (Prell, 1976). Obviously, there was confusion as to the difference between a test method and a scale of measurement that was a part of that test method. To some extent, this confusion still exists, along side other information that ratio scaling (and specifically magnitude estimation) is not superior to other scales of measurement. It has taken several years for most sensory professionals to become aware of this literature (see Anderson, 1970, 1974; Birnbaum, 1982). While it can be argued that this "correction" reflects the strength of the science of sensory evaluation, it should also be noted that some professionals continue to use the scale in the mistaken belief that it is superior. In fairness, some have been using measurement techniques that defy description, so their switch can be understood in that context. However, it is hoped that texts such as these will be of help to those seeking alternatives for measuring perceptions covering all possible variables, known and unknown.

Multivariate methods including factor analysis, multiple regression, discriminant analysis, etc. have had a major impact in sensory evaluation (Kline, 1994; Korth, 1982; Lawless and Heymann, 1999; MacFie and Thomson, 1988; Manly, 1986; Smith, 1988). Sensory professionals welcomed the availability of the methods because of their direct applications. They provide a basis for summarizing large databases, and the ability to uncover potential underlying relationships not obvious when data are examined in a univariate way. In some environments, their use is synonymous with "cutting edge" sensory evaluation. As noted in Chapter 8, optimization and related techniques rely on use of multivariate analyses hence their importance for the health of a sensory program. However, this comes with a price; the price being a working knowledge of the methods and their limitations. Misuse of multivariate analyses is common because of the ease with which they can be used on a PC, and the availability of software that often does not come with detailed tutorials about the risks. As a result, investigators glibly use various programs that iterate until a solution is obtained without any appreciation for how it was obtained, only that a significant effect was determined. The analyses are applied to data obtained from three or four products and someone is left to implement a change that may have statistical merits but no practical value what so ever. Some of the programs will transform the data through use of normalization techniques; identify and exclude outliers and the experimenter has no way of knowing what the behavioral effects will be. This is not to intimate that the computations for these transformations are incorrect, rather they are potentially dangerous because they will lead to conclusions that are impossible to implement. In any complex analysis, there are numerous decision points that can have a significant impact on results. Investigators cannot afford to become so enamored with a specific multivariate program, that they lose sight of their limitations when extolling the virtues.

Multivariate designs and analyses enable one to study the mathematical relationships between products, sensory characteristics, and consumer attitudes that cannot be achieved by other means easily and as cost effective. The application of neural networks to sensory problems is an example of a multivariate methodology that has not yet proven itself. The methodology provides a means by which very large data sets from disparate sources (about an array of products) can be analyzed to identify relationships not realized by other means (see Bomio, 1998). The methodology incorporates fuzzy logic and essentially "learns" from previous analyses, adjusting as more data are analyzed. Such an approach will likely prove more useful in repetitive analysis situations, such as quality control, but must first prove its reliability and applicability to each situation. However, such systems do not replace the human input, as noted by Bomio. That said, it is important to remember the price for such sophistication; significantly more effort (and cost) and time at the outset. No investment is without some risk, and this risk must be assessed before making any commitment. The relative importance of this risk cannot be ignored, yet the sensory professional who has not learned the principle of sensory evaluation will probably rush to use more popular multivariate methods without taking the time to understand them, with embarrassing consequences.

Developments in the science of perception and in sensory evaluation as well as in allied sciences will continue. The sensory professional must be able to assess these developments and determine the extent to which they are applicable to their specific needs rather than adopting them with appreciating the consequences. Knowledge of the basic principles of sensory evaluation is essential to ensure that the risk of an incorrect or premature decision to incorporate these developments into their test program is minimized.

Finally, some additional comments are necessary with regard to the importance of educating managers about the science on which sensory evaluation is based. As mentioned in Chapter 2, the sensory professional must establish the basis on which a program is developed; however, information is communicated to managers, and power of sensory information. Sensory professionals must think strategically, be aware of changes in business plans, and their impact on technology, which in turn, impacts available sensory resources. Managers receive information regularly about new developments from external as well as internal sources; yet they cannot always assess the value without additional background knowledge. The externally derived development, because it comes from a manager, can put the sensory professional in a defensive situation and/or it raises questions about internal resources. Sensory professionals must keep current with the literature (made easy by access to the Internet) and with new developments that have potential applications.

New developments are often presented in workshops. As previously mentioned, one can offset lack of a formal education through workshop participation. For more than three decades, programs have been offered and have usually attracted a diverse audience. Workshops enable the individual to become familiar with the principles of testing, with appropriate tests for a particular problem, and with the potential value of new developments.

III. The Future

The future for sensory evaluation is bright, judging from the number of industry openings and the many companies that are expanding their sensory test capabilities.

While mergers and cutbacks have significantly changed the landscape, the need for product sensory information remains strong.

If sensory evaluation is to become more successful, it must move from a passive, service-oriented program to an active, results-oriented resource. This metamorphosis will require a conscious effort on the part of each sensory professional to anticipate needs and to be able to respond with minimal delay. Sensory professionals need to think and act according to their company's business plans and especially in relation to brand strategies. At the same time, those individuals who could be users of sensory evaluation must be made aware of its potential. Thus, the sensory professional not only must acquire new knowledge but also must educate others about the science. Sensory evaluation has proven beneficial for many companies and we can hope that this experience will continue to work its magic.

There is no question that sensory evaluation is a profitable investment. We think of it in terms of a one-to-ten ratio; that is, for every dollar invested in sensory, it will return ten. This kind of success occurs when sensory professionals actively participate in the business of sensory evaluation. The development and use of predictive models of consumer-product behavior has had and will continue to have a salutary impact, not only because of the specific and immediate value to a company but also because of effectiveness in demonstrating a higher degree of sophistication than was realized possible for sensory evaluation. For these reasons, we can be optimistic about the future for sensory evaluation in business and as a science. It is hoped that this book will continue to provide the impetus for the continued growth of the science, that it will stimulate more academic growth of the science, and especially that it will stimulate more recognition for the science of sensory evaluation.

References

Aaker, D. A., Kumar, V. and Day, G. S. (1995). 'Marketing Research', 5th ed. John Wiley, New York, NY.

Aaker, D. D. (1995). 'Developing Business Strategies', 4th ed. John Wiley, New York, NY.

Aaker, D. A. (1996). 'Building Strong Brands', The Free Press, New York, NY.

Alder, H. L. and Roessler, E. B. (1977). 'Introduction to Probability and Statistics,' 6th ed. Freeman, San Francisco, CA.

Amerine, M. A. and Roessler, E. B. (1983). 'Wines: Their Evaluation'. Freeman, San Francisco, CA.

Amerine, M. A., Roessler, E. B. and Filipello, F. (1959). Modern sensory methods of evaluating wine. *Hilgardia* **28**, 477–565.

Amerine, M. A., Pangborn, R. M. and Roessler, E. B. (1965). 'Principles of Sensory Evaluation of Food', Academic Press, New York, NY.

American Meat Science Association (AMSA) (1978). 'Guidelines for Cookery and Sensory Evaluation of Meat', American Meat Science Association, Chicago, IL.

American Society for Testing and Materials (ASTM) (1968). 'Manual on Sensory Testing Methods', STP 434. American Society Testing Materials, Philadelphia, PA.

Andani, Z., Jaeger, S. R., Wakeling, I. and MacFie, H. J. H. (2001). Mealiness in apples: towards a multilingual consumer vocabulary. *J. Food Sci.* **66**(6), 872–879.

Anderson, N. H. (1970). Functional measurement and psychological judgment. *Psychol. Rev.* **77**, 153–170.

Anderson, N. H. (1974). Algebraic models in perception. *In* 'Handbook of Perception' (E. C. Carterette and M. P. Friedman, eds), Vol. 2, pp. 215–298. Academic Press, New York, NY.

Anonymous (1968). 'Basic Principles of Sensory Evaluation', ASTM STP 433. American Socitey of Testing and Materials, Philadelphia, PA.

Anonymous (1975). Minutes of Division Business Meeting. Institute of Food Technologists – Sensory Evaluation Division, IFT, Chicago, IL.

Anonymous (1981a). 'Guidelines for the Selection and Training of Sensory Panel Members', STP 758. American Society Testing and Materials, Philadelphia, PA.

Anonymous (1981b). Sensory evaluation guide for testing food and beverage products. *Food Technol.* **35**(11), 50–59.

Anonymous (1984). Overview. Outstanding Symposia in Food Science & Technology. Use of computers in the sensory lab. *Food Technol.* **38**(9), 66–88.

Anonymous (1989). Playing it safe with new products. *Food Business* **March 20**, 40–42.

ASTM (1998). Standard guide for sensory claim substantiation, E-1958-98. ASTM Book of Standards, Volume 15.08, November 2003, ASTM International, West Conshohoken, PA.

ASTM (2002). Standard test method for sensory analysis – triangle test, E1985–97. 'Annual Book of ASTM Standards. 15.08., 160165', ASTM International, West Conshohoken, PA.

Aust, L. B. (1984). Computers as an aid in discrimination testing. *Food Technol.* **38**(9), 71–73.

Baker, G. A., Amerine, M. A. and Roessler, E. B. (1954). Errors of the second kind in organoleptic difference testing. *Food Res.* **19**, 205–210.

Baker, R. C., Hahn, P. W. and Robbins, K. R. (1988). 'Fundamentals of New Food Product Development'. Elsevier, Amsterdam.

Bartlett, P. N., Elliot, J. M. and Gardner, J. W. (1997). Electronic noses and their application in the food industry. *Food Technol.* **51**(12), 44–48.

Baten, W. D. (1946). Organoleptic tests pertaining to apples and pears. *Food Res.* **11**, 84–94.

Baumgardner, M. and Tatham, R. (1988). 'No preference' in paired-preference testing. *Quirk's Market. Res. Rev.*, June/July, 18–20.

Bell, R. (1993). Some unresolved issues of control in consumer tests: the effects of expected monetary reward and hunger. *J. Sensory Stud.* **8**, 329–340.

Bendig, A. W. and Hughes, J. B. (1953). Effect of amount of verbal anchoring and number of rating-scale categories upon transmitted information. *J. Exp. Psychol.* **46**, 87–90.

Bengtsson, K. and Helm, E. (1946). Principles of taste testing. *Wallerstein Lab. Commun.* **9**(28), 171–181.

Bennet, G. B., Spahr, M. and Dodds, M. L. (1956). The value of training a sensory test panel. *Food Technol.* **10**, 205–208.

Bi, J. and Ennis, D. M. (2001). Statistical models for the A–not A method. *J. Sensory Stud.* **16**, 215–237.

Bi, J. and Ennis, D. M. (2001). Exact beta-binomial tables for small experiments. *J. Sensory Stud.* **16**, 319–325.

Bi, J., Ennis, D. M. and O'Mahoney, M. (1997). How to estimate and use the variance of d' from difference tests. *J. of Sensory Studies*, **12**, 87–104.

Billmeyer, B. A. and Wyman, G. (1991). Computerized sensory evaluation system. *Food Technol.* **45**(7), 100–101.

Birnbaum, M. H. (1982). Problems with so-called 'direct' scaling. *In* 'Problems and Approaches to Hedonics' (J. T. Kuznicki, R. A. Johnson and A. F. Rutkiewick, eds) American Society for Testing and Materials, Philadelphia, PA.

Blake, S. P. (1978). 'Managing for Responsive Research and Development', Freeman, San Francisco, CA.

Bleibaum, R. N., Stone, H., Tan, T., Labreche, S., Saint-Martin, E. and Isz, S. (2002). Comparison of sensory and consumer results with electronic tongue sensors for apple juices. *Food Qual. Pref.* **13**, 409–422.

Blom, G. (1955). How many taste testers? *Wallerstein Lab. Commun.* **18**(62), 173–177.

Bock, R. D. and Jones, L. V. (1968). 'The Measurement and Prediction of Judgment and Choice', Holden-Day, San Francisco, CA.

Boelens, M. and Boelens, H. (2002). Main verbal responses during human olfaction. *Perfumer & Flavorist* **27**, 34–43.

Boggs, M. M. and Hansen, H. L. (1949). Analysis of foods by sensory difference test. *Adv. Food Res.* **2**, 219–258.

Bomio, M. (1998). Neural networks and the future of sensory evaluation. *Food Technol.* **52**(8), 62–63.

Bone, R. (1987). The importance of consumer language in developing product concepts. *Food Technol.* **41**(11), 58–60, 86.

Boring, E. G. (1950). 'A History of Experimental Psychology', 2nd ed. Appleton, New York, NY.

Box, G. E. P. (1954). The exploration and exploitation of response surfaces: some general considerations and examples. *Biometrics* **10**, 16–61.

Box, G. E. P. and Draper, N. R. (1987). 'Empirical Model-Building and Response Surfaces', John Wiley, New York, NY.

Box, G. E., Hunter, W. G. and Hunter, J. S. (1978). 'Statistics for Experimenters', John Wiley, New York, NY.

Brady, L. P. (1984). Computers in sensory research. *Food Technol.* **38**(9), 81–83.

Brady, L. P., Ketelsen, S. M. and Ketelsen, L. J. P. (1985). Computerized system for collection and analysis of sensory data. *Food Technol.* **39**(5), 82, 84, 86, 88.

Bradley, R. A. (1953). Some statistical methods in taste testing and quality evaluation. *Biometrics* **9**, 22–38.

Bradley, R. A. (1963). Some relationships among sensory difference tests. *Biometrics* **19**, 385–397.

Bradley, R. A. (1975). 'Science, Statistics, and Paired Comparisons', ONR Tech. Rep. No. 92 (Contract N00014-67-A-0235-0006). Office of Naval Research, Washington, DC.

Bradley, R. A. and Harmon, T. J. (1964). The modified triangle test. *Biometrics* **20**, 608–625.

Bradley, R. A. and Terry, M. E. (1952). The rank analysis of incomplete block designs. I. The method of paired comparison. *Biometrika* **39**, 324–345.

Brandt, F. I. and Arnold, R. G. (1977). Sensory tests used in food product development. Prod. Dev. **8**, 56.

Brandt, M. A., Skinner, E. and Coleman, J. (1963). Texture profile method. *J. Food Sci.* **28**, 404–410.

Bressan, L. P. and Behling, R. W. (1977). The selection and training of judges for discrimination testing. *Food Technol.* **31**(11), 62–67.

Bruning, J. L. and Kintz, B. L. (1987). 'Computational Handbook of Statistics', 3rd ed. Scott, Foresman & Co., Glenview, IL.

Buchanan, B., Givon, M. and Goldman, A. (1987). Measurement of discrimination ability in taste tests: an empirical investigation. *J. Market. Res.* **24**, 154–163.

Byer, A. J. and Abrams, D. (1953). A comparison of the triangular and two-sample taste-test methods. *Food Technol.* **7**, 185–187.

Cain, W. S. (1977). Differential sensitivity for smell: 'Noise' at the nose. *Science* **195**, 796–798.

Cain, W. S. and Marks, L. E. (1971). 'Stimulus and Sensation: Readings in Sensory Psychology', Little, Brown, Boston, MA.

Cairncross, W. E. and Sjöström, L. B. (1950). Flavor profile – a new approach to flavor problems. *Food Technol.* **4**, 308–311.

Cardello, A. V., Maller, D., Kapsalis, J. G., Segars, R. A., Sawyer, F. M., Murphy, C. and Moskowitz, H. R. (1982). Perception of texture by trained and consumer panels. *J. Food Sci.* **47**, 1186–1197.

Cardello, A. V. and Schutz, H. G. (1996). Food appropriateness measures as an adjunct to consumer preference/acceptability evaluation. *Food Qual. Pref.* **7**, 239–249.

Cardello, A. V. and Schutz, H. G. (2004). Sensory science II: consumer acceptance. In "Handbook of Food Science" (M. Shafiur Rahman, ed.) Marcel Dekker, New York, in press.

Carlson, K. D. (1977). New products – problems or opportunities? *Food Prod. Dev.* **11**, 34, 36–37.

Carter, C. and Riskey, D. (1990). The roles of sensory research and marketing research in bringing a product to market. *Food Technol.* **44**(11), 160–162.

Carterette, E. C. and Friedman, M. P. (1974). 'Handbook of Perception', Vol. 2, Academic Press, New York, NY.

Caul, J. F. (1957). The profile method of flavor analysis. *Adv. Food Res.* **7**, 1–40.

Chambers, E., IV and Wolf, M. B. (1996). 'Sensory Testing Methods', ASTM Manual Series: MNL 26. ASTM International, West Conshohoken, PA.

Chen, A. W., Resurreccion, A. V. A. and Paguio, L. P. (1996). Age appropriate hedonic scales to measure food preferences of young children. *J. of Sensory Studies*, **11**, 141–163.

Christensen, C. M., Vickers, Z., Fahrenholtz, S. K. and Gengler, I. M. (1988). Effect of questionnaire design on hedonic ratings. Paper No. 388, presented at the 48th Annual Meeting of the Institute of Food Technologists, New Orleans, LA, June 19–22.

Civille, G. V. and Lawless, H. T. (1986). The importance of language in describing perceptions. *J. Sensory Stud.* **1**, 203–215.

Clapperton, J. R., Dalgliesh, C. E. and Meilgaard, M. C. (1975). Progress towards an international system of beer flavor terminology. *MBAA Tech. Q.* **12**, 273–280.

Clark, R. (1991). Sensory–texture profile analysis correlation in model gels. *In* 'Fronteirs in Carbohydrate Research', 2. Purdue University.

Cloninger, M. R., Baldwin, R. E. and Krause, G. F. (1976). Analysis of sensory rating scales. *J. Food Sci.* **41**, 1225–1228.

Clurman, A. (1989). Kids are consumers. *Market. Res.* **June**, 70–71.

Cochran, W. G. and Cox, G. M. (1957). 'Experimental Designs', 2nd ed. Wiley, New York, NY.

Cohen, J. (1977). 'Statistical Power Analysis for the Behavioral Sciences', revised ed. Academic Press, New York, NY.

Cohen, E. (1993). TURF analysis. *Quirk's Market. Res. Rev.* **7**(6), 10.

Cohen, J. and Cohen, P. (1983). 'Applied Multiple Regression/Correlation Analysis for the Behavioral Sciences', 2nd ed. Lawrence Erlbaum Associates, Hillsdale, NJ.

Coombs, C. H. (1964). 'A Theory of Data', Wiley, New York, NY.

Cover, S. (1936). A new subjective method of testing tenderness in meat – the paired-eating method. *Food Res.* **1**, 287–295.

Cox, E. P., III (1980). The optimal number of response alternatives for a scale: a review. *J. Market. Res.* **17**, 407–422.

Crask, M., Fox, R. and Stout, R. G. (1995). 'Marketing Research, Principles and Applications', Prentice-Hall Inc., Englewood Cliffs, NJ.

Cross, H. R., Moen, R. and Stanfield, M. S. (1978). Training and testing of judges for sensory analysis of meat quality. *Food Technol.* **32**, 48–54.

Daniel, W. W. (1978). 'Applied Nonparametric Statistics', Houghton Mifflin, Boston, MA.

Davenport, K. (1994). NBC's television advertising review procedures and guidelines. *Food Technol.* **48**(8), 83–84.

Dawson, E. H. and Dochterman, E. F. (1951). A comparison of sensory methods of measuring differences in food qualities. *Food Technol.* **5**, 79–81.

Dawson, E. H., Brogdon, J. L. and McManus, S. (1963a). Sensory testing of differences in taste. I. Methods. *Food Technol.* **17**(9), 45–48, 51.

Dawson, E. H., Brogdon, J. L. and McManus, S. (1963b). Sensory testing of differences in taste. II. Selection of panel members. *Food Technol.* **17**(10), 39–41, 43–44.

Day, R. L. (1974). Measuring preferences. *In* 'Handbook of Marketing Research' (R. Ferber, ed.), Part A. pp. 31-101–3-125.

Dember, W. N. (1963). 'The Psychology of Perception', Holt, New York, NY.

Dorland, W. E. and Rogers, J. A., Jr. (1977). 'The Flavor and Fragrance Industry', W. E. Dorland, Mendham, NJ.

Downs, P. A., Anderson, E. O., Babcock, C. T., Herzer, F. H. and Trout, G. M. (1954). Evaluation of collegiate student dairy products judging since World War II. *J. Dairy Sci.* **34**, 1021–1026.

Draper, N. and Smith, H. (1981). 'Applied Regression Analysis', 2nd ed. Wiley, New York, NY.

Duncan, A. J. (1974). 'Quality Control and Industrial Statistics', 4th ed. R. D. Irwin, Inc., Homewood, IL.

Edelstein, J. S. (1994). Supporting and challenging advertising claims with consumer perception studies. *Food Technol.* **48**(8), 79–80, 82.

Eggert, J. (1989). Sensory strategy for success in the food industry. *J. Sensory Stud.* **3**, 161–167.

Eggert, J. and Zook, K. (eds) (1986). 'Physical Requirement Guidelines for Sensory Evaluation Laboratories', ASTM STP 913. American Society Testing and Materials, Philadelphia, PA.

Eisler, H. (1963a). How prothetic is the continum of smell? *Scand. J. Psychol.* **4**, 29–32.

Eisler, H. (1963b). Magnitude scales, category scales, and Fechnerian intergration. *Psychol. Rev.* **70**, 243–253.

Ekman, G. and Sjöberg, L. (1965). Scaling. *Annu. Rev. Psychol.* **16**, 451–474.

Ellis, B. H. (1966). 'Guide Book for Sensory Testing', 2nd ed. Continental Can Co., Chicago, IL.

Engel, J. F., Blackwell, R. D. and Miniard, P. W. (1995). Consumer Behavior, 8th Ed., Harcourt Brace & Co., Orlando, FL 32887.

Engen, T. (1960). Effect of practice and instruction on olfactory thresholds. *Percept. Motor Skills* **10**, 195–198.

Engen, T. (1971). Psychophysics. II. *In* 'Scaling Methods in Experimental Psychology', 3rd ed. (J. W. Kling and L. A. Rigg, eds), pp. 47–86. Holt, New York, NY.

Ennis, D. M. (1993). The power of sensory discrimination methods. *J. Sensory Stud.* **8**, 353–370.

Ennis, D. M. and Bi, J. (1998). The beta-binomial model: accounting for inter-trial variation in replicated difference and preference tests. *J. Sensory Stud.*, **13**, 389–412.

Ennis, D. M., Boelens, H., Haring, H. and Bowman, P. (1982). Multivariate analysis in sensory evaluation. *Food Technol.* **36**(11), 83–90.

Ennis, D. M. and Mullen, K. (1985). The effect of dimensionality on results from the triangular method. *Chem. Senses* **10**, 605–608.

Ennis, D. M. and Mullen, K. (1986). Theoretical aspects of sensory discrimination. *Chem. Senses* **11**, 513–522.

Ferdinandus, A., Oosterom-Kleijngeld, I. and Runneboom, A. J. M. (1970). Taste testing. *MBAA Tech. Q.* **7**, 210–227.

Fern, E. F. (1982). The use of focus groups for idea generation: The effects of group size, acquaintanceship and moderator on response quantity and quality. *J. Market. Res.* **19**, 1–13.

Ferrier, J. G. and Block, D. E. (2001). Neural-network-assisted optimization of wine blending based on sensory analysis. *Am. J. Enol. Vitic.* **52**(4), 386–395.

Fisher, C. and Scott, T. R. (1997). 'Food Flavours: Biology and Chemistry', The Royal Society of Chemistry, Cambridge, UK.

Fleiss, J. L. (1981). 'Statistical Methods for Rates and Proportions', 2nd ed. Wiley, New York, NY.

Friedman, M. (1990). Twenty-five years later and 98,900 new products later. *Prep. Foods New Products Ann.* **159**(8), 23–25.

Fritjers, J. E. R. (1980). Three-stimulus procedures in olfactory psychophysics: an experimental comparison of Thurstone-Ura and three-alternative forced-choice models of signal detection theory. *Percept. Psychophys.* **28**, 390–397.

Fritjers, J. E. R. (1988). Sensory difference testing and the measurement of sensory discriminability. *In* 'Sensory Analysis of Foods', 2nd ed. (J. R. Piggott, ed.), pp. 131–153. Elsevier Applied Science, London.

Fritjers, J. E. R. Blauw, Y. H. and Vermoaat, S. H. (1982). Incidental training in the triangular method. *Chem. Senses* **7**, 63–69.

Fulks, F. T. (1991). Total quality management. *Food Technol.* **45**(6) 96, 98, 99–101.
Fuller, G. W. (1994). 'New Food Product Development: From Concept to Marketplace'. CRC Press, Boca Rotan, FL.
Gacula, M. C., Jr. (1975). The design of experiments for shelf life study. *J. Food Sci.* **40**, 399–403.
Gacula, M. C., Jr. (1978). Analysis of incomplete block designs with reference samples in every block. *J. Food Sci.* **43**, 1461–1466.
Gacula, M. C., Jr. (1993). 'Design and Analysis of Sensory Optimization'. Food and Nutrition Press, Trumbull, CT.
Gacula, M. C., Jr. and Kubala, J. J. (1975). Statistical models for shelf life failures. *J. Food Sci.* **40**, 404–409.
Gacula, M. C., Jr. and Singh, J. (1984). 'Statistical Methods in Food and Consumer Research.' Academic Press, Orlando, FL.
Garner, W. R. (1960). Rating scales, discriminability, and information transmission. *Psychol. Rev.* **67**, 343–352.
Garner, W. R. and Hake, H. W. (1951). The amount of information in absolute judgments. *Psychol. Rev.* **58**, 446–459.
Geldard, F. A. (1972). 'The Human Senses', 2nd ed. Wiley, New York, NY.
Giovanni, M. E. and Pangborn, R. M. (1983). Measurement of taste intensity and degree of liking of beverages by graphic scales and magnitude estimation. *J. Food Sci.* **48**, 1175–1182.
Giradot, N. E., Peryam, D. R. and Shapiro, R. (1952). Selection of sensory testing panels. *Food Technol.* **6**, 140–143.
Goldman, A. E. and McDonald, S. S. (1987). 'The Group Depth Interview', Prentice-Hall, Inc. Englewood Cliffs, NJ.
Gordin, H. H. (1987). Intensity variation descriptive methodology: development and application of a new sensory evaluation technique. *J. Sensory Stud.* **2**, 187–198.
Gorman, B. (1990). New products for a new century. *Prep. Foods New Products Ann.* **159**(8), 16–18.
Graf, E. and Saguy, I. S. (1991). 'Food Product Development: From Concept to the Marketplace' (E. Graf and I. S. Saguy, eds), Van Nostrand, New York, NY.
Granit, R. (1955). 'Receptors and Sensory Perception', Yale Press, New Haven, CT.
Green, D. M. and Swets, J. A. (1966). 'Signal Detection Theory and Psychophysics', Wiley, New York, NY.
Green, B. G., Shaffer, G. S. and Gilmore, M. M. (1993). Derivation and evaluation of a semantic scale of oral sensation magnitude with apparent ratio properties. *Chem. Senses.* **18**, 683–702.
Greene, P. E. and Carmone, F. J. (1970). 'Multidimensional Scaling and Related Techniques in Marketing Analysis', Allyn & Bacon, Inc., Boston, MA.
Gridgeman, N. T. (1955a). The Bradley–Terry probability model and preference testing. *Biometrics* **11**, 335–343.
Gridgeman, N. T. (1955b). Taste comparisons: two samples or three. *Food Technol.* **9**, 148–150.
Gridgeman, N. T. (1958). Psychophysical bias in taste testing by pair comparison, with special reference to position and temperature. *Food Res.* **23**, 217–220.

Gridgeman, N. T. (1959). Pair comparison, with and without ties. *Biometrics* **15**, 382–388.

Gridgeman, N. T. (1964). Sensory comparisons: The 2-stage triangle test with sample variability. *J. Food Sci.* **29**, 112–117.

Gridgeman, N. T. (1984). Tasting panels: sensory assessment in quality control. *In* 'Quality Control in the Food Industry' (S. M. Herschdeorfer, ed.), pp. 299–349. Academic Press, London.

Guilford, J. P. (1954). 'Psychometric Methods', 2nd ed. McGraw-Hill, New York, NY.

Guinard, J. -X., Pangborn, R. M. and Shoemaker, C. F. (1985). Computerized procedure for time-intensity sensory measurements. *J. Food Sci.* **50**, 543–544, 546.

Gunst, R. F. and Mason, R. L. (1980). 'Regression Analysis and Its Application: A Data-Oriented Approach', Dekker, New York, NY.

Hall, R. L. (1958). Flavor study approaches at McCormick and Co., Inc. *In* 'Flavor Research and Food Acceptance', (A. D. Little, ed.), pp. 224–240. Reinhold-Van Nostrand, Princeton, NJ.

Hanson, J. E., Kendall, D. A., Smith, N. F. and Hess, A. P. (1983). The missing link: correlation of consumer and professional sensory descriptions. *Beverage World* **Nov.** 108–115.

Harper, R. M. (1950). Assessment of food products. *Food* **19**, 371–375.

Harper, R. M. (1972). 'Human Senses in Action', Churchill-Livingstone, Edinburgh and London.

Harper, R. M. (1982a). Art and science in the understanding of flavour. *Food Flavour Ingredients Pack. Process.* **4**(1), 13–15, 17, 19, 21.

Harper, R. M. (1982b). Art and science in the understanding of flavour. *Food Flavour Ingredients Pack. Process.* **4**(2), 17–19, 21, 23.

Harries, J. M. (1956). Positional bias in sensory assessments. *Food Technol.* **10**, 86–90.

Harrison, S. and Elder, L. W. (1950). Some applications of statistics to laboratory taste testing. *Food Technol.* **4**, 434–439.

Hays, W. L. (1973). 'Statistics for the Social Sciences', 2nd ed. Holt, New York, NY.

Helm, E. and Trolle, B. (1946). Selection of a taste panel. *Wallerstein Lab. Commun.* **9**(28), 181–194.

Henika, R. G. (1972). Simple and effective system for use with response surface methodology. *Cereal Sci. Today* **17**(10), 309–314, 334.

Henika, R. G. (1982). Use of response-surface methodology in sensory evaluation. *Food Technol.* **36**(11), 96–101.

Henry, J. and Walker, D. (1994). 'Managing Innovation', Sage, Thousand Oaks, CA.

Herschdoerfer, S. M. (1984). Quality Control in the Food Industry. Vol. 1, 2nd Ed., Academic Press, London NW1 7DX.

Hinreiner, E. H. (1956). Organoleptic evaluation by industry panels – the cutting bee. *Food Technol.* **31**(11), 62–67.

Hollander, M. and Wolfe, D. A. (1973). 'Nonparametric Statistical Methods', Wiley, New York, NY.

Hootman, R. C. (ed.) (1992). Manual on Descriptive Analysis Testing for Sensory Evaluation. *Amer. Soc. For Test. & Materials.* MNL 13, Philadelphia, PA 19103.

Hopkins, J. W. (1954). Some observations on sensitivity and repeatability of triad taste difference tests. *Biometrics* **10**, 521–530.

Hopkins, J. W. and Gridgeman, N. T. (1955). Comparative sensitivity of pair and triad flavor intensity difference tests. *Biometrics* **11**, 63–68.

Horsfield, S. and Taylor, L. J. (1976). Exploring the relationship between sensory data and acceptability of meat. *J. Sci. Food Agric.* **27**, 1044–1053.

Hubbard, M. R. (1996). 'Statistical Quality Control for the Food Industry', 2nd ed., pp. 161–173. Van Nostrand Reinhold, New York, NY.

Hughes, G. D. (1974). The measurement of beliefs and attitudes. *In* 'Handbook of Marketing Research' (R. Ferber, ed.), pp. 3–16. McGraw-Hill, New York, NY.

Huitson, A. (1989). Problems with procrustes analysis. *J. Appl. Stat.* **16**, 39–45.

Inglett, G. E. (1974). 'Symposium: Sweeteners', Avi Publishing Company, Wesport, CT.

Ishii, R. and O'Mahony, M. (1990). Group taste concept measurement: verbal and physical definition of the umami taste concept for Japanese and Americans. *J. Sensory Stud.* **4**, 215–227.

Ishii, R. and O'Mahony, M. (1991). Use of multiple standards to define sensory characteristics for descriptive analysis: aspects of concept formation. *J. Food Sci.* **56**, 838–842.

Jackson, R. A. (2002). 'Wine Tasting: A Professional Handbook', Academic Press, San Diego, CA.

Jellinek, G. (1964). Introduction to and critical review of modern methods of sensory analysis (odour, taste and flavour evaluation) with special emphasis on descriptive sensory analysis (flavour profile method). *J. Nutr. Diet.* **1**, 219–260.

Joanes, D. (1985). On a rank sum test due to Kramer. *J. Food Sci.* **50**, 1442–1444.

Johnson, P. B. and Civille, G. V. (1986). A standard lexicon of meat WOF descriptors. *J. Sensory Stud.* **1**, 99–104.

Johnson, R. M. (1973). 'Simultaneous Measurement of Discrimination and Preference', Market Facts, Inc., Chicago, IL.

Jones, F. N. (1958). Prerequisites for test environment. *In* 'Flavor Research and Food Acceptance' (A. D. Little, ed.), pp. 107–111. Van Nostrand-Reinhold, Princeton, NJ.

Jones, L. V., Peryam, D. R. and Thurstone, L. L. (1955). Development of a scale for measuring soldiers' food preferences. *Food Res.* **20**, 512–520.

Kamen, J. M., Peryam, D. R., Peryam, D. B. and Kroll, B. J. (1969). Hedonic differences as a function of number of samples evaluated. *J. Food Sci.* **34**, 475–479.

Kamenetzky, J. (1959). Contrast and convergence effects in ratings of foods. *J. Appl. Psychol.* **43**, 47–52.

Kimmel, S. A., Sigman-Grant, M. and Guinard, J- X. (1994). Sensory testing with young children. *Food Technol.* **48**(3), 92–94, 96–99.

Kline, P. (1994). 'An Easy Guide to Factor Analysis', Routledge, London.

Korth, B. (1982). Use of regression in sensory evaluation. *Food Technol.* **36**(11), 91–95.

Kramer, A. (1960). A rapid method for determining significance of differences from rank sums. *Food Technol.* **10**, 576–581.

Kramer, A. (1963). Revised tables for determining significance differences. *Food Technol.* **17**, 124–125.

Kramer, A. and Twigg, B. A. (1970). 'Quality Control for the Food Industry', 3rd ed. Vol. I. Avi Publishing Company, Westport, CT.

Kroll, B. J. (1990). Evaluating rating scales for sensory testing with children. *Food Technol.* **44**(11), 78–86.

Krzanowski, W. J. (1988). 'Principles of Multivariate Analysis', Oxford University Press, Oxford.

Labovitz, S. (1970). The assignment of numbers to rank order categories. *Am. Soc. Rev.* **36**, 515–524.

Laming, D. (1986). 'Sensory Analysis', Academic Press, Orlando, FL.

Land, D. G. and Shepherd, R. (1988). Scaling and ranking methods. *In* 'Sensory Analysis of Foods', 2nd ed. (J. R. Piggott, ed.), pp. 155–185. Elsevier Applied Science, London.

Larson-Powers, N. and Pangborn, R. M. (1978). Descriptive analysis of the sensory properties of beverages and gelatins containing sucrose or synthetic sweeteners. *J. Food Sci.* **43**, 42–51.

Laue, E. A., Ishler, N. H. and Baltman, G. A. (1954). Reliability of taste testing and consumer testing methods. *Food Technol.* **8**, 387–388.

Lawless, H. T. (1989). Logarithmic transformation of magnitude estimation data and comparisons of scaling methods. *J. Sensory Stud.* **4**, 75–86.

Lawless, H. T. and Malone, G. J. (1986a). The discriminative efficiency of common scaling methods. *J. Sensory Stud.* **1**, 85–98.

Lawless, H. T. and Malone, G. J. (1986b). A comparison of rating scales: sensitivity, replicates and relative measurement. *J. Sensory Stud.* **1**, 155–174.

Lawless, H. T. and Heymann, H. (1999). 'Sensory Evaluation of Food Principles and Practices', Aspen Publishers, Inc. Gaithersburg, MD.

Lawless, H. T., Horne, J. and Spiers, W. (2000). Contrast and range effects for category, magnitude and labeled magnitude scales in judgements of sweetness intensity. *Chem. Senses* **25**, 85–92.

Lieb, M. E. (1989). Playing it safe with new products. *Food Business* **2**, (March 20) 40–42.

Lindquist, E. F. (1953). 'Design and Analysis of Experiments in Psychology and Education', Houghton Mifflin, Boston, MA.

Lockhart, E. E. (1951). Binomial systems and organoleptic analysis. *Food Technol.* **5**, 428–431.

Lotong, V., Chambers, D. H., Dus, C., Chambers, E., IV and Civille, G. V. (2001). Matching results of two independent highly trained panels using different descriptive analysis methods. Presented at The 4th Pangborn Sensory Science Symposium '2001: A Sense Odyssey. Dijon, France.

Luce, R. D. and Edwards, W. (1958). The derivation of subjective scales from just noticeable differences. *Psychol. Rev.* **65**, 222–237.

Lyon, B. G. (1987). Development of chicken flavor descriptive attribute terms aided by multivariate statistical procedures. *J. Sensory Stud.* **2**, 55–67.

Lyon, C. E., Lyon, G. B., Townsend, W. E. and Wilson, R. L. (1978). Effect of level of structured protein fiber on quality of mechanically deboned chicken meat patties. *J. Food Sci.* **43**, 1524–1527.

Lyon, D. H., Francombe, M. A., Hasdell, T. A. and Lawson, K. (1992). 'Guidelines for Sensory Analysis in Food Product Development and Quality Control'. Chapman & Hall, London.

MacFie, H. J. H. and Thomson, D. M. H. (1988). Preference mapping and multidimensional scaling. *In* 'Sensory Analysis of Foods', 2nd ed. (J. R. Piggot, ed.), pp. 381–409. Elsevier Applied Science, London.

Mackey, A. O. and Jones, P. (1954). Selection of members of a food tasting panel: Discernment of primary tastes in water solution compared with judging ability for foods. *Food Technol.* **8**, 527–530.

Mahoney, C. H., Stier, H. L. and Crosby, E. A. (1957). Evaluating flavor differences in canned foods. I. Genesis of the simplified procedure for making flavor difference tests. *Food Technol.* **11**, 29–41.

Manly, B. F. J. (1986). 'Multivariate Statistical Methods: A Primer', Chapman and Hall, New York, NY.

Manoski, P. and Gantwerker, S. (2002a). Managing the new product development process. Part 1. Food Process., **64**(5), 48, 50–51.

Manoski, P. and Gantwerker, S. (2002b). Managing the new product development process. Part 2. Food Processing, **64**(6), 40, 42, 44, 46.

Marks, L. E. (1974). On scales of sensation: Prolegomena to any future psychophysics that will be able to come forth as science. *Percept. Psychophys.* **16**, 358–376.

Martens, M. and Martens, H. (1986). Partial least squares regression. *In* 'Statistical Procedures in Food Research', (J. R. Piggott, ed.), Elsevier Applied Science, London.

Marshall, R. J. and Kirby, S. P. J. (1988). Sensory measurement of food texture by free-choice profiling. *J. Sensory Stud.* **3**, 63–80.

Marx, M. H. and Hillix, W. A. (1963). 'Systems and Theories in Psychology', McGraw-Hill, New York, NY.

McBride, R. L. and Hall, C. (1979). Cheese grading versus consumer acceptability: an inevitable discrepancy. *Aust. J. Dairy Technol.* **34**, 66–68.

McBride, R. L. and Laing, D. G. (1979). Threshold determination by triangle testing: effect of judgmental procedure, positional bias and incidental training. *Chem. Senses Flav.* **4**, 319–326.

McBride, R. L. (1983). A JND-scale/category-scale convergence in taste. *Percept & Psychophys.* **34**, 77–83.

McBride, R. (1990). 'The Bliss Point Factor', Macmillan Company of Australia, South Melbourne.

McBride, R. L. and MacFie, H. J. H. (eds) (1990). 'Psychological Basis of Sensory Evaluation', Elsevier Science Publishing, New York, NY.

McCall, R. B. (1975). 'Fundamental Statistics for Psychology', 2nd ed. Harcourt Brace Jovanovich, Inc., New York, NY.

McDaniel, M. R. and Sawyer, F. M. (1981). Preference testing of whiskey sour formulation: magnitude estimation versus the 9-point hedonic. *J. Food Sci.* **46**, 182–185.

McDermott, B. J. (1990). Identifying consumers and consumer test subjects. *Food Technol.* **44**(11), 154–158.

McLellan, M. R. and Cash, J. N. (1983). Computerized sensory evaluation: a prototype data-collection system. *Food Technol.* **37**(1), 97–99.

McNemar, Q. (1969). 'Psychological Statistics', 4th ed. Wiley, New York, NY.

Meilgaard, M., Civille, G. V. and Carr, B. T. (1999). 'Sensory Evaluation Techniques', 3rd ed. CRC Press, Inc. Boca Raton, FL.

Meiselman, H. L., Waterman, D. and Symington, L. E. (1974). 'Armed Forces Food Preferences', Tech, Rep. 75-63-FSL. US Army Natick Dev. Cent., Natick, MA.

Meiselman, H. L. and MacFie, H. J. H. (eds) (1996). 'Food Choice, Acceptance and Consumption', Chapman & Hall, New York, NY.

Meiselman, H. L. and Schutz, H. G. (2003). History of food acceptance research in the US Army. *Appetite*, **40**(3), 199–216.

Mela, D. J. (1989). A research note: a comparison of single and concurrent evaluations of sensory and hedonic attributes. *J. Food Sci.* **54**, 1098–1100.

Meyer, R. S. (1984). Eleven stages of successful new product development. *Food Technol.* **38**(7), 71–78, 98.

Miller, I. (1978). Statistical treatment of flavor data. *In* 'Flavor: Its Chemical, Behavioral and Commercial Aspects' (C. M. Apt, ed.), pp. 149–159. Westview Press, Boulder, CO.

Moncrieff, R. W. (1951). 'The Chemical Senses', Leonard Hill, London.

Morgan, C. T. and Stellar, E. (1950). 'Physiological Psychology', 2nd ed. McGraw-Hill, New York, NY.

Morrison, D. F. (1990). Multivariate Statistical Methods, 3rd ed. McGraw-Hill Publishing Co., New York, NY.

Morrison, D. G. (1981). Triangle taste tests: are the subjects who respond correctly lucky or good? *J. Market.* **45**, 111–119.

Mosher, H. A., Dutton, H. J., Evens, C. D. and Cowan, J. C. (1950). Conducting a taste panel for the evaluation of edible oils. *Food Technol.* **4**, 105–109.

Moskowitz, H. R. (1972). Subjective ideals and sensory optimization in evaluating perceptual dimensions in food. *J. Appl. Psychol.* **56**, 60–66.

Moskowitz, H. R. (1975). Applications of sensory measurement to food evaluations. II. Methods of ratio scaling. *Lebens.-Wiss. Technol.*, **8**, 249–254.

Moskowitz, H. R. (1980). Product optimization as a tool in product planning. *Drug Cosmet. Ind.* **126**(6), 48, 50, 52, 54, 124–126.

Moskowitz, H. R. and Sidel, J. L. (1971). Magnitude and hedonic scales of food accept ability. *J. Food Sci.* **36**, 677–680.

Moskowitz, H. R., Jacobs, B. and Firtle, N. (1980). Discrimination testing and product decisions. *J. Market. Res.* **17**(2), 35–43.

Mullen, K. and Ennis, D. M. (1979). Rotatable designs in product development. *Food Technol.* **33**(7), 74–75, 78–80.

Mullet, G. M. (1988). Applications of multivariate methods in strategic approaches to product marketing and promotion. *Food Technol.* **42**(11), 145, 152, 153, 155, 156.

Muñoz, A. M. (1986). Development and application of texture reference scales. *J. Sensory Stud.* **1**, 55–83.

Myers, J. L. (1979). 'Fundamentals of Experimental Design', 3rd ed. Allyn & Bacon, Inc., Boston, MA.

Nakayama, M. and Wessman, C. (1979). Application of sensory evaluation to the routine maintenance of product quality. *Food Technol.* **33**(9), 38–39.

Newell, G. J. and MacFarlane, J. D. (1987). Expanded tables for multiple comparison procedures in the analysis of ranked data. *J. Food Sci.* **52**, 1721–1725.

Noble, A. (1975). Instrumental analysis of the sensory properties of food. *Food Technol.* **29**(11), 56–60.

Noble, A. C., Arnold, R. A., Buechsenstein, J., Leach, E. J., Schmidt, J. O. and Stern, P. M. (1987). Modification of a standardized system of wine aroma terminology. *Am. J. Enol. Vitric.* **38**, 143–151.

Nunnally, J. C. (1978). 'Psychometric Theory', 2nd ed. McGraw-Hill, New York, NY.

O'Mahony, M. (1979). Short-cut signal detection measures for sensory analysis. *J. Food Sci.* **44**, 302–303.

O'Mahony, M. (1982). Some assumptions and difficulties with common statistics for sensory analysis. *Food Technol.* **36**(11), 75–82.

O'Mahony, M. (1986). 'Sensory Evaluation of Food', Marcel Dekker, Inc, New York, NY.

O'Mahony, M., Kulp, J. and Wheeler, L. (1979). Sensory detection of off-flavors in milk incorporating short-cut signal detection measures. *J. Dairy Sci.* **62**, 1857–1864.

O'Mahony, M., Garske, S. and Klapman, K. (1980). Rating and ranking procedures for short-cut signal detection multiple difference tests. *J. Food Sci.* **45**, 392–393.

O'Mahony, M., Rathman, L., Ellison, T., Shaw, D. and Buteau, L. (1990). Taste descriptive analysis: concept formation, alignment and appropriateness. *J. Sensory Stud.* **5**, 71–103.

O'Mahony, M., Thieme, V. and Goldstein, L. R. (1988). The warm-up effect as a means of increasing the discriminability of sensory difference tests. *J. Food Sci.* **53**, 1848–1850.

Orne, M. T. (1981). The significance of unwitting cues for experimental outcomes: toward a pragmatic approach. *In* 'The Clever Hans Phenomenon: Communication with Horses, Whales, Apes, and People', *Ann. NY Acad. Sci.* **364**, 152–159.

Pangborn, R. M. (1964). Sensory evaluation of foods: a look backward and forward. *Food Technol.* **18**(9), 63–67.

Pangborn, R. M. (1979). Physiological and psychological misadventures in sensory measurement or the crocodiles are coming. *In* 'Sensory Evaluation Methods for the Practicing Food Technologists' (M. R. Johnson, ed.), pp. 2-1–2-22. Institute of Food Technologists, Chicago, IL.

Pangborn, R. M. (1980). Sensory science today. *Cereal Foods World* **25**(10), 637–640.

Pangborn, R. M. and Dunkley, W. L. (1964). Laboratory procedures for evaluating the sensory properties of milk. *Dairy Sci. Abs.* **26**, 55–62.

Pangborn, R. M. Guinard, J. X. and Meiselman, H. L. (1989). Evaluation of bitterness of caffeine in hot chocolate drink by category, graphic, and ratio scaling. *J. Sensory Stud.* **4**, 31–53.

Passman, N. (1994). Support advertising superiority claims with taste tests. *Food Technol.* **48**(8), 71–72, 74.

Payne, S. L. (1965). Are open-ended questions worth the effort? *J. Market. Res.* **10**, 417–419.

Pearce, J. H., Korth, B. and Warren, C. B. (1986). Evaluation of three scaling methods for hedonics. *J. Sensory Stud.* **1**, 27–46.

Pecore, S. D. (1984). Computer-assisted consumer testing. *Food Technol.* **38**(9), 78–80.

Perfetti, T. A. and Gordin, H. H. (1985). Just noticeable difference studies of mentholated cigarette products. *Tob. Sci.* **57**, 20–29.

Peryam, D. R. and Haynes, J. H. (1957). Prediction of soldiers' food preferences by laboratory methods. *J. Appl. Psychol.* **41**, 2–6.

Peryam, D. R. and Pilgrim, F. J. (1957). Hedonic scale method of measuring food preferences. *Food Technol.* **11**(9), 9–14.

Peryam, D. R. and Swartz, V. W. (1950). Measurement of sensory differences. *Food Technol.* **4**, 390–395.

Peryam, D. R., Pilgrim, F. J. and Peterson, M. S. (eds) (1954). 'Food Acceptance Testing Methodology', National Academy of Sciences – National Research Council, Washington, DC.

Peryam, D. R., Polemis, B. W., Kamen, J. M., Eindhoven, J. and Pilgrim, F. J. (1960). 'Food Preferences of Men in the Armed Forces', Quartermaster Food and Container Institute of the Armed Forces, Chicago, IL.

Peryam, D. R. (1991). A history of ASTM Committee E-18. ASTM Standard. *News* **19**(3), 28–35.

Petty, M. F. and Scriven, F. M. (1991). The use of Fourier analysis to compare the sensory profiles of products. *J. Sensory Stud.* **6**, 17–23.

Pfaffman, C., Schlosberg, H. and Cornsweet, J. (1954). Variables affecting difference tests. *In* 'Food Acceptance Testing Methodology' (D. R. Peryam, F. J. Pilgrim and M. S. Peterson, eds), pp. 4–17. National Academy of Sciences – National Research Council, Washington, DC.

Phillips, J. L., Jr. (1973). 'Statistical Thinking', Freeman, San Francisco, CA.

Piggot, J. R. (ed.) (1988). 'Sensory Analysis of Foods', 2nd ed. Elsevier Applied Science, London.

Pilgrim, F. J. and Wood, K. R. (1955). Comparative sensitivity of rating scale and paired comparison methods for measuring consumer preference. *Food Technol.* **9**, 385–387.

Popper, R. and Kroll, J. J. (2003). Conducting sensory research with children. *Food Technol.* **57**(5), 60–65.

Powers, J. J., Warren, C. B. and Masurat, T. (1981). Collaborative trials involving three methods of normalizing magnitude estimations. *Lebensm.-Wiss. Technol.* **14**, 86–93.

Powers, J. J. (1988). Current practices and applications of descriptive methods. *In* 'Sensory Analysis of Foods', 2nd ed. (J. R. Piggot, ed.), pp. 187–266. Elsevier Applied Science, London.

Poynder, T. M. (ed.) (1974). 'Transduction Mechanisms in Chemoreception', Information Retrieval Ltd., London.

Prell, P. A. (1976). Preparation of reports and manuscripts which include sensory evaluation data. *Food Technol.* **30**(11), 40–47.

Prince, G. M. (1970). 'The Practice of Creativity', Harper & Row, New York, NY.

Radkins, A. P. (1957). Some statistical considerations in organoleptic research: triangle, paired, duo–trio tests. *Food Res.* **22**, 259–265.

Radkins, A. P. (1958). Sequential analysis in organoleptic research: triangle, paired, duo–trio tests. *Food Res.* **23**, 225–234.

Rainey, B. A. (1986). Importance of reference standards in training panelists. *J. Sensory Stud.* **1**, 149–154.

Read, J. (1994). Role of marketing research in claims testing. *Food Technol.* **48**(8), 75–77.

Resurreccion, A. V. A. (1988). Applications of multivariate methods in food quality evaluation. *Food Technol.* **42**(11), 128, 130, 132–134, 136.

Resurreccion, A. V. A. (1998). 'Consumer Sensory Testing for Product Development', Aspen Publishers, Inc., Gaithesburg, MD.

Roessler, E. B., Warren, J. and Guymon, J. F. (1948). Significance in triangular taste tests. *Food Res.* **13**, 503–505.

Roessler, E. B., Baker, G. A. and Amerine, M. A. (1953). Corrected normal and chi-square approximations to the binomial distribution in organoleptic tests. *Food Res.* **18**, 625–627.

Roessler, E. B., Baker, G. A. and Amerine, M. A. (1956). One-tailed and two-tailed tests in organoleptic comparisons. *Food Res.* **21**, 117–121.

Roessler, E. B., Pangborn, R. M., Sidel, J. L. and Stone, H. (1978). Expanded statistical tables for estimating significance in paired-preference, paired-difference, duo–trio and triangle tests. *J. Food Sci.* **43**, 940–943.

Roper, G. (1989). Research with marketing's paradoxical subjects: children. *Market. Res.* **June**, 16–23.

Rousseau, B. and Ennis, D. M. (2001). A Thurstonian model for the dual pair (4IAX) discrimination method. *Percept. Psychophys.* **63**, 1083–1090.

Rousseau, B., Meyer, A. and O'Mahony, M. (1998). Power and sensitivity of the same–different test: comparison with triangle and duo–trio methods. *J. Sensory Stud.* **13**, 149–173.

Rousseau, B., Stroh, S. and O'Mahony, M. (2002). Investigating more powerful discrimination tests with consumers: effects of memory and response bias. *Food Qual. Pref.* **13**, 39–45.

Russell, G. F. (1984). Some basic considerations in computerizing the sensory laboratory. *Food Technol.* **38**(9), 67–70, 77.

Rutledge, K. P. and Hudson, J. M. (1990). Sensory evaluation: method for establishing and training a descriptive flavor analysis panel. *Food Technol.* **44**(12), 78–84.

Ryan, T. A. (1959). Multiple comparisons in psychological research. *Psychol. Bull.* **56**, 26–47.

Ryan, T. A. (1960). Significance tests for multiple comparisons of proportions, variances, and other statistics. *Psychol. Bull.* **57**, 318–328.

Savoca, M. R. (1984). Computer applications in descriptive testing. *Food Technol.* **38**(9), 74–77.

Sawyer, F. M., Stone, H., Abplanalp, H. and Stewart, G. F. (1962). Repeatability estimates in sensory-panel selection. *J. Food Sci.* **27**, 386–393.

Scheffé, H. (1952). An analysis of variance for paired comparisons. *J. Am. Stat. Assoc.* **47**, 381–400.

Schiffman, S. S., Reynolds, M. L. and Young, F. W. (1981). 'Introduction to Multidimensional Scaling: Theory, Methods, and Applications', Academic Press, New York, NY.

Schlich, P. (1993). Risk tables for discrimination tests. *J. Food Qual. Pref.* **4**, 141–151.

Schlosberg, H., Pfaffmann, C., Cornsweet, J. and Pierrel, R. (1954). Selection and training of panels. *In* 'Food Acceptance Testing Methodology'. (D. R. Peryam, J. J. Pilgrim and M. S. Peterson, eds), pp. 45–54, National Academy of Sciences – National Research Council, Washington, DC.

Schutz, H. G. (1954). Effect of bias on preference in the difference–preference test. *In* 'Food Acceptance Testing Methodology' (D. R. Peryam, F. J. Pilgrim and M. S. Peterson, eds.), pp. 85–91. National Academy of Sciences – National Research Council, Washington, DC.

Schutz, H. G. (1965). A food action rating scale for measuring food acceptance. *J. Food Sci.* **30**, 365–374.

Schutz, H. G. (1988). Beyond preference: appropriateness as a measure of contextual acceptance of food. *In* 'Food Acceptability' (D. M. H. Thomson, ed.), pp. 115–134. Elsevier Applied Science, London.

Schutz, H. G. (1990). Measuring the relative importance of sensory attributes and analytical measurements of consumer acceptance. *ISHS Acta Hort.* **259**, 173–174.

Schutz, H. G. and Pilgrim, F. J. (1957). Differential sensitivity in gustation. *J. Exp. Psychol.* **54**, 41–48.

Schutz, H. G., Damrell, J. D. and Locke, B. H. (1972). Predicting hedonic ratings of raw carrot texture by sensory analysis. *J. Text. Stud.* **3**, 227–232.

Schutz, H. G. (1983). Multiple regression approach to optimization. *Food Technol.* **37**(11), 46–48, 62.

Schutz, H. G. (1988). Multivariate analyses and the measurement of consumer attitudes and perceptions. *Food Technol.* **42**(11), 141–144, 156.

Schutz, H. G. and Cardello, A. V. (2003). Sensory science II: consumer acceptance. *In* 'Handbook of Food Science', (M. S. Rahman, ed.). Marcel Dekker, New York, NY, in press.

Schutz, H. G. and Cardello, A. V. (2001). A labeled affective magnitude (LAM) scale for assessing food liking/disliking. *J. Sensory Stud.* **16**, 117–159.

Schutz, H. G. (1998). Evolution of the sensory science discipline. *Food Technol.* **52**(8), 42–46.

Seaton, R. (1974). Why ratings are better than comparisons. *J. Adv. Res.* **14**, 45–48.

Shepard, R. N. (1966). Metric structure in ordinal data. *J. Math. Psychol.* **3**, 287–315.

Shepard, R. N. (1981). Psychological relations and psychophysical scales: on the status of 'direct' psychophysical measurement. *J. Math. Psychol.* **24**, 21–57.

Sherman, P. (1969). A texture profile of foodstuffs based upon well-defined rheological properties. *J. Food Sci.* **34**, 458–462.

Sidel, J. L. and Stone, H. (1976). Experimental design and analysis of sensory tests. *Food Technol.* **30**(11), 32–38.

Sidel, J. L., and Stone, H. (1983). Introduction to optimization research – definitions and objectives. *Food Technol.* **37**(11), 36–38.

Sidel, J. L. and Stone, H. (1993). The role of sensory evaluation in the food industry. *Food Qual. Pref.* **4**, 65–73.

Sidel, J. L., Woolsey, A. L. and Stone, H. (1975). Sensory analysis: theory methodology, and evaluation. *In* 'Fabricated Foods' (G. E. Inglett, ed.), pp. 109–126. Avi Publishing Company, Westport, CT.

Sidel, J. L., Stone, H. and Bloomquist, J. (1981). Use and misuse of sensory evaluation in research and quality control. *J. Dairy Sci.* **64**, 2296–2302.

Sidel, J. L., Stone, H. and Bloomquist, J. (1983). Industrial approaches to defining quality. *In* 'Sensory Quality in Foods and Beverages: Its Definitions, Measurement and Control', (A. A. Williams and R. K. Atkin, eds), pp. 48–57. Ellis Horwood Ltd., Chichester.

Sidel, J. L., Stone, H. and Thomas, H. A. (1994). Hitting the target: sensory and product optimization. *Cereal Foods World* **39**(11), 826–830.

Silver, D. (2003). The seven deadly sins of product development. *Food Prod. Des.* **12**(2), 93, 95, 97, 99.

Sjöström, L. B. and Cairncross, S. E. (1954). The descriptive analysis of flavor. *In* 'Food Acceptance Testing Methodology' (D. R. Peryam, F. J. Pilgrim and M. S. Peterson, eds), pp. 25–30. National Academy of Sciences – National Research Council, Washington, DC.

Smith, G. C., Savell, J. W., Cross, H. R. and Carpenter, Z. L. (1983). The relationship of USDA quality grade to beef flavor. *Food Technol.* **37**(5), 233–238.

Smith, G. L. (1981). Statistical properties of simple sensory difference tests: confidence limits and significance tests. *J. Sci. Food Agric.* **32**, 513–520.

Smith, G. L. (1988). Statistical analysis of sensory data. *In* 'Sensory Analysis of Foods', 2nd ed. (J. R. Piggot, ed.), pp. 335–379. Elsevier Applied Science, London.

Smithies, R. H. (1994). Resolving advertising disputes between competitors. *Food Technol.* **48**(8), 68, 70.

Stagner, R. and Osgood, C. E. (1946). Impact of war on a nationalistic frame of reference: I. changes in general approval and qualitative patterning of certain stereo types. *J. Soc. Psychol.* **24**, 187–215.

Stampanoni, C. R. (1993). The quantitative flavor profiling technique. *Perfumer Flavorist* **18**, 19–24.

Steiner, E. H. (1966). Sequential procedures for triangular and paired comparison tasting tests. *J. Food Technol.* **1**, 41–53.

Stevens, S. S. (1951). Mathematics, measurement and psychophysics. *In* 'Handbook of Experimental Psychology'(S. S. Stevens, ed.), pp. 1–49, Wiley, New York, NY.

Stevens, S. S. (1957). On the psychophysical law. *Psychol. Rev.* **64**, 153–181.

Stevens, S. S. (1960). On the new psychophysics. *Scand. J. Psychol.* **1**, 27–35.

Stevens, S. S. (1962). The surprising simplicity of sensory metrics. *Am. Psychol.* **17**, 29–38.

Stevens, S. S. and Galanter, E. H. (1957). Ratio scales and category scales for a dozen perceptual continua. *J. Exp. Psychol.* **54**, 377–411.

Stewart, R. A. (1971). Sensory evaluation and quality assurance. *Food Technol.* **25**(4), 103–106.

Stone, H. (1963). Determination of odor differences limens for three compounds. *J. Exp. Psychol.* **66**, 466–473.

Stone, H. (1972). 'Food Products and Processes', SRI International, Menlo Park, CA.

Stone, H. (1995). Sensory analysis and individual preferences. How precisely can we measure the pleasure of food? *In* 'Health and Pleasure at the Table' (L. Dubé, J. Le Bel, C. Tougas and V. Troche, eds), EAMAR, Montreal, Canada.

Stone, H. (1999). Sensory evaluation: science and mythology. *Food Technol.* **53**(10), 124.

Stone, H. (2002). Sensory evaluation in the 21st century. Presented at the New Products Conference, Scottsdale, AZ.

Stone, H. and Bosley, J. J. (1965). Olfactory discrimination and Weber's Law. *Percept. Mot. Skills* **20**, 657–665.

Stone, H. and Drexhage, K. A. (1985). Use of computers in sensory evaluation. *Tragon Newsletter* **1**, 1–5.

Stone, H. and Oliver, S. (1969). Measurement of the relative sweetness of selected sweeteners and sweet mixtures. *J. Food Sci.* **34**, 215–222.

Stone, H. and Pangborn, R. M. (1968). Intercorrelations of the senses. *In* 'Basic Principles of Sensory Evaluation', ASTM STP 433, pp. 30–46. American Society for Testing Materials, Philadelphia, PA.

Stone, H. and Sidel, J. L. (1978). Computing exact probabilities in sensory discrimination tests. *J. Food Sci.* **43**, 1028–1029.

Stone, H. and Sidel, J. L. (1981). Quantitative descriptive analysis in optimization of consumer acceptance. Presented at Eastern Food Science and Technology Conference on 'Strategies of Food Product Development.' Lancaster, PA.

Stone, H. and Sidel, J. L. (1995). Strategic applications for sensory evaluation in a global market. *Food Technol.* **49**(2), 80, 85–89.

Stone, H. and Sidel, J. L. (1998). Quantitative descriptive analysis: developments, applications, and the future. *Food Technol.* **52**(8), 48–52.

Stone, H. and Sidel, J. L. (2003). Descriptive analysis. *In* 'Encyclopedia of Food Science', 2nd ed., pp. 5152–5161. Academic Press, London.

Stone, H., Sidel, J., Oliver, S., Woolsey, A. and Singleton, R. C. (1974). Sensory evaluation by quantitative descriptive analysis. *Food Technol.* **28**(11), 24, 26, 28, 29, 32, 34.

Stone, H., McDermott, B. J. and Sidel, J. L. (1991). The importance of sensory analysis for the evaluation of quality. *Food Technol.* **45**(6), 88, 90, 92–95.

Swartz, M. L. and Furia, T. E. (1977). Special sensory panels for screening new synthetic sweetners. *Food Technol.* **31**(11), 51–55, 67.

Szczesniak, A. S. (1963). Classification of textural characteristics. *J. Food Sci.* **28**, 385–389.

Szczesniak, A. S. (1998). Sensory texture profiling – historical and scientific perspectives. *Food Technol.* **52**(8), 54–57.

Szczesniak, A. S., Brandt, M. A. and Friedman, H. H. (1963). Development of standard rating scales for mechanical parameters of texture and correlation between the objective and the sensory methods of texture evaluation. *J. Food Sci.* **28**, 397–403.

Taguchi, G. (1987). 'System of Experimental Design (English Ed.)' vols. I and II. Unipub/Kraus International Publications, White Plains, New York, NY.

Tamar, H. (1972). 'Principles of Sensory Physiology', Thomas, Springfield, IL.

Thorngate, J. H. III. (1995). Power analysis of sensory taste panels. Presented at 2nd International Pangborn Sensory Symposium, Davis, CA.

Thurstone, L. L. (1927). The law of comparative judgement. *Psychol. Rev.* **34**, 273–286.

Thurstone, L. L. (1959). 'The Measurement of Values', University of Chicago Press, Chicago, IL.

Tilgner, D. J. (1962). Dilution tests for odor and flavor analysis. *Food Technol.* **16**, 47–50.

Tilgner, D. J. (1965). Flavor dilution profilograms. *Food Technol.* **19**(12), 25–29.

Tilgner, D. J. (1971). A retrospective view of sensory analysis and some considerations for the future. *Adv. Food Res.* **19**, 216–277.

Tobias, R. D. (1999). 'An introduction to partial least squares regression', SAS Institute. Cary, N Ca.

Tourangeau, R. and Fasinski, K. A. (1988). Cognitive processes underlying context effects in attitude measurement. *Psychol. Bull.* **103**, 299–314.

Trant, A. S., Pangborn, R. M. and Little, A. C. (1981). Potential fallacy of correlating hedonic responses with physical and chemical measurements. *J. Food Sci.* **46**, 583–588.

Tushman, M. L. and Anderson, P. (1997). 'Managing Strategic Innovation and Change', Oxford University Press, New York, NY.

Vickers, Z. M. (1983). Magnitude estimation vs. category scaling of the hedonic quality of food sounds. *J. Food Sci.* **48**, 1183–1186.

Vie, A., Gulli, D. and O'Mahony, M. (1991). Alternative hedonic measures. *J. Food Sci.* **56**, 1–5.

Warren, C., Pearce, J. and Korth, B. (1982). Magnitude estimation and category scaling. *ASTM Stand. News* **10**, March, 15–16.

Weiss, D. J. (1972). Averaging: an empirical validity criterion for magnitude estimation. *Percept. Psychophys.* **12**, 385–388.

Wenzel, B. M. (1949). Differential sensitivity in olfaction. *J. Exp. Psychol.* **39**, 129–143.

Wiley, R. C., Briant, A. M., Fagerson, I. S., Murphy, E. F. and Sabry, J. H. (1957). The Northeast regional approach to collaborative panel testing. *Food Technol.* **11**, 43–49.

Williams, A. A. and Arnold, G. (1985). A comparison of the aromas of six coffees characterized by conventional profiling, free-choice profiling and similarity scaling methods. *J. Sci. Food Agric.* **36**, 204–214.

Williams, A. A. and Atkins, R. K. (eds) (1983). 'Sensory Quality in Foods and Beverages: Definition, Measurement and Control', Ellis Horwood Limited, Chichester, UK.

Williams, A. A. and Langron, S. P. (1984). The use of free-choice profiling for the evaluation of commercial ports. *J. Sci. Food Agric.* **35**, 558–568.

Winer, R. J. (1971). 'Statistical Principles in Experimental Design', 2nd ed. McGraw-Hill, New York, NY.

Winn, R. L. (1988). Touch screen system for sensory evaluation. *Food Technol.* **42**(11), 68–70.

Wolfe, K. A. (1979). Use of reference standards for sensory evaluation of product quality. *Food Technol.* **33**(9), 43–44.

Woodward, W. A. and Schucany, W. R. (1977). Combination of a preference pattern with the triangle taste test. *Biometrics* **33**, 31–39.

Yandell, B. S. (1997). 'Practical Data Analysis for Designed Experiments', Chapman & Hall, London.

Young, P. T. (1961). 'Motivation and Emotion', Wiley, New York, NY.

Zelek, E. F., Jr. (1990). Legal aspects of sensory analysis. Presented at the IFT Annual Meeting and Food Expo, June 16–20, Anaheim, CA.

Zook, K. and Wessman, C. (1977). The selection and use of judges for descriptive panels. *Food Technol.* **31**(11), 56–60.

Index

Page numbers in *italics* refer to figures or tables

Food Science and Technology
International Series

Maynard A. Amerine, Rose Marie Pangborn, and Edward B. Roessler, *Principles of Sensory Evaluation of Food*. 1965.

Martin Glicksman, *Gum Technology in the Food Industry*. 1970.

Maynard A. Joslyn, *Methods in Food Analysis*, second edition. 1970.

C. R. Stumbo, *Thermobacteriology in Food Processing*, second edition. 1973.

Aaron M. Altschul (ed.), *New Protein Foods:* Volume 1, *Technology, Part A* – 1974. Volume 2, *Technology, Part B* – 1976. Volume 3, *Animal Protein Supplies, Part A* – 1978. Volume 4, *Animal Protein Supplies, Part B* – 1981. Volume 5, *Seed Storage Proteins* – 1985.

S. A. Goldblith, L. Rey, and W. W. Rothmayr, *Freeze Drying and Advanced Food Technology*. 1975.

R. B. Duckworth (ed.), *Water Relations of Food*. 1975.

John A. Troller and J. H. B. Christian, *Water Activity and Food*. 1978.

A. E. Bender, *Food Processing and Nutrition*. 1978.

D. R. Osborne and P. Voogt, *The Analysis of Nutrients in Foods*. 1978.

Marcel Loncin and R. L. Merson, *Food Engineering: Principles and Selected Applications*. 1979.

J. G. Vaughan (ed.), *Food Microscopy*. 1979.

J. R. A. Pollock (ed.), *Brewing Science*, Volume 1 – 1979. Volume 2 – 1980. Volume 3 – 1987.

J. Christopher Bauernfeind (ed.), *Carotenoids as Colorants and Vitamin A Precursors: Technological and Nutritional Applications*. 1981.

Pericles Markakis (ed.), *Anthocyanins as Food Colors*. 1982.

George F. Stewart and Maynard A. Amerine (eds.), *Introduction to Food Science and Technology*, second edition. 1982.

Malcolm C. Bourne, *Food Texture and Viscosity: Concept and Measurement*. 1982.

Hector A. Iglesias and Jorge Chirife, *Handbook of Food Isotherms: Water Sorption Parameters for Food and Food Components*. 1982.

Colin Dennis (ed.), *Post-Harvest Pathology of Fruits and Vegetables*. 1983.

P. J. Barnes (ed.), *Lipids in Cereal Technology*. 1983.

David Pimentel and Carl W. Hall (eds.), *Food and Energy Resources*. 1984.

Joe M. Regenstein and Carrie E. Regenstein, *Food Protein Chemistry: An Introduction for Food Scientists*. 1984.

Maximo C. Gacula, Jr., and Jagbir Singh, *Statistical Methods in Food and Consumer Research*. 1984.

Fergus M. Clydesdale and Kathryn L. Wiemer (eds.), *Iron Fortification of Foods*. 1985.

Robert V. Decareau, *Microwaves in the Food Processing Industry*. 1985.

S. M. Herschdoerfer (ed.), *Quality Control in the Food Industry*, second edition. Volume 1 – 1985. Volume 2 – 1985. Volume 3 – 1986. Volume 4 – 1987.

F. E. Cunningham and N. A. Cox (eds.), *Microbiology of Poultry Meat Products*. 1987.

Walter M. Urbain, *Food Irradiation*. 1986.

Peter J. Bechtel, *Muscle as Food*. 1986.

H. W.-S. Chan, *Autoxidation of Unsaturated Lipids*. 1986.

Chester O. McCorkle, Jr., *Economics of Food Processing in the United States*. 1987.

Jethro Japtiani, Harvey T. Chan, Jr., and William S. Sakai, *Tropical Fruit Processing*. 1987.

J. Solms, D. A. Booth, R. M. Pangborn, and O. Raunhardt, *Food Acceptance and Nutrition*. 1987.

R. Macrae, *HPLC in Food Analysis*, second edition. 1988.

A. M. Pearson and R. B. Young, *Muscle and Meat Biochemistry*. 1989.

Dean O. Cliver (ed.), *Foodborne Diseases*. 1990.

Marjorie P. Penfield and Ada Marie Campbell, *Experimental Food Science*, third edition 1990.

Leroy C. Blankenship, *Colonization Control of Human Bacterial Enteropathogens in Poultry*. 1991.

Yeshajahu Pomeranz, *Functional Properties of Food Components*, second edition. 1991.

Reginald H. Walter, *The Chemistry and Technology of Pectin*. 1991.

Herbert Stone and Joel L. Sidel, *Sensory Evaluation Practices*, second edition. 1993.

Robert L. Shewfelt and Stanley E. Prussia, *Postharvest Handling: A Systems Approach*. 1993.

R. Paul Singh and Dennis R. Heldman, *Introduction to Food Engineering*, second edition. 1993.

Tilak Nagodawithana and Gerald Reed, *Enzymes in Food Processing*, third edition. 1993.

Dallas G. Hoover and Larry R. Steenson, *Bacteriocins*. 1993.

Takayaki Shibamoto and Leonard Bjeldanes, *Introduction to Food Toxicology*. 1993.

John A. Troller, *Sanitation in Food Processing*, second edition. 1993.

Ronald S. Jackson, *Wine Science: Principles and Applications*. 1994.

Harold D. Hafs and Robert G. Zimbelman, *Low-fat Meats*. 1994.

Lance G. Phillips, Dana M. Whitehead, and John Kinsella, *Structure-Function Properties of Food Proteins*. 1994.

Robert G. Jensen, *Handbook of Milk Composition*. 1995.

Yrjö H. Roos, *Phase Transitions in Foods*. 1995.

Reginald H. Walter, *Polysaccharide Dispersions*. 1997.

Gustavo V. Barbosa-Cánovas, M. Marcela Góngora-Nieto, Usha R. Pothakamury, and Barry G. Swanson, *Preservation of Foods with Pulsed Electric Fields*. 1999.

Ronald S. Jackson, *Wine Science: Principles, Practice, Perception*, second edition. 2000.

R. Paul Singh and Dennis R. Heldman, *Introduction to Food Engineering*, third edition. 2001.

Ronald S. Jackson, *Wine Tasting: A Professional Handbook*. 2002.

Malcolm C. Bourne, *Food Texture and Viscosity: Concept and Measurement*, second edition. 2002.

Benjamin Caballero and Barry M. Popkin (eds), *The Nutrition Transition: Diet and Disease in the Developing World*. 2002.

Dean O. Cliver and Hans P. Riemann (eds), *Foodborne Diseases*, second edition. 2002.

Martin Kohlmeier, Nutrient Metabolism. 2003.